Contents

Introduction

Teachers from a variety of subjects are increasingly being asked to participate in sex education lessons, which may be included in everyday classwork in primary schools, or in such curriculum areas as child care, religious studies, biology, health education or home economics, or be part of the tutorial group work or pastoral care system, at secondary level. In spite of recommendations for more help for schools undertaking this work, many members of staff will still not have had any training to help them cope with teaching in this sensitive and sometimes controversial field.

To gain the confidence necessary to participate in sex education courses, it is essential teachers acquire both knowledge of human sexuality, and the absolute assurance they are doing the right thing in teaching children about it.

Parents also are concerned about the sex education of their children, both at home, and at school, so it would seem a sensible and profitable approach for teachers and parents to liaise, to discuss the many factors involved when this subject is considered. These include the earlier maturation of children, the increase in sexual activity of young people, the impact of the mass media on sexual expectations, the changing roles of women and men, and the urgent need to increase parenting and family relationship skills.

After consulting with parents in this way, and with advice from the local education authority, health education officers and other interested members of the community, schools may be able to develop realistic sex education programmes, structured to help children cope in our modern society.

In planning this work teachers will be able to take into account the very relevant research of the Goldmans [53], showing there is in fact no 'latent' period of sexual disinterest between the ages of 5–11, as postulated by Freud, so children are able to absorb facts and ideas about sex throughout their developmental stages, and in the absence of such information they invent their own explanations, which are often misleading and may be anxiety promoting.

With support and encouragement from responsible and caring members of the community, parents will be able to get help for their own role as sex educators, and teachers will be able to continue and extend this work in school, presenting material and ideas in a knowledgeable and professional way, as an acceptable and normal part of the school curriculum.

Some guidelines for teachers

Dilys Went

Lecturer in Science Education
University of Warwick

Consultant Editor **M.K. Sands, BSc, PhD**

Bell & Hyman

First published 1985 by
Bell & Hyman Limited
Denmark House
37–39 Queen Elizabeth Street
London SE1 2QB

Went, Dilys Janet
  Sex education: some guidelines for teachers.
  ——(Modern teaching series)
  1. Sex education
  I. Title   II. Series
  613.9′5′07   HQ57.3

ISBN 0 7135 1436 1 Limp
ISBN 0 7135 2468 5 Cased

Typeset by MS Filmsetting Limited, Frome, Somerset.
Printed in Great Britain by The Thetford Press, Thetford, Norfolk.

Chapter 1

SEX EDUCATION IN CONTEXT

Factors affecting sex education

We have learnt much about human sexuality in the last few decades. The pioneer work of Freud and Kinsey and later of Masters and Johnson, has shown it to be a far more variable phenomenon than was previously appreciated. It is also now known that sexual acts, though natural, are by no means entirely instinctive. They are modified by psychosomatic effects influenced by learning, sometimes at a very early age.

Very many factors are involved in this learning process, so the biological, historical, economic and political, as well as sociological and psychological aspects of sex should all have consideration in school.

Some of the basic principles in education such as starting curriculum development by first considering what the children already know and relating material to real life situations and allowing full time for questions and discussion, seem in some cases not to be applied to sex education. This is probably a reflection of some unease about the subject, so one major question must now be fully considered.

Does sex education increase promiscuity?

Many people, including some teachers and parents, still fear that talking about sex, and hence 'telling them how to do it', will increase 'promiscuity', or 'experimentation'. Evidence on this point is reassuring.

i)   Farrell [2] discovered the age at which sexual information was given did not affect the age at which sex was first experienced: 'there is no clear causal relationship between early information sources and teenage sexual behaviour'.

ii)   Rogers [20] summarising the evidence on the effects of sex education says, 'the available data give us no reason to believe that sexual instruction of itself will either "turn the individual on" or "turn him off"'.

iii)   In a study of the effects of courses for college age students in the USA Kirby [9] writes 'programs appear to have little effect on the amount of various types of sexual behaviour.'

iv)   Reid [17] summarises many evaluations saying 'In general we can be confident about the benign effects of school sex education courses, since the conclusions reached by a number of reviewers in this field are remarkably similar', that is that they had no effect on the sexual activity of the recipients.

v)   Zelnik and Kim [4], in a statistical analysis of USA data, confirm previous findings providing 'overwhelming support for the claim that the decision to engage in sexual activity is not influenced by whether or not teenagers have had sex education at school'.

To link sex education with the increase in the incidence of sexually transmitted diseases, and to school-girl pregnancies is unwarranted as surveys of individuals in both categories have found a high proportion of them had not received any kind of sex education in school (see page 9). In fact Francome [25] suggests the sharp drop in actual births to teenagers in Great Britain from 51 per thousand in 1971 to 28 per thousand in 1982 is not fully accounted for by the rise in the number of abortions to the same group. Assuming the level of sexual activity has not been reduced, he suggests that birth control methods have been used effectively, thus refuting the idea that more sex education for teenagers leads to more pregnancies.

All responsible teachers will continually be on the look out for evidence showing any adverse effects of sex education programmes in school and be able to adapt them at once in response to valid criticism.

The increase in sexual activity of young people

Farrell's [2] research into the way young people learn about sex and birth control, is of major importance to sex educators. She found there has been a definite increase in teenage sexual activity since the previous report by Schofield (1965), and that 12% of girls and 31% of boys, had had some sexual experience before they were 16. She says, 'the possibility that over a third of all teenagers in the sample had had some sexual experience before or by the age of 16 has some important implications for sex education and medical services'.

Further evidence of the increase comes in a study *Family Formation* (Dunnell, 1979 [33]) which found 20% of sixteen year old girls and 50% of nineteen year old girls had had intercourse. On a rather different, journalistic, level of research, results from a survey of 1000 girls for the magazine *Loving* (18th Feb. 1984) suggested 50% had had sex before they were 16. It might perhaps be thought unlikely that all these sexual experiences would be negative ones, and necessarily damaging to the young people concerned.

However, the adverse effects of increased sexual activity in young people must be considered fully, and they should be made aware of what these could be, so their choice of behaviour is at least based on a realistic knowledge of the possible consequences.

Medical considerations

Catterall [54] has documented those he considers most serious, which include an overall rise in the number of sexually transmitted diseases, with clinical effects ranging from mild discomfort, to severe pain, infertility, ectopic pregnancies, and possible damage to a foetus. Some antibiotics have now become less effective against some of these infections. He states 'public health education about sexual matters in general and sexually transmitted diseases in particular, is inadequate'. Singer (1981) and others, have shown a correlation between age of first intercourse, particularly at puberty, the number of sexual partners and the subsequent incidence of cervical cancer, which is now on the increase. Some doctors are concerned about the possible effects of hormonal contraception on young girls whose natural cycle has not become established.

Adolescents who do become pregnant are more at risk, both mother and child being affected (see chapter 10).

It is very important to give adolescents an explanation of the many medical reasons why adults are uneasy about teenage sex. These facts should not be used as shock tactics for a blanket disapproval of their sexuality however, or communication on sexual matters may speedily come to an end.

The effects of witholding information on sex

An alternative approach, that of witholding information about sexual matters, has not been shown to be an effective method of reducing either the amount or the traumas of teenage sexual behaviour. The following examples may illustrate this point:

i)   In 1976 the British Pregnancy Advisory Service [46] reported that nearly 300 of the 446 pregnant school girls attending that year had thought they were too young to become pregnant.

ii)   Ashken & Soddy [5] in a study of pregnant teenage girls found 29% of them had had no sex education at all, at home or at school, whereas this applied to only 4% of the control group, who had not become pregnant.

iii)   Farrell [2] found those who had learnt about sex primarily from their friends, and not from their school or parents, were in fact more likely to be sexually experienced.

iv)   Rogers [20] says 'Once we see learning as an active process, lack of adequate knowledge reaching the child can lead not just to a knowledge gap, but to inaccurate knowledge that may take considerable effort to unlearn.' The research of the Goldmans [53] and Kreitler [44] confirms this view. See page 54 for wrong concepts in childhood.

v)   Paragraph 47 of the *Pregnant at School* report [7] says 'In spite of criticisms and fears expressed about possible consequences of explicit sex education, the Working Party are convinced that to leave our young people in ignorance and confusion is to leave them at greater risk.'

It appears there is no evidence so far that sex education either increases the amount of sexual activity, or is damaging in any way to the children receiving it. There is evidence that without sex education irresponsible sexual behaviour takes place and that ignorance can be both humiliating and harmful.

The situation in the classroom

Within any one age group a teacher may be faced with a class of children at very different levels of maturity and with very different life styles. There is a danger that some pseudosophisticated members may give the impression they already 'know it all'. Very little investigation is usually needed, however, to detect their ignorance, sometimes even of the most basic facts. If the veneer of worldliness can then be gently prised aside such children may be able to allow themselves to learn and understand more, providing this can be done without any loss of face on their part. '

An entirely different type of child to that depicted above also deserves careful consideration, those who have absolutely no wish to be sexually active at this stage in their life. The right not to involve oneself in sexual behaviour needs strong reinforcement and support to counteract the pressures from peer groups and the media, which can be considerable. These pupils too need to learn about human sexuality with dignity, but the implication that everyone in their age group must be pre-occupied with sex, and they are somehow getting left behind in the sexual market must be positively refuted. A case illustrating this situation came from Valerie. She thought she must be 'a "Fridgidair" person' because when a boy stroked her she 'didn't feel a thing'. She said the other girls constantly called her a 'virgy' and said they could tell she was by the way she walked across a room. 'What is a "virgy" anyway?' she eventually asked.

There were complex factors involved in her case, but the feeling she had at 14, gained from her peers, of being sexually inadequate has implications for all educators. It needs considerable skills on the part of a teacher to keep the balance right when teaching any subject to a class which includes such diverse pupils as those outlined above. Sex education requires an even greater awareness of the subcultures represented, as attitudes and needs can be so very different.

An integrated approach
Ideally the various areas categorised as sex education should be integrated into a much wider programme of health education, pastoral care or education for parenthood and be truly interdisciplinary. Care must be taken, however, that both sexes have equal time for the subject. Boys can be a very deprived group where sex education is concerned [7, 23].

Questions on sexual matters can arise spontaneously (overtly or covertly) at any time, and in any subject. It is very reassuring if teachers feel they can cope with these queries confidently and without embarrassment. In turn this can help lessen fear of 'danger areas' in class discussion which can cause extra tension and strain in teaching. Once the children know staff are prepared to give time and consideration to topics often uppermost in their media-primed minds, experience in many schools has shown they are then more willing to concentrate on the non-sexual parts of the curriculum, and the 'endless innuendoes, excitement, nudging and winking' syndrome so well known to teachers, quietens down or even disappears.

Children's views on sex education in school
Children in general do feel school is a good place to learn about sex. Farrell [2] found many in her sample said they would prefer school as a source of information about sex, and in Balding's survey [11] in over 40 schools in England, of importance ratings for 28 health education topics, 'Sex' was ranked very high by children, as well as by teachers and parents. The research by the Goldmans [53] involved interviews with 1000 children aged 5–15 in England, Australia, North America and Sweden, and showed the great majority of children in all countries felt they should be taught about sex at school.

If sex education is in context and at the right level for the children concerned the evidence is that they then accept it willingly and sensibly.

Parents and sex education

Teachers are very concerned about the views of parents on sex education. They are naturally reticent about intruding into what might be considered a private aspect of family life, and the image of an irate parent storming up to the school is a very disconcerting one. In fact this fear is very exaggerated, as many schools discovered once they started their sex education programme. The vast majority of parents at parent-teacher meetings show they are both pleased and relieved the school is prepared to accept some of the responsibility for the sex education of their children and often say they have learnt much from the evening. The parents in return have a lot to offer the school in contributing to the mutual understanding of the children concerned. Such co-operation between parents and staff is of major importance in successful sex education, as both groups gain in confidence if they feel they have shared aims, and a line of communication should any problems arise.

Farrell [2] showed that no fewer than 96% of parents of secondary school children were in favour of them receiving sex education at school. It does seem likely the 4% apparently not in favour, exert a negative influence out of all proportion to their actual numbers. There may be some rather vociferous people among them of course, who do not hesitate to make their feelings known. Their views should always be considered carefully, and it is usually possible to sympathise and agree with them to some extent as they are only expressing worries we all have about the physical and moral well-being of our children. If such people are able to voice their fears at parent-teacher meetings in this way the other parents can often explain the reality of the situation as they see it, and together with members of staff help allay misgivings and worries. If this is not possible, then such parents are seen to be expressing a minority view, which though respected, should not be allowed to radically alter the proposed programme. If they wish to withdraw their child from certain sessions, then although they do not have any statutory right to do so, it is wisest to allow this to happen. It can be done in a tactful way so as not to focus attention on the absence of that particular pupil.

If all parents have been consulted about the sex education programme, are aware of its content and presentation, and have met the staff involved, cases of requests for the withdrawal of children from classes will be very rare. The other group of parents of concern to staff, are those who never come to meetings at all, and there are many reasons why this may be the case. It is sometimes possible to make contact with them by arranging small social events on an informal basis. We have a lot to learn here from Community Schools, who are expert in fostering links between school and home.

Differences in culture and hence to attitudes about human sexuality can raise particular issues which need careful consideration. These are discussed later (page 31).

The parents' role in sex education

Parents do, obviously, have great responsibilities as sex educators, and many studies have shown this role is perceived by parents, teachers and children. They start even before the child is born.

It is helpful to discuss with parents and children, their opinions on how far these parental responsibilities extend. Which three areas of those listed below might be considered most important for example?

i)   Parents should be responsible for planning the conception of their children, so parenthood is a chosen occupation and not a side effect, and good pre-conception and antenatal care can then be obtained for both partners.

ii)   They should be able to accept the sex of their children, and not try to channel them into the opposite one, nor voice their preference for one sex or the other. They should also accept that children are naturally sexual beings, and love both ends of them with equal enthusiasm. At adolescence they should acknowledge their children's developing sexuality and help them cope with the physical and emotional consequences.

iii)   Parents should ensure their children do know the truth about 'the facts of life' when they are ready for this information (often before they attend school) and not give them false stories of baby deliveries by storks, in hospital bags or under gooseberry bushes and so on. They should answer questions on sex when they arise, thus developing good communication on sexual matters within the family.

iv)   Parents should be prepared to co-operate with school sex education programmes by attending discussion meetings, and reinforcing their messages at home when appropriate, particularly perhaps, those concerning sexist attitudes, and the need to try and develop all the children's talents equally.

v)   They should provide a caring and loving home background where parents show respect and affection for each other, and help their children develop a good self image and overall physical and mental health. They should also provide moral guidelines and codes of behaviour in accordance with their race and religion but be able to accept these may need adaptation to meet changing world conditions.

Parents' difficulties

The home would seem an ideal environment for sex education to take place 'naturally', with knowledge being gained gradually, and questions answered as they arise. However, this state of affairs does not always exist, perhaps because of some of the following factors:

i)   The parents' own knowledge of sexual matters may be lacking, even though they have produced children. They may not have had sex education at school themselves of course. They may also lack the necessary education skills, as not everyone is good at explaining things to other people. The children's questions may come up much earlier than expected, when the parents are quite unprepared for them so they may be too embarrassed to answer perhaps because they have not yet fully accepted their own sexuality.

ii) They may be unsure what vocabulary to use, the vernacular or the latinate? In either case they are afraid the child will repeat these new words, loudly, at the bus stop, or in front of Grandma or the neighbours. They usually do. To overcome this fear, a family code language may develop, for genital parts and behaviour. This does not disturb the general public when used outside the home, but has its limitations when communication with peers, teachers or hospital staff becomes desirable and necessary.

iii) They may believe that children do not need to know 'these things', and are trying to keep them 'innocent'. Again, this shows a lack of acceptance of the fundamental nature of human sexuality, and understanding that children may be far more shocked when discovering certain facts from 'friends', than if they are explained in a caring and sensitive way by their own parents. If children formulate a question they may already have some idea of an answer, or will invent one for themselves if not provided with the information [20, 53, 44]. It is not necessary however to tell children all the facts as soon as they ask any questions about sex. This is rather misguided and boring for the child. It is better to restrict the answer to the question, or ask a supplementary question to find out more about what *is* actually being asked, which may be on a much simpler level than first thought. Parents should also be prepared to answer the same question many times, children forget facts in this field just as in any other.

iv) Parents may have deeper fears that the child will immediately relate the information back to them and ask personal questions, or even want to watch the sex act itself. The follow-up from small children after hearing the facts of life is in fact much more likely to be of the 'do you have to lift your nightie?' variety, and it is possible to gently explain the private nature of sexual love, and that onlookers are not appreciated. Young children can have no concept of adult sexual arousal, nor is it appropriate to try and explain it to them. They have to take on trust that this amazing procedure is something grown ups do when they love each other, and that it gives them pleasure. Some parents go to great lengths to conceal any physical attraction for each other from their offspring, in the fear the children will think they are leading on to full intercourse. The opposite situation occurs where parental love making can be heard or seen by a child, who may find it frightening and inexplicable. For pubertal and post-pubertal children, knowledge of their parents' sexuality can create an uncomfortable awareness of the sexual attraction between parents and child, or even be perceived as a threat. The rationalisation sometimes developed to alievate this feeling is 'my parents are far too old still to be having sex', and conversely 'he/she is far too young to be interested in sex'. Both are protective mechanisms, for family life together, but if parents deny the sexual development of their children they cannot help them to accept the responsibility which goes with it, nor make the right decisions about their sexual behaviour.

v) Parents can feel hurt if in spite of previously good communication, their child goes to another adult for information on sex. It helps perhaps to realise there is a time when children will need other sources of help, and that they are going through a phase of needing extra privacy, both for the growth of new feelings and for adapting to new curves and hairs. Personal development does require some degree of detachment from parental overseeing.

vi)   In a one parent family, problems may arise when a child learns about the father or mother side of procreation and asks why the other parent isn't there. Under these circumstances it is helpful if the parent has already given some thought as to how to answer this question, perhaps consulting with the class teacher, so they can co-operate in helping the child accept the one parent situation. One in seven children now live in one parent families, so this will be an increasing consideration. The same type of question arises when adopted or foster children learn about human reproduction, and again these need to be handled very sensitively by both parents, foster parents and school. Foster children often need extra love, affection and cuddling, even when adolescent. This can put rather a strain on the opposite sex foster parent.

Finally the parents' own views on sex education may conflict with those of the school, either of them being more liberal than the other. The need for communication is particularly high in these cases.

Families and sex education

Because of the problems outlined above, relating largely to the sex education of younger children, some parents are never able to discuss sexual matters freely with their family. It does not 'become easier' as children grow older, as they will already have detected the reluctance to provide information in this area and learnt to take questions elsewhere, to save both themselves and their families from embarrassment.

Parents have the difficult task then, of trying to provide accurate information about sex in a sensitive way, while at the same time maintaining their childrens' social acceptability.

I have used the term 'parents' throughout this section, but it is usually the mother who is the home sex educator. Fathers frequently show a great reluctance to take up this role.

64% of parents in Farrell's study [2] thought that mothers were the 'right people' to tell children where babies come from. Children too rate mothers highly as a source of information on sex (Goldman [53]), Walters and Walters [22] detail the powerful influence of the family on the development of children's attitudes towards sex, and subsequent sexual behaviour. Negative attitudes are formed when the subject is avoided, and they stress the benefits gained by families talking more about sexual matters, and communicating positive values, particularly if the fathers are involved in this process. Information will be sought from parents if they do not in return probe into their children's private lives, or seem shocked or alarmed at facts given to them. Above all they suggest parents should indicate in advance their willingness to support their children, even if not necessarily agreeing with their views and behaviour. Children who can discuss sex with their parents are more prepared for, and can cope better with subsequent sexual encounters, and it has been shown that these are then likely to take place later rather than earlier in their adolescence.

Help for parents

It can perhaps be appreciated from the formidable list of considerations outlined above, that parents need help in the sex education of their children, in increasing their own knowledge and understanding of human sexuality, and in developing their own teaching and discussion skills and overcoming the specific difficulties mentioned. Some of this help can be obtained from their children's school, if the staff are sympathetic and have the insight to realise it is often easier to do sex education for other people's children than your own, as there is less emotional involvement.

Other possible sources of help for parents include health visitors, health education officers, doctors and nurses, who are increasingly involved in sex education. Particular local groups such as Young Wives, the National Housewives Register, Mother and Toddler Groups etc. may arrange talks and discussions on sex education hopefully extending the invitation to fathers as well, so they too, if they wish, can develop their skills in talking to their children.

Courses in sex education specifically designed for parents can be arranged by the FPA, NMGC, BAC, and by Regional or District Health Authorities.

Chapter 2

SEX EDUCATION IN SCHOOLS

It cannot be over emphasised that schools are not trying to usurp the parents' role in sex education. The need for this both at home and at school is acknowledged [1, 3, 7, 182] etc and the two should complement and enhance each other.

A school can however offer facilities and expertise not available to most families. These include staff skills in teaching techniques and educational theory, and their awareness of the general level of sexual knowledge and behaviour of each age group of children. The school may have a variety of teachers who can demonstrate an ease in talking about sexual matters, and who can present a range of views and ideas within the context of their own subject areas, or who may choose to make use of outside expert speakers and advisors. The teachers themselves may be able to increase their knowledge and skills, by participating in in-service courses, or attending conferences with relevance to sex education. They also have an opportunity in school, to assess childrens' knowledge and attitudes by testing, so discovering potential misunderstandings. Some staff may have counselling skills enabling them to help pupils and their families with any special problems.

The school can provide a neutral environment in which to discuss personal relationships, and can organise discussion groups of peers, from any one class or year group. It also has access to material for the sex education curriculum giving planned sequences linked with the children's concept levels, and making use of appropriate audio visual aids.

Overall, as explained in the introduction, a school can seek a broad based community support, enabling the subject to be approached with confidence and treated in a fully professional manner.

Official recommendations
Senior administrators may be asked to justify time spent on sex education. They will find it helpful to know about

i) The Education Act 1980: Publication of Information (Section 8) [1] requires local education authorities to publish details about each school within their jurisdiction including information on 'the ways and context in which sex education is provided'.

ii) The Newsom Report, *Half our Future*, (Central Advisory Council for Education [England]) HMSO 1963, 'Positive guidance to boys and girls in sexual behaviour is essential. This should include the biological, moral, social and personal aspects.'

iii) DES, *Health Education in Schools*, HMSO 1977 p112

'The main point (of the development of the "permissive society") which affects the work of the schools is that they can no longer avoid their responsibilities in sex education because information, often misleading, is thrust at children out of school.'

iv) *Pregnant at School* Joint Working Party on Pregnant Schoolgirls and Schoolgirl mothers, National Council for One Parent Families 1979. Chapter 2, *Responsibility for Prevention* (of schoolgirl pregnancies) ends with six recommendations, the following three being particularly relevant:

a) Girls and boys, including those over 16, of all levels of ability should receive education in personal development and relationships, social responsibility and preparation for family life throughout their primary and secondary schooling.

b) Appropriate teaching about responsible sexual behaviour should start in the first years of the secondary school curriculum and should include specific and accurate information about contraception.

c) Schools should involve parents in health education. There should be close co-operation between parents and teachers in developing an understanding of adolescents and in giving them guidance and information.

v) The report quotes from the National Union of Students evidence requesting a more comprehensive approach to integrating sex education and child care into both the school curriculum and the training of teachers, as in their experience the majority of newly-trained teachers had received no guidance on this subject.

vi) The Department of Education and Science and the Welsh Office *The School Curriculum* March 1981. Moral, health, and sex education are identified as subjects more effectively covered if they are distributed across the curriculum. Paragraph 26:

'Schools are responding in a variety of ways to the need for sound sex education. Sex education is one of the most sensitive parts of broad programmes of health education, and the fullest consultation and co-operation with parents are necessary before it is embarked upon. In this area offence can be given if a school is not aware of, and sensitive to, the cultural background of every child. Sex education is not a simple matter and is linked with attitudes and behaviour.'

vii) Local education reports. Many local education authorities have produced guideline reports on personal relationship education, or more specifically on sex education, recognising the concern felt by teachers about these subjects. All acknowledge the need for them to become part of a normal school curriculum. The following are particularly helpful.

a) *Sex Education*. 1974. Liverpool Education Department, 14, St Thomas Street, L1 6B.

b) *How are you Man?* 1979, a detailed strategy for health education in schools. City Education Department, Civic Centre, Barras Bridge, Newcastle on Tyne, NE1 8PU

c) *Education for Personal Relationships*. 1972. Wiltshire County Council Education Committee.

d) *Pastoral Work and Education in Personal Relationships in Lancashire Secondary Schools*. 1979.

What exactly is sex education?

It is easier to start by considering what it is not. In the past, sex education has often been confined to facts about reproduction in animals. These were given in the first year at secondary school, some mention of human reproduction possibly coming at the end of the session on mammals. Biology teachers were thus required and expected to cope with all the questions and emotions arising from such lessons, often without any help, and without the time for the full implications of the work to be considered. A quiescent period followed until just before leaving school. There was then a burst of activity, several 'one-off' sessions being arranged in the hall, 100 or more children watching a film shown by an outside speaker whose role was to '*tell* them all they need to know', about contraception or sexually transmitted diseases, in one frenetic hour. Would any other important subject requiring on-going learning processes have been treated in such a way?

Happily this pattern is now not so often found [17] as many schools have developed much broader programmes, accepting human sexuality involves far more than crisis situations of unwanted pregnancies or damaging infections. Sexuality can then be viewed as an integral part of an individual's total personality and not as an isolated piece of sexual behaviour.

Every subject and teacher is already involved in sex education in its widest sense. It proceeds all the time, everywhere that socialisation processes take place, expressed in values, attitudes, personal relationships, and in all feelings about sex, expressed or hidden. The decision to be made is not whether to do sex education or not, but how to do it.

Is it right to try and help our children make some sort of sense out of the information on sex, positive and negative coming to them all the time? Or is it preferable to leave them to find their own paths in the general minestrone of conflicting facts and fallacies, and merely condemn them when they are not successful?

Every human being has to make decisions about sex, even if one of these decisions is not to become actively involved. Young people have the right to information which will help them make the best decisions for the particular circumstances they are in at the time; develop skills enabling them to take responsibility for their own behaviour and gain understanding and insight into the emotional, social and moral factors involved in human sexuality. The next consideration is 'when do these rights begin?' The Goldmans [53] found children wanted sex education in the primary school (5–11 years) yet on average less than 50% of the English-speaking sample had been to schools providing it below the age of 12. A survey by HM inspectors of 15 primary schools in the Avon area [188] found few had actually planned programmes for sex education, but dealt with the subject as it arose.

If information is to be given before decisions have to be taken, then surely we have to respond to evidence of earlier puberty and earlier sexual activity, and supply more sex education in the first years in secondary school, rather than leave it all to the last two? One strategy might be to find out from the children themselves what their needs are, and plan lessons accordingly, after consultation with teachers, parents etc. A suitable questionnaire for doing just this is provided in Appendix E of the Schools Council Paper 57 (1976) [41] .

The aims of sex education

Because of the very wide scope of sex education programmes it is difficult to summarise the aims of a whole course. Individual parts can, and should have very specific objectives, related to knowledge, attitudes, communication skills, decision making processes, sensitivity to others and so on.

However, it might be salutory first to consider the overall effect we have when teaching boys or girls, and the attitudes we show to them as male and female teachers. This is what will actually constitute much of 'sex education', whatever is actually on the curriculum. Michelle Stanworth in her study *Gender and Schooling* [24], found teachers, particularly male ones, are more attached to and concerned for boys, and more often actually reject girls. She says 'When boys are more outspoken and manifestly confident, and especially when teachers take more notice of boys, pupils tend to see this as evidence that boys in general are more highly valued, and more capable, than girls.' This research obviously has far reaching implications for schools.

One well established aim of sex education is to provide factual information. At the moment we do not seem to be succeeding even at this level, as the Goldmans [53] found many English children in their sample did not understand the fundamentals of sex. The aims might be as follows:

i)   To combat ignorance and increase understanding. To provide full, honest information about the physical, emotional and social aspects of human sexual development from conception to old age, including the nature of love, personal relationships and family life. This may enable people to have a positive and happy acceptance of their own sexuality, thus increasing self value and esteem. To increase sensitivity to the sexual nature of oneself, and members of both sexes, so insight may be gained into the potential for fulfilling sexual relationships and enjoyment.

ii)   To reduce guilt and anxiety. To provide knowledge and acceptance of the variety and variability of human sexual behaviour, and by seeking not to establish unrealistic 'norms', improve the quality of sexual relationships, and encourage better mental health.

iii)   To promote responsible behaviour. To increase individual responsibility for sexual behaviour so that neither one's own, nor one's partner's body or feelings are hurt. This includes not passing on sexually transmitted diseases, initiating unwanted pregnancies, nor forcing unwanted sexual activity on other people.

iv)   To combat exploitation. To promote an awareness of the misuse of sex, both for commercial profit, and in personal relationships, so enabling people to protect themselves from exploitation. To become aware of dual codes of sexual behaviour, and work towards their elimination.

v)   To promote the ability to make informed decisions. To help young people develop the ability to determine their own values within a moral framework, and to make decisions about their behaviour which will be beneficial to themselves and their partner, and to enable children to recognise the pressures on groups or individuals to behave in certain ways, and develop strategies for coping with them.

vi)   To facilitate communication on sexual matters. To provide an acceptable vocabulary for discussing sex, and to enable this to be used without embarrassment in a group, class or clinic situation.

vii)   To develop educational skills for future parents and child carers. To further understanding of the sex education needs of small children, so as parents, nurses, doctors, police, social workers, friends or relations, can provide explanations of sex without embarrassment, and at the right level for the child concerned.

As in all health education we are working for attitude and behaviour changes away from negative damaging ones, towards positive helpful ones. This involves the most difficult skills ever required of teachers, and as some of the changes will be slow, they are often difficult to evaluate in the short term. It is important not to lose heart at the enormity of the task, but do the best possible under the circumstances, and be aware of the many variables involved, some of which are quite out of the control of the school.

Setting up a programme for health and sex education
A suggested sequence might be:

i)   Head and Senior staff, in consulation with LEA adviser, Health Education Officer etc., decide to introduce, (or extend) the programme, and all staff are informed of this decision, and the reasons behind it.

ii)   A course coordinator is designated and leads a small working party to map out a broad course outline, (see curriculum suggestions) and discover the attitudes of staff, parents and children to these proposals. Use could be made here of the General Health Topic Questionaire, 'Just one minute', a survey document devised by J. W. Balding, available from the Schools' Health Education Unit, University of Exeter. (See also TACADE *Monitor* Autumn 1979 No. 52).

iii)   Using the survey results, the working party revise the course and determine to which part various departments would be prepared to contribute. The course is now filled out in more detail and any weaknesses, or 'deprived' groups of children identified.

iv)   A meeting, whole or half day conference is arranged for all the staff, to present the current state of the course, the rationale behind it and the involvement of departments, and to ask for further suggestions and ideas of possible contributors from outside the school. The course is adjusted as necessary in the light of comments from this meeting.

Suitable staff willing to be involved are identified and approached, and their particular needs discovered.

These might be training:

a)   as a course co-ordinator (see below)

b)   in informal teaching methods (contact TACADE or LIFESKILLS [55])

c)   in personal relationship teaching (contact NMGC or FPA or BAC)

d)   in specific subject areas (see list of national organisations, resource centres and local help page 45)

e)   in counselling techniques in school, (NMGC, LEA Courses in Pastoral Care or RHA courses etc).

Local specialists in the above areas, perhaps suggested by the Health Education Officer, could be invited to talk to the staff team.

v)   A PTA meeting is arranged to explain the proposals to the parents and gain their support and involvement (see page 29).

The co-ordinator

At the moment sex education is rarely defined as such on the timetable, but is covered in a variety of subject areas across the curriculum or in tutorial group work or in pastoral care. The designation of a co-ordinator is therefore of paramount importance if the subject is not to become fragmented, repetitive or sporadic and a spiral syllabus adapted to the different ages, abilities and needs of the children is to be developed and maintained.

The Schools Council with the HEC has produced two kinds of material in Health Education 13–18 [9]. The first is related to curriculum development in health education at secondary school level, and the training of school co-ordinators for such work. In association with LEAs or RHAs the project can offer two-day workshops for teachers in each of three terms. School-based work between the sessions forms an integral part of the course. Details can be obtained from the Director at the Health Education Unit, Department of Education, the University of Southampton.

The role of a health education co-ordinator is clearly defined in the Newcastle LEA health education report 'How are you man?' (see page 17).

Self help for in-service training

In addition to in service courses, the sex education team will find it helpful to have informal meetings to discuss specific areas of the curriculum, to view audio visual material, and to extend their own understanding of human sexuality. This last aim might be achieved in some measure by viewing the film *Sexuality and Communication.*

This film shows a symposium in Ontario on adolescent sexuality. Two doctors, the married couple Avinoam and Beryl Chernick demonstrate by role play of doctor/patient and husband/wife relationships, how attitudes and feelings affect sexual performance, and how the pressures and anxieties of daily living interfere with family relationships. The physical aspects of sex are explained in context. The film is suffused with good humour and wit, and is an excellent example of how human sexuality can be presented to an audience in a comfortable and acceptable way. The film (50 minutes, sound and colour) is on free loan from Ortho-Pharmaceutical Ltd. It would be suitable for showing to all the staff, perhaps with a speaker from the NMGC or RHA or FPA to help lead discussion groups afterwards. For suitable background books, see page 35.

Selection of staff

The choice of members of staff is central to the success of any sex education programme. It is the personality of the teacher chosen however, rather than their main subject area or responsibilities, which is all important. The selection of suitable teachers should be considered so critical that their availability takes priority over other curriculum restraints when designing the programme. This may well cause some problems, but the alternative strategy, of delegating staff to teach in this area because they are the only ones free when all other courses have been arranged, could be unsatisfactory for all concerned.

No member of staff should be pressurised into taking part in sex education work if not fully prepared to do so. Children are quick to detect when a teacher is not perfectly at ease with a subject, so it is defeating one of the main aims of the course to impose it on a reluctant member of staff. Non-verbal communication can be more indicative of true feelings than what is actually spoken, and a class can be very perceptive about contradictory messages conveyed in this way. It is not only what is said but how it is said that constitutes sex education.

This brings us to the question of 'over enthusiastic' volunteers for this work. Such people should be viewed with suspicion, as their motives may be questionable. Would they take sex out of context as one aspect only, of personal relationship education, and be unable to talk of anything else? Might they relate their own sexual experiences to a class, in the mistaken idea that this is what sex education is all about? Would they cause distress by ignoring the varied backgrounds and family life of the pupils, teaching in a biased or dogmatic way? Would they fail to distinguish between facts and opinions, or teach without reference to any moral codes? Such people, who show themselves to be unbalanced on sexual matters, are present in all walks of life. When, rarely, they are found in a school, they are easily identifiable in whatever subject area they teach. They are not suitable candidates for a team involved in sex education.

Qualifications of sex educators

So what are the positive characteristics to look for in a sex educator? The following guidelines were formulated by a pioneer in the sex education field, Nathaniel N. Wagner, Ph. D., Professor of Psychology in the Department of Obsteterics & Gynaecology and Director of Clinical Psychology at the University of Washington, Seattle, during the time he spent in the UK, working with the Family Planning Association.

In many ways these desirable qualities are those of any competent teacher. It is, however, essential to develop the highest level of responsibility in those involved in sex education. Qualified sex educators should have the qualities listed below.

i)   A genuine and sincere concern for other human beings.
ii) A comfortable acceptance of their own and other people's sexuality.
iii) Sensitivity to and respect for the views of other people.
iv) Knowledge of techniques of curriculum development and education which involve student participation.
v)   A non-defensive attitude which facilitates cooperation with parental and other interested groups.
vi) A professional attitude which protects the student against any form of exploitation.
vii) A commitment to confidentiality concerning any personal information obtained directly or indirectly in the role of sex educator.
viii) An ability to recognise and refer those matters that require professional assistance beyond the competence of the sex educator.
ix) Mastery of the basic facts of human sexuality and a commitment to continuing professional education.
x)   Communication skills involving instructional, discussion and role-playing methods and knowledge of audio-visual and other teaching aids.

Each of these qualities deserves serious consideration, and most can be developed by further training.

In addition they should be teachers with a particular ability to relate well to their classes, and to create a relaxed, non-threatening atmosphere, where questions can be asked without fear of ridicule or humiliation. A sense of humour is also a great asset.

It does not matter whether the staff involved are old or young, male or female, married or unmarried, heterosexual or homosexual. There is absolutely no evidence to suggest that homosexual teachers, male or female, are any more likely to act unprofessionally towards the children in their care than a heterosexual.

The main subject area of the team member is irelevant as teachers trained in different subjects will have different skills to offer and different areas of knowledge to draw upon.

Biologists are sometimes thought to have particular advantages as sex educators, but not many B.Sc., B.Ed., or PGCE Biology courses have a component in human sexuality, so they themselves often feel the need for more training in this area. See the Institute of Biology's guidelines on sex education.

The team approach
A number of potential difficulties mean it is important to have a team of teachers in the sex education programme, rather than just one or two being used as 'willing horses'. This avoids any one person being labelled 'sex queen or king' by pupils, staff or parents. It also provides some guarantee of the continuity of the programme, as so often when only a few teachers are involved, if they leave, or are promoted the whole programme declines. The

team can include members from many different subject areas and administrative levels as well as possibly the school medical officer, nurse or health visitor. It is helpful to have senior members of staff involved, as this draws on their high teaching skills and understanding of young people, gives confidence to others and confers status on the subject.

Team members can give each other moral support when teaching in one of the few subjects which sometimes attracts negative feelings or active criticism.

Regular discussions about human sexuality greatly increase ease in talking about sexual matters and help the team 'think through' the total rationale of the work, develop communication skills, and consolidate belief in the value of the programme.

This committed approach can also demonstrate it is perfectly respectable to be interested in teaching about human sexuality!

Sex education is an enormous subject in its own right. It does require study and 'homework' by the team teaching it. Merely being 'grown up' does not, alas, equip one adequately for the task. When meetings and discussions are held with parents, the team can present an obviously considered approach to sex education, which is thus seen to have full professional backing. This is reassuring for all. Other members of staff can refer parent's queries to team members, who will be able to handle them with diplomacy, from a full knowledge of the overall aims of the programme.

Overall staff support

Although relatively few teachers will be actively involved in the sex education programme, it is very important to gain the support of all the staff for the general approach planned. Unless this happens there may well be misunderstandings and feelings of resentment, and children could receive quite different messages from different teachers or subject areas. The staff most involved in the work might well fear criticism or condemnation from their colleagues. To prevent this situation occurring the suggested sequence in setting up the programme could be followed (see page 20). Personal relationship education starts in the staff room perhaps, and an harmonious staff at least lends credibility to the system.

The concerns teachers have

As soon as teachers move away from their traditionally accepted information-giving role, and enter into more widely ranging discussions, they may feel more vulnerable, as their control of the classroom situation requires new and different skills.

Fear of personal questions

There is absolutely no obligation to answer personal questions on sex, and it can be counter-productive to do so. If children ask for example, 'Are you a virgin Miss?', 'What sort of contraceptive do you use then?' 'Do you fancy girls with big boobs Sir?'. The answer could be to the effect 'I don't really think that information would be much use to you! We started this course agreeing everyone has a right to privacy in their sex lives, and that goes for me as well. I shan't ask you about your sex life, and I don't expect you to ask me about mine', or a similar formula for avoiding answering, while indicating the reason is the private nature of such information, and that no offence has been taken. Even if the question has been asked out of genuine interest rather than just to 'test' the teacher, it really is not a good idea to answer directly, because:

i) it might set an ideal or 'norm' of behaviour which would not be possible for that youngster,
ii) it could be followed up by even more personal questions,
iii) the information gained might eventually be distributed widely, probably in a distorted form and certainly out of the context of the original discussion.

A consistent, pleasant but firm refusal to be drawn on personal matters will soon be accepted, and is in itself a valid way of showing how to cope with an invasion into one's sexual privacy.

Confidentiality

Ways of conducting discussions and answering questions without the danger of children revealing their own sexual behaviour, will be found in the section on methodology (page 37). When involved in sex education teachers may be given information about their personal lives by many people, ranging from school cleaners to governors. This certainly increases one's knowledge of the range of human sexuality, and feelings about it, but it is obviously essential that absolute confidentiality be maintained. If a pupil talking privately to a teacher reveals a situation where they may need some help, there are procedures for enabling this to be sought in confidence. These are outlined in later chapters.

Fear of embarrassment

Familiarity with the subject matter really does help here. Most of us have not had occasion to use sexual words out loud 'in public', so there can be a sense of shock when hearing your own voice saying these things for the first time in a class situation. Lead up to increasing this skill by practice, first of all perhaps in front of a mirror. Say all the dreaded words out loud. Answer hypothetical questions, again out loud or tape record them. Then practice with a small group of friends from the sex education team. Ask each other difficult questions, role play children asking personal questions and get used to the way of answering fluently, or of asking a question back to make sure the original question is fully understood.

If still apprehensive about the first occasion with a sex education class, use a film strip or slides so it is possible to stand at the back behind the children, thus avoiding full eyeball confrontation to begin with. The use of any good visual aids always helps as it is much easier to lose one's self-consciousness when explaining them, than when giving a straight forward verbal account, or conducting a discussion from the front of the class.

The children might work in small groups to start with, as this makes it easier both for them and the teacher. Work up to whole class involvement slowly. Ease of discussing sexual matters often follows the sequence: self and thoughts, best friend or spouse/partner, small group of friends, larger group, class, large meeting etc. Some people progress along these stages quickly, others would never be happy addressing a large gathering, but are perfectly at ease with smaller groups. This is just another example of human variation, but one which should be allowed for with children as well as staff. Start with the sex education areas you are most comfortable with, and as confidence is gained, on finding how sensible children are, move on to the ones originally thought more difficult. Try and go at your own pace; it does take time to assimilate ideas and develop new skills.

Not knowing the answer to a question

Why should anyone, even a teacher (!) be expected to know all the answers? Be non-defensive 'I'm not sure of the best way to answer that question for you. Does anyone have any idea where we could find out? We can discuss it next time'.

Don't forget to follow it up at the next session, even if the 'immediacy' has gone. Sex education should involve an exchange of ideas, it is not merely a 'telling' process. Of course if teachers are not able to discuss from the basis of a substantial knowledge of the subject, then they really have not done their homework and should not be attempting the work anyway. Fears about specific questions such as on oral sex, homosexuality or abortion should be talked out with the other sex education team members, and an overall approach decided. Some help is given later, on how such questions might best be considered.

Giggling and larking around from the children

This type of behaviour happens far less than teachers anticipate, if the subject is approached in a low key manner, and is not built up as an exciting event. When it does occur it is a symptom of the 'uncomfortableness' of the children with the topic, and should be treated as such. The comment might be 'Isn't it strange how talking about sex in public makes us want to laugh? Don't worry, you'll soon feel better about it, and won't feel the need to giggle.' Then introduce some humour so everyone can justifiably have a good laugh, and the air is cleared. Telling people not to giggle or 'titter' directly, only makes things much worse, as we all know! It will soon die down after such an approach, and as the children get more involved in the work.

One kind of behaviour which should be stopped early on is any jeering at the person asking a question. Stop the discussion at once. 'Let's get one thing very clear, we are talking about these things as sensible adults and I expect you to behave as such. You may all in the future be asked these questions by other people yourselves, so it's a good idea to find out the right answers now, and we should all respect those who admit they don't know everything but are willing to learn more.'

Fear of upsetting children

A survey done by Ripley et al [26] in secondary schools included asking first and fourth year pupils what worries they had about growing up. Of the younger girls one third had worries about menstruation, one tenth about sexual intercourse and no fewer than one half about childbirth.

Such worries were expressed very clearly in the free writing done by twelve year old Claire, during a series of lessons at school on human growth and development (see FIG 1). The fact that she was able to express her anxieties in this way, enabled her to get much needed reassurance from her teachers. It did take a while to allay her fears, but she was comforted by knowing they were taken seriously, and that other girls had had similar worries. It is surely far better to provide opportunities to reveal such disturbed feelings in this way, than that they should be suppressed, causing distress, and perhaps more serious problems later. 18% of the older girls in the Ripley study still expressed worries about childbirth. The boys in the study were more concerned about marriage, finding the right partner, and work prospects.

If material used in sex education work is carefully chosen and presented and is at the right level for the age group, there is no evidence that children are

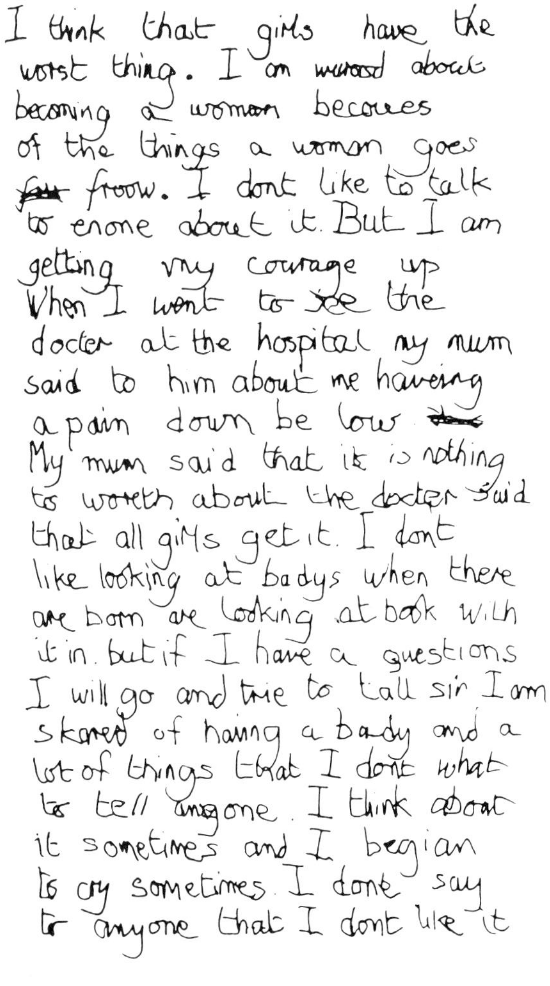

I think that girls have the worst thing. I am worried about becoming a woman becaues of the things a woman goes froow. I dont like to talk to enone about it. But I am getting vuy courage up Vhen I wont to see the docter at the hospital my mum said to him about me haveing a pain down be low My mum said that it is nothing to woreth about the docter suid that all gills get it. I dont like looking at badys when there are born are looking at book with it in. but if I have a questions I will go and trie to tall sir I am skared of haning a badly and a lot of things tbat I dont what to tell anyone. I think about it sometimes and I begian to cry sometimes. I dont say tr anyone that I dont like it

Figure 1　Free writing from a twelve year old.

upset primarily by its use. The anxieties they have are likely to be from incidents and information gained outside school, as Farrell [2] confirmed the findings of Gagnon and Simon [27], and Schofield [28] that 'friends' are the most frequent sources of information. Openness in talking about sex is not yet the norm in our society, so a few children may feel disturbed when sexual matters, raising thoughts and fears supressed over the years, are brought into the open. It is extremely important for a teacher to be sensitive to this possibility, and however great the general acceptance of the subject matter by the rest of the class, be always on the look out for children who may need further reassurance and help. This could be given in a small group situation, or in private. It is not possible to counter long felt anxieties with one or two 'sensible' lessons, so if there are any signs that a child is disturbed (looking away, seeming withdrawn and unhappy, not answering questions nor talking to other children, or conversely, too excitable and chatty and full of bravado) then the matter should be followed up tactfully by the teacher. As shown, free writing, in confidence, can be a method of expressing anxieties. If a teacher feels the child's worries are deep then he/she must be encouraged to get help from parents, a school counsellor or specialists. Cases like this are uncommon, but if staff are aware of such possibilities arising then help can be obtained early on.

The angry parent?

If the team approach is adopted it is extremely unlikely that individual teachers would ever be faced with an angry parent. However the thought is a worry to some, so, if it does arise teachers should remember their professional training and that they are working with the full support of the head and other members of staff. They should not take the complaint personally, but remain calm and non-defensive, welcoming the chance of hearing another point of view. They should first decide whether to refer the parent to a senior colleague or the head, ask a colleague to join them, or, if they wish to find out more about the problem first.

The parent could be asked to explain in detail what it is that has concerned him or her, whilst the teacher checks his or her understanding by summarising from time to time 'Does that mean that you feel ...?' 'Am I correct in thinking that ...?'

It may turn out to be a misunderstanding which can easily be cleared up, if not explain this point of view will be brought to the staff team, who will discuss it fully, and would then welcome another chance to talk to the parent.

The parent could be asked if they had been at the PTA meeting outlining the rationale behind the work. If not, it could be explained what other parents felt, and an invitation offered for the next session.

If the discussion has taken place alone with the parent a colleague could be asked to join in at the end – to hear a summary of the conversation, so there is agreement on what has been said. It also helps to provide a cup of tea and remember it is unlikely anyone will be able to please all the people all of the time! Afterwards a full report of the meeting should be given to the head and the staff team, so the parent's view may be considered, and action taken if necessary.

Parent-teacher meetings about sex education

It is not usual to involve parents in course work development in school, but this can be a very rewarding approach where sex education is concerned. Many official reports (page 16) advocate such co-operation.

Some of the difficulties parents face, have been outlined previously, so it can be appreciated that to continue with their role as the home members of the sex education team, they need to understand the aims of sex education in the school context.

Aims and Benefits

An informal series of staff parent meetings could enable parents to increase their own knowledge of human sexuality, so gaining confidence in discussing matters with their families, as nobody likes to appear ignorant in front of their children. They can also become aware of what topics *will* have been discussed at school, and this is very necessary as children are not renowned for communication on lesson content at home. The parents will be helped by having the development of their own child put in the context of the peer group known to the teachers. They often only see one side of their offspring, who may seem very different when in 'the gang' or class. The views of other parents can be heard and it can be reassuring to find that *not* 'everyone else' allows their offspring to go to all night discos, 'adult only' films etc!

The normality of adolescent turmoils can be explained and insight gained in how to help their children during this time. By the end of the meetings parents should feel they would be able to approach one of the teachers if they wished, to discuss their child's behaviour, and feel confident the school does understand parents' problems, is sympathetic to them, and can offer support and help for the family as a unit. In turn they may be more able to appreciate the very varied problems a school has, when coping with large numbers of children of different backgrounds, temperaments, and stages of maturity.

Organisation of the meeting

The way in which parents are invited to the meeting is important. Stress they will be able to meet the staff involved, join in discussion, ask questions, view material and their opinions will be welcomed.

It can be reassuring if a visiting speaker with a specialist expertise in sex education is also invited, perhaps from an academic or medical establishment. However, it may be advisable for such a person to take a subsidiary role in the proceedings and for the teachers to make the course presentation and lead discussions. By seeing them take an active role in this way parents can get to know the staff better, and gain confidence in their approach. The head could first introduce the sex education team, and outline the reasons for the school's involvement in personal development education. If the parents are then asked for their views on, for example, sex on television, 'girlie' magazines, 'adult' videos, etc the ensuing discussion usually shows clearly that young people today face situations the older generation did not have to cope with, and they may well need the combined help of home and school in determining values in a changing society.

Teachers from the team could explain how the school approached the course and outline its aims and methodology. The emphasis here would be the on-going nature of the programme, its adaptation to the maturity and ability level of the children, and the encouragement given to develop decision-making skills and personal responsibility. Some of the visual aid materials for the course could then be shown, with emphasis on the way in which they were to be used; the carefully planned lead in, the follow up work and so on. If the course had already run, collected comments from children could be read out (or could have been recorded) and would confirm it was realistic, and also reveal the questions and issues likely to be raised. If the parents were of 12 and 13 year old children the film *Then One Year* [15] would be most suitable for showing. It stresses the wide variation in rates of adolescent growth, which of course can be of concern to parents as well as children.

The viewing of audio-visual material really is very valuable to parents. It enables them to learn or revise sex education without loss of face, and it gives them confidence to know exactly what their children will be shown and what discussion may arise. It would be appropriate however, to explain they are experiencing a very concentrated version of the course, which when taken with the children would allow time to assimilate new facts, ideas and feelings. After questions and comments on the session so far, everyone would appreciate a break for refreshments, however simple. This may seem very obvious but it is important to have an informal stage in the evening, where any tension can be dissipated and parents can talk freely to each other and approach members of staff, or the visiting expert, to ask questions they would not feel able to raise in front of the full meeting. If they have not had sex education themselves at school, it may be a little shocking to hear and see sexual material being discussed in such a hallowed environment, and time to adjust to the new circumstances will be appreciated.

A selection of books to be used on the course, and those specifically written to help parents could be on display. If some of these are available for sale, one hurdle in sex education can be overcome, possible embarrassment when looking for material in bookshops. Most people confess to some such unease, so to be 'given permission', to take an open interest in books on sex, and get advice on their suitability for different age groups can be very useful. Local booksellers, or libraries may be able to help here, or each FPA region has a book centre and can provide a stall with a wide selection of books.

After the break one of the short trigger films from the *Loving and Caring* series [16] might be shown. *Mother and Daughter* or *Parents Talk* would be appropriate, and the teaching points that arise from them could be discussed. This would demonstrate that family relationships are of great concern, and helping parents and children to communicate with each other, and with teachers, is an important aim of the course.

Parents' feelings
Most parents will be fully supportive of the school programme, but a range of the concerns sometimes raised are given below, together with possible ways of dealing with them.

'My child is too young for this course'

'The teachers know from the general maturity of the children, and the questions they have already asked, that the class as a whole is ready for this material. If any particular children are not particularly interested, in the school's experience they just forget the information. The staff feel it protects children to hear the true facts nicely presented and this certainly won't hurt, but will mean the children are not so vulnerable to worrying stories they may hear later.'

'I have already told my child the facts of life and feel it is the parents' right to do so.'

'From the teaching point of view that is indeed most helpful, and the course will reinforce the message of caring and loving already given. Unhappily some parents are not as fortunate in being able to talk freely to their children, or they prefer the work to be done in school, so the teachers feel there is a need to help pupils who will have no help from their parents at all.'

'It is not right to do this work in school.'

'In fact research has shown children *do* accept sex education in school. They find it helpful to find out what their friends are thinking, have a chance to discuss their own feelings, and to ask questions of adults other than their parents, sometimes.'

'They're country children and they'll learn it from the animals.'

'Indeed, they do then have a great advantage. However, mating animals do not show much affection for each other. The process can be impersonal and quick, so it might be rather devastating if that was the only picture of sexual love ever presented. The mating of animals, flies, frogs, gerbils or dogs etc should always be explained when seen by children, but does not alone provide enough information. Human courtship and love is a far more complex matter – we are not after all "just like rabbits".'

'My religion has reservations on talking about sex to children'

'The teachers fully understand that different religions vary in their attitudes to human sexuality, and discussion of these differences will form part of the course. Staff do emphasise the right of each person to keep to the values of their own religion but also feel they should be aware of the beliefs of other religions and societies. The school would very much welcome help from you and your church leaders in presenting your particular beliefs.'

Cultural differences of approach

In multicultural schools pupils may come from families with very differing views on human sexuality. It is very important to find out exactly what the attitudes are of the particular culture, as represented in the area. The views of groups of people, including the leaders, should be sought, as these can vary, and stereotype classification is best avoided. Some help can be obtained:

i) *Discovering life through Growing Up* [31]. The religious and cultural differences in approaches to sex education in the Christian, Muslim, Hindu,

Sikh, Jewish and West Indian cultures are explained;

ii) *Report on the Study Day on Culture and Sexuality* prepared for the West Midlands Regional Health Authority, 146, Hagley Road, Birmingham. B16 9PA;

iii) Christopher's *Sexuality and Birth Control in Social & Community Work* 1980 Temple Smith, Chapter 14. 'The influence of Religion & Culture.' A most useful analysis of the attitudes of Catholics, Irish Catholics, Hindus, Muslims, Greek Cypriots, Turkish Cypriots and West Indians, to sex, marriage and contraception.

iv) *Guidelines on Muslim Pupils* (ILEA) includes reference to changing, swimming, dancing and sex education. Copies from EO/CEC7, County Hall, London.

The language problem

If the parents are unable to speak much English this particularly limits communication for sex education, where there are often restrictions within the culture. If only the fathers speak and understand English, it will be their views which will be put forward most strongly and tend anyway to dominate culturally. It may require some diplomacy to discover the views of the mothers.

Cultural changes

If the parents left their country some time ago, their views may now be somewhat old fashioned. Their own culture may be in the process of change, particularly with regard to the role of women.

The traditional extended family system may not be established in this country, so historically developed patterns of information giving, and support for the children may not be fully available.

There may also be a considerable 'generation gap' between school children and their parents, related to the culture clash. This can build up resentment particularly in girls, who may wish for more 'freedom' like their European friends. The children may need help in understanding the very great importance of 'family honour' which parents see as intrinsically involved when personal relationships are under consideration.

There may be differences in attitude within one culture, related to race, religion, rural or urban life, education level, cast, language spoken and past experience. Very generally, the lower the socio-economic class of any culture, the more traditional and rigid are their ideas about modesty, sex and marriage.

General attitudes of Asian cultures

Girls are seen to be particularly vulnerable, and daughters need to be protected from 'taking the wrong steps', i.e. developing an emotional or physical involvement with a member of the opposite sex. Girls are not allowed to learn about personal relationships by having a series of boyfriends as is more common in European cultures. Virginity for girls is necessary for a good marriage. The followers of Islam are most strict in enforcing this behaviour. Girls of some cultures are extremely restricted in their activities out of school, and their social behaviour is watched carefully.

Boys are also expected to behave in an appropriate manner, but they are sometimes given more freedom of movement and involvement in relationships than the girls. They may also be valued more highly in a family, particularly as they will not need a dowry on marriage.

Sex is not talked of openly within the family, ignorance is thought of as being protective, and information, when provided, is often at or after the event e.g. menarche or marriage.

Marriages are often 'arranged' ones. The family takes responsibility for finding a suitable partner and the matching of backgrounds and status etc. is seen as more important than the emotions of the individuals. There is an increasing trend for couples in Britain to be allowed to meet before the final decision is made. There is very great support for the marriage from within the family, children are expected, and may be financed by the extended family.

'Love' marriages are sometimes allowed if the couple have similar backgrounds, but as the choice of partner has been theirs, should the marriage break down there might be less support given by the family in this situation.

West Indians

West Indians differ entirely from the attitudes explained above, as they have a greater acceptance of sex, marital and extra-marital, for both men and women. Because of their social history, illegitimacy is not considered a social stigma for mother or child and in fact may be used to show fertility or a 'love bond', and men and boys do not necessarily accept responsibility for their children. Patterns of marriages vary, but generally real marriage is viewed as an important step which may come after several 'common law marriages', and then responsibility is taken for children both from and outside the marriage. Girls are sometimes very restricted by their parents who fear they will become pregnant too early and chastise them severely if they do. Boys do not come under the same kind of social control. The mother is often the central person for the family and the parent best known to the children.

It is obviously impossible to summarise complex historical, sociological and cultural factors in a few sentences, and it is essential that schools find out for themselves exactly what the values and attitudes to sex, and sex education, are of the parents of the children they are teaching.

Parent-Teacher meetings in multicultural areas

It is extremely important that parental support be gained for the sex education programme. This is by no means an impossible task, given good will and more understanding of the nature of the beliefs of both the families and the schools.

The letter of invitation to such an occasion could be in the native language, sent by post, with the promise that an interpreter will be present at the meeting. Again, it is very important to remember that parents are individuals and not stereotypes.

At the meeting the role of sex education in the school could be explained as previously suggested, but the parents' confidence increased by emphasising that the course is aimed at promoting understanding and knowledge of the human body, so anxiety, worry and distress (for example about menstruation) can be avoided. It can be explained that this is knowledge other children will have and the course will counter media implications that free love is the norm in 'our' society.

The course will try to increase understanding between men and women and hence eventual domestic harmony and happiness and cultural differences in attitudes to the role of women and marriage will be examined, including the consequences in all cultures of foregoing family support and approval. The overall aim is to increase knowledge of sexuality, without increasing social problems. It can be explained that it might be possible for girls and boys to be taken in separate groups for this work, and by a teacher of their own sex. (It may be more acceptable if that person is not of the same culture as the children, because of historical taboos on talking about the subject.)

It can be explained that requirements for modesty are appreciated and special arrangements have been made for changing for physical education and swimming.

Children in cross cultural situations are sometimes in a very difficult position and deserve our sympathy and help. The knowledge that their parents are aware of what they are being taught in school can be a great relief to them, and can lessen any feelings of guilt and anxiety. Each area in the country has a unique blend of circumstances, and every school has to develop its own systems of communication and feel confident it has majority support for the sex education programme.

Books suitable for parents, and teachers
i) *Goodbye to the Stork* Kenner J. 1973 National Marriage Guidance Council. A general introduction to sex education.
ii) *How did I grow? A parents' guide to children's questions* Gwynne Jones E. 1977 BBC Excellent background information and sound advice on answering questions from 8–10 year old children.
iii) *Parents listen* Pickering L. 1981 Cassell Ltd Helpful advice on relationships and sex education for all ages. (My only reservation is the explanation of homosexuality). Companion book to '*Girls talk*' and '*Boys talk*'
iv) *Answering a Child's Questions* HEC Health Education Council leaflet with questions from all ages of children.
v) *Adolescent Sex – its difficulties and dangers, an outline for clinic personnel, parents and teachers.* Kleinman R. L. (Ed.) 1978. Not as problem orientated as it sounds, this has some useful advice. IPPF International Planned Parenthood Federation.
vi) *The Facts of Love* Comfort A & J 1979 Mitchell Beazley. A superbly illustrated book, honest enough to tackle the realities of adolescent sexuality and written in a sensitive way. All parents should read this while their children are still young, so they are prepared for using it with them before and during puberty.

Books suitable for children, parents and teachers
(For books for pre-school and infant children see page 55)
i) *How did I grow?* Chovil C. 1977 BBC. A well illustrated book for 8–10 year old children, follow-up to the BBC sex education TV programmes.

ii) *Girls Talk* Pickering L. 1981 Cassell Ltd. For girls of about 10 & 12

iii) *Boys Talk* Pickering L. 1981 Cassell Ltd. For boys of about 10 & 12
These two books, companions to *Parents listen*, put a full explanation of growing up and being married within a natural story line emphasising relationships.

iv) *Girls' and Boys' Questions Answered* NMGC 1980 National Marriage Guidance Council. Straightforward answers to all usual questions from teenagers.

v) *Knowing about sex – Growing up* Hemming J. & Maxwell Z. (Ed.) Macmillan. A story of a brother and sister approaching puberty. Beautifully illustrated partly by black and white photographs, loving family context throughout.

vi) *Learning to live with sex* Burkitt A. 1980 FPA. A glossary of the words teenagers want to know about.

vii) *Knowing about Sex – Achieving Sexual Maturity* Hemming J. & Maxwell Z. (Ed.) Macmillan. A lavishly illustrated book with many beautiful photographs. All aspects of sex and responsibility are considered. Suitable for children from 13 and 14 on.

Please also see book lists in each curriculum section.

Books useful for the sex education team background reading

1 *Sexuality and birth control in social and community work.* Elphis Christopher. 1980 Temple Smith. An invaluable guide for understanding a wide range of common problems causing emotional and physical difficulties for families.

2 *Making sense of sex.* Helen Kaplan. 1979 Quartet Books. An excellent account of human sexuality, in a most readable form.

3 *Pregnant at School.* Joint Working Party on Pregnant Schoolgirls and Schoolgirl Mothers. Sept. 1979. National Council for One Parent Families.
A most valuable survey of the many issues involved when girls at school become pregnant.

4 *Understanding Human Sexual Inadequacy.* Fred Belliveau & Lin Richter 1971. Hodder Paperback. This provides an interpretation of the work of the pioneer research into human sexuality done by Masters & Johnson.

5 *Children's Sexual Thinking.* Ronald and Juliette Goldman, 1982. Routledge and Kegan Paul. Absolutely essential for sex educators, this fascinating book details in-depth research into children's perception, knowledge and understanding of the sexual world.
Their next book *Readiness for Sex Education* will give further information on children's conceptual development in sex education.

6 *Journal of Research and Development in Education.* Vol 16 No 2. 1983. The whole issue is devoted to sex education.

7 *My Mother said . . .* Christine Farrell. 1978. Routledge and Kegan Paul. See page 8.

Chapter 3

THE METHODOLOGY OF SEX EDUCATION

Affective teaching

Over the past few years in health education there has been a move away from the fact-giving topic-based approach, towards 'affective' or 'informal' teaching, demanding different methods and skills. Behind this shift in emphasis is a growing awareness that knowledge by itself does not enable people to change their attitudes or behaviour. For this to happen much more understanding is needed of the social pressures acting against free choice. Individuals need help to enable them to recognise what factors are operating and to link 'school knowledge' with its use in real life [3].

The aim of affective education is 'self empowerment' or 'autonomy' where individuals, by understanding the consequences of their actions can take responsibility for controlling their own lives, and enhancing their own self esteem, but not at the expense of others. A 'considerate' way of life is the ultimate goal. Affective teaching involves consideration of the social side of each issue, often by using 'situations' or 'scenarios'. Children are encouraged to discover by writing, role play and discussion etc., why the characters portrayed are behaving as they are, what the pressures on them have been, and so on.

This leads to increased awareness of the reasons behind a person's behaviour, and hence to the possibility of changing that behaviour, if appropriate.

Help available

Keith Tones has provided an extensive analysis of the methods used in affective teaching in Chapter 1 of *Health Education in Schools* [30] and another most helpful publication is *Informal methods in Health and Social Education* by Bill Rice. TACADE 1981. This book explains the skills used in informal teaching, and contains many practical suggestions.

Life Skills Associates have produced teaching programmes, books, and a quarterly journal for those involved in teaching social skills, including those of parent/teacher and teacher/parent interactions.

Discussion Techniques

The use of group discussion methods is fundamental to affective teaching. Help for developing these skills is available from:

i) TACADE see details of specific interest courses
ii) *Health Education in Secondary Schools* Schools Council Working Paper 57, [41] Part 2. VI has details on how to organise discussion groups effectively.

iii) *Learning to teach through discussion* [49] This book and associated tape investigate discussion techniques, have advice on the role of a 'neutral' chairperson, and on handling difficulties such as non-contributors, or over dominant children. 'Discussion' needs careful preparation and lead in, as if attempted too soon in a session, opinions may polarise and harden.

Affective education is one of the most difficult areas teachers have ever been asked to participate in, but the benefits of doing it could be tremendous. It is inappropriate for young children to make major decisions about their life styles so the development of decision making skills, by affective education, is a long process linked with the increasing maturity, concept development and responsibility of the children. Both SCHEP 5-13 and Health Education 13-18 are based on this type of approach as is the excellent TACADE project *Free to choose*, [32].

The crisis approach to sex education
Often in the past the only permissable sex education has been designed to prevent sexual activity altogether, by threats of unwanted pregnancies, disabling diseases or emotional rejection. The technique using fear as a disincentive does not have a very good track record however. Tones [30] finds clear evidence that the arousal of fear is counterproductive. This confirms Dallas [48] who suggests that to cope with the arousal of great fear, individuals reject the given information as irrelevant, (the 'it can't happen to me' feeling) and do not in fact change their behaviour. Emery [34] suggests it is a great mistake to exaggerate consequences in order to make a greater impression, because when found out, credibility is lost. It seems a more positive approach is likely to be effective, and a problem orientated curriculum may well be self defeating.

A realistic approach is therefore needed. Small amounts of fear, which can be coped with, can be valuable motivators, but gloom and doom scenarios build up resistance and rejection.

Self-revelation
One of the hazards of an informal approach to health and sex education is the potential threat to the privacy of both children and staff. Ways in which a teacher's privacy can be maintained have already been suggested (page 24). In a class situation great care must be taken a pupil does not pour out a personal or family experience. Methods which can be used to avoid this situation are as follows:

i) Work through a third party; the boy, girl or adult presented in a situation or story. This allows feelings to be expressed through them, in a way which does not threaten personal or family relationships. So the suggestion ... 'If you were Jane/Simon how would you feel about ...' is used, rather than the direct 'If *you* were in that situation ...'. This protective technique can be used in discussion groups and role play, to prevent the revelation of information which might be regretted later, or used by other class members to bring pressure on the person concerned.

ii)   Personal data such as the length of menstrual cycles can be collected anonymously and presented as overall class statistics, showing variations, but *not* relating these to individuals.

iii) Dalzell-Ward [50] suggests the use of a multiple choice system. Children are given items to place under various headings, as a small group, thus when their choices are discussed, individuals cannot be identified.

iv)   To avoid personal identification when asking questions (which can reveal a great deal about the questioner) the anonymous question box can be used. Identical slips of paper are given out, and everyone hands them in folded, with a question or comment or just left blank. This method can also be used later to evaluate the course, or for suggestions for future work.

v)   Some degree of self revelation is helpful when young people are sorting out ideas and feelings, but only in a one to one teacher/pupil situation within the teacher's overall counselling role. Again care is needed to prevent confidences being made which might afterwards be regretted, and no member of staff will imagine themselves to be an instant sex therapist however much reading they have done! If the problem seems serious, referral to a specialist counsellor may be necessary.

Vocabulary to be used

To facilitate communication on sexual matters, it is necessary to provide an acceptable vocabulary.

There are many highly descriptive vernacular words for sexual parts and acts, and it is helpful if a teacher has some knowledge of these. The Goldmans [53] give lists of more than 60 pseudonyms for a penis and 40 for a vagina for example, and Burkitt [42] provides a glossary of more usual expressions. Some children may not have any other way of expressing themselves, so it is important a teacher is not shocked by their use. However, because of the enormous variation in regional and local expressions it is wisest to set up a universal language and use accepted Latin terms, at their simplest level. The class confidence will be increased by using them and communication with the medical profession and understanding of leaflets and books, will be promoted.

When starting a course at secondary level for example it is vital that everyone does understand exactly what is being talked about, so using charts of the human body, the Latin names for parts are provided, and variations asked for. The Goldmans' lists could be used here. This usually causes much mirth, and is a lead in to discussing the sociology of language and how some words can be used to shock or show aggression. When 'translated' they lose their sting and, hopefully, some of the fear associated with them. The words little children use for sexual parts could be talked about too, and the use of 'codes' within families, to save themselves and others from embarrassment. The advantages and disadvantages of vernacular and family languages could be discussed, leading to an appreciation of the advisability of using terms everyone understands.

Many children use 'bad language' without realising what it means, just knowing they can get a reaction from adults by using it. 'He even said "knickers" in the Post Office!' said one mother, verbally terrorised by her four year old son.

Don't be afraid of words in themselves. A 'non-reaction' if they are being used to shock is the most effective strategy. Making a fuss and forbidding their use only enables them to be developed as weapons.

Mixed sex classes or not?

In co-education schools some staff feel teaching separate sex classes defeats one of the objectives of sex education, increasing ease of communication with the opposite sex. Others argue this is too embarrassing and that single sex groups are the only ones possible. I have found *both* can be appropriate at various times for the following reasons.

Advantages

Where mixed sex classes are usual, to split boys and girls as soon as sex education is considered, puts this subject immediately into a 'special' category and may raise the anticipation level of the children unduly. To hear sex talked about in a sensible and relaxed way to a mixed group is in itself an aid to acceptability, and it is also valuable for one sex to hear the opinions of the other, thus promoting a greater understanding of the feelings and attitudes involved.

Disadvantages

There are perhaps three main reasons why single sex classes are sometimes appropriate. The first of these is sexism.

There is evidence [24] that in mixed classes in any subject, girls are more reticent about answering than boys, even if they know the answer, and boys tend to dominate the answering and discussion sessions. This phenomenon is even more apparent when sex education classes are taken. Is it equally socially acceptable for boys and girls to talk about sex in public? Is it acceptable for a girl to tell a sexual joke or make a 'witty' comment? Is there more fear in the girls of giving away information about themselves? If boys and girls are to be helped to talk about their feelings without the need to 'show off' or impress each other, this is much more likely to happen in single sex small group situations than in a full mixed class. Different sorts of discussion take place in single sex and mixed groups, as everyone with experience of both will know. Even basic questions about the opposite sex, can be raised in the former without loss of face, and information and reassurance provided.

The second reason for arranging single sex classes might be because of cultural differences. If a large proportion of the pupils are Asian or other cultures where the children may have been brought up to feel talking about sexual matters in mixed sex classes is embarrassing or even degrading, then it may be advisable to arrange for single sex classes, and that only women teachers talk with the girls and men with the boys. Finally the maturity difference in the children should be considered. Because of very great differences in the age of puberty between boys and girls, it can happen that a class of 12 to 13 year old children has a majority of post-pubertal girls, but pre-pubertal boys. The girls being more 'mature' in every way, benefit from a different approach and this can be provided in a single sex situation.

Organisation within a class

Some mixed sex classes organise themselves into single sex groups – and to be forced to work 'with the girls' or 'join the boys group' is seen as an imposition. This situation can be taken advantage of, if the children are asked to work in 'friendship' groups. The teacher can circulate and more delicate questions can be asked within the smaller groups. Some of these can then be raised with the whole class but without disclosing their origin. It would be encouraging if the children realised eventually why they felt the need to keep in single sex groups initially, and were then able to tolerate each other better. The Goldmans [53] stress the need to reduce antipathy between boys and girls of all ages.

Timetabled single sex classes

Physical education is one subject where boys and girls are taken separately as a norm in secondary schools. Some sex education may already be included. If this could be co-ordinated with the core course, it would be a most helpful way of allowing discussion to take place in single sex groups, without making a great issue of their separation. Some schools separate boys and girls temporarily for subjects, such as mathematics. The strategy would be very suitable for some stages of the sex education curriculum. The groups are re-united when confidence has developed.

The use of outside speakers in sex education

Outside visitors can be of great value (Clarke [59]) particularly if they are integrated into an overall programme, and not used as the only method of 'covering' the particular issue. They can add variety and interest to the programme and offer specialist knowledge and training and a different approach. Some have practical clinical experience and a first hand knowledge of human variation, giving high credibility and a link with 'real life' situations. People coming in from the community show health education is an on-going team effort, involving many different 'caring' groups and the speakers themselves can help to give teachers confidence, by showing an ease in talking about sexual matters with children.

The pupils may in fact feel freer to ask a speaker questions, as the event is seen as more confidential, the child can be anonymous, the visitor does not 'know the parents' and is not seen as part of the authoritarian establishment.

Class involvement in inviting and welcoming the visitor, and in organising the session, is a most useful exercise. Advice on this is given in the first sections of each of the *Active Tutorial Work Books* [35].

Many visitors will not have been trained in education skills so it is extremely helpful if they can contact the teacher before their visit and discuss such matters as the exact nature of the proposed presentation, i.e. whether this is to be factual only, or perhaps even more usefully about their experiences in the health care system. Previous work done by the class can be explained including the anti-sexist approach being taken and any link up and lead on points that might be possible in the time available, realistically! The visitor will need to know the ability range, vocabulary level and idiom of the class and the format of the session, discussion group arrangements, visual aid facilities etc. The procedure for feedback to the visitors about the effectiveness of the session can be arranged together with discussion of any recent incident, e.g. a pregnancy or sexual assault, which could have affected the class.

Should the teacher stay in the session?

An opportunity might be provided at some stage for children to speak to the visitor privately, or in small groups, without the teacher present. However, if staff have already gained the pupils' confidence, by doing some of the work themselves, it will not be embarrassing if they stay in. There are many advantages in doing so. Consider the effect if teachers disappear after introducing the speaker.

Do they already know it all?

Aren't they interested in what the visitor has to say?

Are they too embarrassed by the occasion?

Are they having a 'feet up' cup of tea in the staffroom?

The hidden curriculum works powerfully on such occasions, so the temptation to catch up on urgent marking or reports is perhaps best resisted. By remaining in the session, teachers can account for what has been said, give the speaker confidence in good discipline, and also increase their own understanding of the subject. They will be able to note the reaction of the class and use this in later lessons and can assess whether the visitor is making contact with the children or misunderstandings are developing. Finally, and most importantly, by staying in the session teachers will be more able to answer questions from pupils later, as these can arise days or even weeks after the visit.

Ideally, when visitor and teacher get to know one another, a 'team teaching' session can be set up, profiting from the teacher's expert knowledge of the children, and the visitor's expertise in the subject.

Useful visitors

The most useful kind of visitor would be someone involved in the social side of health care, for example

i)   a health visitor involved in domicilliary visiting, explaining the difficulties some have in getting to clinics

ii) a nursery school teacher able to talk about the reactions of small children 'left' for the first time by their parents

iii) a nurse or receptionist from a preparation for pregnancy, ante-natal or family planning clinic, who could describe how the clinic was run, the welcome given couples seeking advice together etc.

iv) a contact tracer from a special clinic, on the need to help those who may not know they might have an infection.

This approach is probably more productive than asking such people to give straight talks on 'the facts', of ante natal care etc. which could be covered in other ways. However, the need for such information would arise from the sessions and would then appear more relevant.

The Health Education Officer or LEA Advisor could make suggestions for suitable people to ask as visitors. National organisations providing speakers are detailed at the end of this chapter.

Visits by pupils

If visits to clinics, nurseries or maternity homes could be arranged for small groups of pupils over the weeks following a talk about them, this would emphasise links with the community and help to lower any barriers to using such services later.

General points on methodology

The approach to teaching sex education should be to provide *varied* methods and media, not relying exclusively on films for example, though these do have their place of course. Sex education can be as boring as any other if not well taught and it might be agreed that there is no miraculous process of education for this subject alone which ensures children, when 'told' the facts once, will remember them for ever, understand all the implications immediately and never make mistakes!

A spiral syllabus building up information relevant to the needs and concept levels of the children is essential (see next section). Regular testing for understanding is needed, as for any other subject. Teachers will realise that being 'preached at' is strongly resisted by children and, as previously discussed (page 37) problem-based sex education is unlikely to be effective. Time is needed however to learn about and discuss positive feelings about human sexuality. Talking about sexual parts of the body in a non-sexual context can be helpful. For example, if slides of cheek cells are made in biology classes, the opportunity could be taken to compare this process with the cervical smear test, and the nature of the cervix discussed. Pupils could explain this procedure to other small groups perhaps.

The need for all women to have this test done at some stage could be emphasised and the ease and speed of the procedure itself, linked with the pupils' own experience of examining human cells. Cancer of the cervix can be diagnosed and completely cured if detected early. Tragically 90% of women found to have invasive cervical cancer have never had a smear test done at all (Observer 5. 2. 84).

Visual aid material

This can be very powerful, so great care is needed in the choice and use of suitable material which often tends to be too complicated. Use clear, simple pictures and charts and lead up to more explicit material carefully, and then lead down again, within the lesson. Variation is a norm in human sexuality, so beware of focussing attention on *one* body shape or piece of behaviour in the visual aids used as if this was a standard we should all aspire to. Interpretation of visual aid material also needs care as the traditional 'half' people, with various cut ends of gut, bones and tubes can be confusing to adults as well as children. Always use material which relates the part in question to the whole body, and shows it in three dimensions, using models if possible. If a section view is needed, keep relating this back to the 3D version, or make a plasticine model and cut it, to show which view is being presented. Always give the actual range of dimensions of the organs under consideration, and reinforce the understanding of these. How many children think that sperm cells are 1cm long and black, I wonder, (despite evidence to the contrary for some, from wet dreams!)?

Try also to give some idea of the true colour and texture of the organs being described. It is amazing how many hard, blue, purple and green uteri there are, apparently! Hardly any visual aids are perfect in all respects but suggestions for those which come nearest to these standards are given later, in context.

The use of 'wrong' information

One useful technique is to gather myths, about any sex education topic. Discussion on how these could have arisen, the associated fear, and the barriers to communication they create, and the risks taken by those believing in them, can be illuminating. However, presenting wrong information as fact and *then* trying to unscramble truth from half truth presents some hazards. This is the method used in the second sequence of the 'Trigger' [56] films on venereal diseases for example. If it is explained the characters believe wrong things and the class is being asked to 'collect' them for discussion, that would be a valid approach. If this warning is not given, the tremendous impact of film material, particularly that depicting individuals the children readily identify with, may mean the less able pupil firmly fixes on wrong information initially, and this may be difficult to unlearn. It is advantageous, however, to use such films, and other material, to demonstrate that some people, including adults, can talk nonsense confidently and with some persuasion. Sources of accurate information can then be discussed. Who can you trust?

The pre-viewing of all audio-visual material for sex education is absolutely essential, and will enable it to be selected at the right level and for lead up and follow on sessions to be prepared. This could include discussion of the feelings of the characters involved before and after the sequence shown, or of an 'added' character e.g. mother, brother or friend. Full time must be allowed for discussion, which is probably the most important part of the lesson. Stop the film or tape, use half the slides only. The materials sometimes seem to exert a 'take over bid' for the whole lesson! The short, 10–12 minute 'Trigger' films [67] are very useful and have good teachers' notes. Material can be used more than once, of course, as long as this is planned. It takes several viewings sometimes to extract full value from some resources.

Varied activities

The lesson activities can be varied, by the children not only writing about feelings associated with growing up in letter or short article form, but small groups of pupils could interview other children, staff or visitors, on tape perhaps as 'reporters' collecting views on 'family limitation' or 'Women's lib'. They might then be able to prepare a 5 minute local radio programme from the results.

Research could be undertaken by groups or individuals for specified project work (which could include finding addresses, sending off to the FPIS for information, reading leaflets, summarising them or listening to radio and TV programmes) on subjects such as the local welfare services for young families. The findings could be reported back to the group or class, verbally or in writing and the information displayed, in pie chart diagram, or collage form, on for example, 'a history of women's rights'. Similar visual aids could be made about such things as growth rates in young children or attitudes to housework. Family groups and activities, people of different ages, non-stereotyped gender role situations could be photographed and a display mounted on 'the changing role of men and women'. Think tank activities and word association sessions in small groups, could sometimes be organised, the 'scribe' charting the progress of ideas on a large sheet of paper. Discussion of the general picture and feelings presented for example about 'going to a clinic', then follows.

Other group work could involve making models, flow charts, leaflets or booklets for use with other groups or classes. The selection of material and information, the clarity and layout of leaflet etc. become factors involved here. Analyse magazines, advertisements, TV and Radio programmes, rock and pop records and book reviews, looking for hidden messages, chauvinistic or sexist.

Arguments for and against an 'age of consent', 'childless by choice, selfish or not?' could be debated. A form magazine could be produced using all the above skills, plus those of an editorial panel who could consider whether we need censorship or sensitivity when presenting material for others.

In controlled situations role play can be invaluable, and a good release for humour, but great care has to be taken in sex education that children are not acting out home situations. Beware also of stereotype portrayals, though these can be used initially to pin-point such tendencies. By reversing boy/girl roles and using parent/child situations, sexist and generation gap conflicts can be explored and solutions sought for their resolution. Positive role play, showing good relationships is needed, as a contrast to the opposite, which tends to be more dramatic of course. Drama teachers will often help in developing role playing skills.

The actual activities such as suggested above are important not just for the skills developed during them, but because they act as 'distractors', and questions on sex can arise naturally and be discussed as they 'surface', without embarrassment, in a relaxed but busy atmosphere. Many people have found it easier to talk about sex when doing something else as well e.g. mending a bike, or washing up, than when in a direct 'face to face' situation. The 'distraction' principle is also working here.

Sex education skills

A most useful lead-in to sex education in secondary schools is to ask teenagers to consider how they might function as sex educators themselves, if and when they become parents, or are in contact with small children. Adolescents find the questions asked by infants amusing and can discuss their own early wrong ideas. The 'allowable' laughter generated considerably eases possible initial tension in introducing the subject. A great deal of sexual knowledge can be covered by this 'non threatening' method, and without the implications about sexual activity in the older age group, which could cause embarrassment if led into straight away. A suggested scheme for such an approach is given later (page 243). This may enable secondary pupils to develop skills in answering young children's questions simply and clearly, both paving the way for additional information for themselves and allowing basic facts to be revised without insult! It will also perhaps help future generations of parents and friends to function more effectively as sex educators.

Evaluation

Evaluation is an important part of any course and no less so for sex education. The methods used will vary according to the different aims of parts of the course. 'Gain in knowledge' is easy to assess, the way in which such knowledge can be applied, less so. Skills of communication, evaluation of materials and more specific ones such as using a telephone, following instructions, reading a thermometer, recording dates, will all need particular evaluation methods. The classic method, is of pre-and post tests and though these involve considerable work when first setting up the course, once established they will only need small modifications from year to year. The Health Education Council has produced a useful collection of summaries of evaluations of health education projects, *Is Health Education Effective?* (HEC 1979). This contains a survey of the theory of evaluation, and seven sections detailing specific programmes. The studies attempt to assess attitude and behaviour change. The discussion of overall findings affirms it is easier to improve factual knowledge than change attitudes, but that changing behaviour is not more difficult than changing attitudes, as had previously been thought. Individual instruction was found to be the best teaching method, followed by group work. Written instructions were inferior to most other methods, so the adage 'not by leaflet alone' would be worth considering, and those who feel sex education is 'giving them a good book' are unrealistic in their expectations.

Another useful paper is *Formative Evaluation of a Sex Education Course for Young Adolescents*. Parcel, Guy Setal. Journal of School Health. June 1979 p.335–339 available from the HEC. This summarises the evaluation techniques used for a sex education programme for 13 and 14 year olds in the USA.

Resources and in-service training for sex education
Family Planning Association (FPA)
National Centre, London, and 11 regional centres.

i) *Courses in personal relationships and sex education.*
    These are held at the National Centre, London, or custom designed and run locally, by arrangement. All courses use participatory methods.
ii) *Visual aid materials.*
    A range of films and teaching cards, and other material is available.
iii) *Speakers*
    Trained speakers on a wide range of sex education subjects, can present information or lead discussion groups with parents, teachers or children. Contact the Regional centres for details.
iv) *Family Planning Information Service (FPIS)*
    The FPIS, with the HEC, provides extensive literature and information on all aspects of family planning and related areas, including free leaflets, posters and fact sheets. They have a central enquiries department and walk in information bureau with an information and resource centre with reference library. They publish '*Family Planning Today*', a quarterly bulletin with news of the latest research, and books, conferences and courses on sex education.

The London centre and book shop are in Mortimer Street. Each of the 11 regional centres of the FPA also has a book shop, and can provide fact sheets, leaflets, booklists, posters, advice and help for teachers.

Table 1   Summary of available resources.

Resources for Sex Education Summary Sheet

	National courses in sex education	Local courses in sex education	Information/Advisory and Resource Centre	Bookshop	Publications	Local Centre
Family Planning Association	Yes	Yes, by arrangement	London 27–35 Mortimer St. (and local)	London and local	Family Planning Today. Quarterly £2. FPIS	11 Regional Centre (see list page)
Health Education Council	—	In conjunction with Schools Council material (see below)	London 78 New Oxford St. (and local)	London limited range for sale	Health Education News. Termly. Free. via HEO. Health Education Journal. Quarterly £3 year	Local District Health Authority Health Education Departments have HEC material
TACADE	—	Yes, by arrangement	Manchester 2 Mount St., and Bournemouth 202 Holdenhurst Rd.	Manchester	'Monitor' Termly. Free on request	—
National Marriage Guidance Council	—	Yes, by arrangement	Rugby Little Church St. (and local)	Rugby and some local	—	Many centres. See telephone directory
Brook Advisory Centres	—	Yes, by arrangement	Birmingham 8–10 Albert St. Bristol 15/17 Bayswater Ave. (and local)	—	—	See telephone directory for local centres
Schools Council Material	—	Dissemination courses, by arrangement and in conjunction with the HEC & LEA	Southampton write to SCHEP, or HEP, Dept. of Education University of Southampton	Teacher and pupil packs SCHEP 5–13, Nelson Health Education 13–18, Forbes	—	Possibly available from local teacher centre or RHA or DHA Depts

TACADE

This organisation incorporates the Health Education Development Unit (HEDU) and the Teachers' Advisory Council on Alcohol and Drug Education. They have wide experience of running in service courses for teachers. One Unit, a workshop on sex education is particularly relevant, as are

i)   Courses run within a local education authority for the coordination of health education in secondary schools. (Now part of Health Education 13–18 [9].)

ii)   Specific interest modules varying in length from two hours to two days, on situation education, teaching decision making skills, the use of visitors in schools, or using structured discussion in the classroom.

iii)   Courses devised specifically for the needs of the group including one on sex education if requested.

TACADE have a leaflet explaining their many services, which include a wide range of publications, a termly bulletin 'Monitor', and research and evaluation projects. Contact the Information officer, TACADE, 2 Mount St, Manchester.

National Marriage Guidance Council (NMGC)

In addition to their confidential counselling services for people with difficulties in marriage or other relationships, the NMGC

i)   provides speakers for discussion groups of young people;

ii)   meets with teachers to help set up programmes for teachers, parents, or children, or groups of all three;

iii)   publishes a wide range of books and leaflets related to marriage and family life, and available from local centres (see the telephone directory) or from the bookshop at Rugby.

For further details contact the Education Projects Officer, NMGC, Little Church Street, Rugby.

The Health Education Council (HEC)

The HEC can offer teachers:

i)   help in developing the school health education curriculum;

ii)   courses such as SCHEP Health Education 13–18 [9] and ATW [35];

iii)   a wide range of free leaflets, posters and books (see publications catalogue, available from HEOs);

iv)   publication of *Health Education News* available from HEOs free and *Health Education Journal*, quarterly £3 per year;

v)   a resources centre, 78, New Oxford Street, London, which is invaluable for curriculum development in sex education, providing an audio visual collection available for reference and pre-viewing, a comprehensive library from which books and journals may be borrowed and an information service, for all enquires, and numerous free information sheets, source lists, film notes etc. Contact the Information Officer, HEC, address above.

Brook Advisory Centres (BAC)
This organisation:

i)   arranges local courses on personal relationships and sex education, for teachers, pupils or parents.
ii) provides speakers on a range of sex education subjects
iii) produces teaching material, information sheets, leaflets and booklets, all detailed in their catalogue.
iv) They also produce *Newsprint*, a monthly collection of press items relating to sex education. A small fee is charged for this service.

The two BAC education and resource centres where teachers can get help, advice and new material are the Education & Publications Unit, 10, Albert Street, Birmingham and the Sex Education Resource Centre, 15/17, Bayswater Avenue, Bristol. Contact the Education Officers at the above addresses.

The British Pregnancy Advisory Service (BPAS)
The BPAS provides the following for teachers:

i)   speakers for talks or courses, on contraception, abortion, infertility, artificial insemination, and the wider issues these raise
ii) free leaflets and posters on these services
iii) loan or hire of films and a range of audiovisual aids (list available)
iv) a library and information service for reference and research or curriculum development.

Contact the Information Officer, Austy Manor, Wootton Wawen, West Midlands.

The International Planned Parenthood Federation (IPPF)
This organisation produces:

i)   a paper *Research into Reproduction* providing summaries of research in reproductive physiology issued free, four times a year which is rather technical but relevant to advanced work in Biology and Chemistry
ii) information on world population figures, and the provision and status of family planning services, in all countries. Contact the Information Officer IPPF, 18–20, Lower Regent Street, London. SW17 4PW

Office of Population Censuses and Surveys (OPCS)
This government statistical service provides 'Monitors', free of charge, on population growth, the incidence of infectious diseases, legal abortions etc. Contact the Information Branch, (Dept M) OPCS, St Catherine's House, 10, Kingsway, London WC28 6JP

Population concern
A fund raising body linked with FPA. Its education work includes providing material on all world population matters, both demographic and social. Contact Population Concern, 27/35 Mortimer Street, London, W1.

The Inner London Education Authority (ILEA)
Many ILEA services and materials are available to all teachers

i)   Centre for learning Resources. Kennington Lane, London. Library, information service, and selection of health education materials.
ii) Catalogue of material from Learning Materials Service. Contact the ILEA Learning Materials Service, Publishing Centre, Highbury Station Road, London. N1 1SB

Schools Council Health Education Projects and Health Education Council Projects
i)   *SCHEP 5–13*, materials from Nelsons publishers, HEOs or local teachers' centre (see pages 72, 106).
ii) Schools' Council Moral Education Project for Middle Schools, *Startline*,
iii) Home Economics Project for Middle Schools *Home and Family, 8–13* (see page 108).
iv) *Health Education Project 13–18* School's Council and Health Education Council Project. The training courses forming part of the dissemination of this project have been referred to (see page 21).
     The teaching pack, HEP 13–18 by Forbes Publications Ltd, is now available from Homes McDougall Ltd. It consists of 2 copies of an Introductory Handbook and 19 booklets of teacher and pupil material.
v)   HEC. Health Education in initial Teacher Education Project. Units on teaching relationships, and on sexuality, are very relevant. Contact the Director, Health Education Unit, University of Southampton, for details.

Local help
Sex education usually comes within health education so help is available from several sources.

Education Advisor for health education
He/she can be contacted through the local education department. He or she has valuable contacts and can help in curriculum planning, location of resources, organisation of in service courses and meetings and in enabling teachers to identify their needs.

Health Education Officer
An HEO can be an extremely valuable contact for teachers as they work interprofessionally. They can be contacted through the District or Regional Health Authority. Their role is to instigate, plan and evaluate health education (and sex education) services for all interested organisations, including schools. HEOs also run resource centres where HEC material is available free, and from which many of the books and visual aid materials can be borrowed with no charge. The arrangements for using these services differ from region to region; a catalogue is usually available.

Health Education Advisors and Health Education Officers often work closely together.

Jargon check: can you remember who or what are the NMGC, IPPF, BAC, FPA, HEC, BPAS, HEO, TACADE, OPCS, SCHEP, HEP, FPIS?!

Chapter 4

THE SEX EDUCATION CURRICULUM: 0–8 YEARS

Pre-school children: 0–5 years

Non-verbal communication

Sex education starts at birth, with parents' reactions to the sex of their child. Loving, caring for, bathing, cuddling, talking to the baby, are all part of education. Soon, non-verbal communication (a disapproving face, and a cold swab?) may indicate to a young child that some parts of his/her body are less acceptable than others.

Non-verbal communication forms a powerful part of sex education from an early age, particularly in conveying sex roles. (See also later sections e.g. page 59.)

Names of parts: Early vocabulary

For a boy a penis is an obvious feature, so winkle, Johnny, etc. give approval and recognition. What about girls, though? Your 'diddy little botty' or similar phrases do not convey much information. It is important to tell a little girl what she *has* got rather than just what she's not got, even though Freud's castration theory is now unsupported (Goldman [53]). She is unlikely to find out for herself otherwise. So, '*you* have vulva, with a special hole for "wee" (or urine) and a vagina and a clitoris.' To aid familiarity these words can be used well before the child can talk, while washing or wiping the relevant parts, as for any other bit of the body. This also helps parents to get used to saying such words out loud. The health visitor could help the parents identify all the structures while the baby is being bathed and weighed perhaps.

Latin names are given here because there are no acceptable everyday words in our language for these parts! As they are hidden, and taboos on talking or knowing about them are very strong, it is possible for some girls to grow through puberty and even into motherhood without any idea of their plumbing arrangements. 'I just leave it all to my husband and the doctor', explained one woman patient at the clinic.

Children reinforce all new ideas and words by talking about them constantly, for a short while. If friends and relatives are told this stage is current, they should be more able to accept it as part of the growing up process. It is possible to explain to children not everybody talks about their bodies in this way, so it might be better to keep questions and comments to family and friends. This at once puts the information in a 'special' category though, which could be seen as counterproductive.

Names for sexual parts *are* needed. It gives them status, acceptability and a means of communication about them. Family words can be used to start with, but 'proper' names should be given as soon as parents find it acceptable to do so. The Goldmans [53] stress the need to introduce a correct vocabulary from an early age, so thought processes can develop and the terms themselves become usable and understandable.

The basis of a first vocabulary could be: penis, testicles, vulva, vagina, clitoris, anus, breasts, nipples. Urethra is a difficult word to say so 'hole for wee' is perhaps more suitable to start with. A full understanding of the nature and use of each organ will gradually develop, as for any other body part. We do not expect children to understand all about ears, for example, as soon as they are first mentioned. Gradually the words sperm, ovum, ovary and womb (or uterus) can be added. These are much more difficult to understand, as they refer to unseen objects, but are essential for explanations of 'where babies come from', and the beginnings of thoughts about this process. We do *need* words to think with. Children at this stage of conceptual development view analogies literally, so care should be taken when using them. 'Seed' is equated with the garden variety and one small boy worried 'The corners of the packet will scratch me.' 'Eggs' are breakfast-sized and shelled. For these reasons 'sperm' and 'ovum' should be used from the beginning and their minute size emphasised.

Word associations are also important, even if not fully understood. The vagina can be described as 'soft and stretchy' to encourage the development of a good feeling about it, and the adjectives lovely, nice, etc. used for genitals rather than dirty, nasty or stoppit! Clitoris, is perhaps the word least likely to be mentioned. It refers to a 'hidden' organ, solely for pleasure, and female, and is often not acknowledge to exist, (even by SCHEP 5–13 [8]!) An interesting comment on the acceptability of female sexuality perhaps.

Adults as visual aids

If parents have, from the first, sometimes been naked in front of their children, this will be accepted as natural, and names for parts and fur trims will be enquired about in due course. 'Wassat?' It is important to check children have the right information even then. One three-year-old girl explained 'My daddy does a wee through his thumbs.' Direct observation is not always accurate!

If parents have not been used to appearing naked, then to suddenly do so might not be such a good idea, as the novelty element could be too much. Children the same age or younger, or slightly older brothers and sisters would be more acceptable as visual aids and a revelation of adult characteristics in the context of sunbathing, washing, etc. would allow information to be absorbed gradually.

After talking about sexual organs in real life, it is helpful to reinforce information by using simple books. At first use just one picture at a time 'Look that girl's got a vulva, just like you have.' 'That daddy's got ...' etc., or 'How do we know that's a little boy baby?'.

Comfort actions

Young children 'explore' all parts of their bodies with devotion. They may discover that holding, rubbing, or rocking on their genitals give them pleasure. So, not surprisingly, they do it. A very small percentage of young children can experience orgasm (4% of girls by the age of 5) but the action is most often just a 'comfort' one, like hugging a soft toy.

Unfortunately many parents react strongly when their children behave in this way. Research has shown masturbation is a normal part of growing up, and is not damaging in any way, either physically or mentally. Many psychosexual experts feel the experience is in fact helpful, particularly in enabling women to develop their full sexual pleasure potential. So parents have to achieve a difficult balancing act, of accepting this behaviour in their children, (if it is forbidden, feelings of guilt and anxiety may be produced, which can colour attitudes to sex later) while enabling them to remain socially acceptable. If children masturbate very often, it may be a sign they are disturbed about something, or, simply, that they like doing it. In the latter case alternative interesting hobbies could be provided perhaps.

Concept development and answering questions

The Goldmans [53] have provided an extensive analysis of children's concepts of human sexuality, see page 54).

Young children develop concepts gradually. 'I am a boy – I have a penis. Daddy has a penis, Michael has a penis ... *all* boys have penises.' Eventually this builds to the wider concept of 'maleness' extending to all mammals, and other animals. Similarly, the concepts form, that babies 'grow inside Mummies, not Daddies; in other ladies, not men; and that most women have the *potential* for having babies.

Another concept, that you do not *have* to have babies unless you wish to, is an important one to reinforce when appropriate as worries about childbirth are very common (see page 26) and the 'children by choice' idea paves the way for later information on contraception. Boys and girls need information about each other, perhaps provided by a sibling, peer or baby of the opposite sex. They may wish to check this from time to time, verbally or visually, as a normal part of growing up, and a good scientific principle!

Children's questions

A sequence of answers, given over several weeks, or months for the first direct questions on sex (apart from body parts) might be as follows.

'Where do babies come from?'

i) 'From inside their Mummy's tummies' (not stomachs, as this would reinforce a common wrong concept, see page 54).
ii) 'From inside their Mummy's tummies from a special place where they grow.'
iii) 'From inside their Mummy's tummies in a special place called a womb, where they grow for a long time until they're ready to come out or be born.'

Further details can be added gradually about the womb (or uterus) being a strong, stretchy, muscle bag at the end of the vagina, just right to keep the baby safe and warm etc. Children's attention can be drawn to pregnant acquaintances and it helps if one would have a small hand, or ear, placed on her bulge, as 'experiencing' is a powerful aid to understanding.

iv) Opportunities to mention the topic again should be taken when possible, so building up understanding and providing a lead for more questions.

'How does the baby get out?'

This question often arises much later, and the answer could be 'When the baby is ready, the strong womb pushes it down the soft, stretchy vagina between the Mummy's legs. The Mummy and Daddy are very pleased and happy.' Differences between boy and girl babies might be appropriately revised at this point. Follow up about the 'hard work' involved; the baby's 'surprise' at the new conditions etc., can be simply explained.

Adults must understand it is vital *not* to talk about negative experiences in front of children. Exaggerated gynaecological chatter can roll over them and give strong impressions of anxiety, pain and crises, which could colour perceptions of birth for a long time. 'Edna had a terrible do with her first you know, the waters broke early and . . .'. or 'You gave me a shocking time when I had you, young man, I was in agony for . . .'.

The question parents find most difficult to answer, comes later, but in the experience of many mothers it can be asked by children of 3 or 4.

'How do babies get in?'

Any explanation should stress the equal contribution of both partners. The Goldmans [53] found girls particularly tend to view the father as the only active initiator of babies, once they realise he has a role to play at all. It is relatively easy to add the new ideas: 'Inside the Mummy are special places (ovaries) close to the womb, which can make an ovum. To make a baby, a sperm from the daddy and an ovum have to join together.'

'When the Mummy and Daddy want to make a baby, the Daddy's penis is hard and he can put it in the Mummy's soft, slippery vagina, so the sperm can come out, and join with the ovum. Then a baby can begin to grow in the womb. The Mummy and Daddy like doing this because it feels very nice, and is part of grown-ups loving each other.' An erection should be mentioned specifically because:

i) the process is physically impossible without it

ii) boys will have experienced it, from birth on, and the explanation thus gives additional recognition and acceptability (but stress that *only* grown up men make sperm)

iii) girls need to know this fact as well, and if learnt early, it will become a naturally integrated piece of information.

N.B. The verb 'put' is used rather than 'pushed' as it is neutral and does not imply aggression. 'Slippery' is a reassuring term to link with vaginas, and will enable lubrication to be understood later.

Children will not comprehend all of this at once, but the information forms a basis for a growth of ideas, is truthful, non frightening, will not require un-learning, and will prevent the formation of potentially damaging wrong concepts (see below). All facts and ideas need reiteration, confirmation and elaboration as the child grows older, and is able to understand more fully.

Children's wrong ideas

If information is not provided early enough, children develop wrong concepts which may be psychosexually damaging in later life. Research by both Kreitler [44] and Goldman [53], undertaken partly to test the theories of Freud and Piaget, on children's ideas of the creation and birth of babies, found the following beliefs were common.

Table 2   Examples of wrong ideas children can have.

Children's Wrong Ideas	
Babies are made . . .	by eating certain (rich) foods by a 'seed' being put into the mother through the mouth, navel, or manually via vagina by swallowing a ready-made baby by an already existing baby inside the mother (a Russian doll idea) by being put in by the doctor by an operation (medical myth – Goldman)
The father's role . . .	is getting money is possibly helping mother in the home is after the birth is having lots of leisure, a high status job is being the dominant authority is *not* looking after the children There are no clues for a child of course, about the father's role in procreation. Even if they saw the act they would not understand what was happening, nor link it with a birth 9 months later.
The mother . . .	is uniquely involved in child care has little leisure and a low status job or stays at home, "and does not work" (Goldman).
babies in the womb . . .	kick, play, grow, sleep and 75% of Western girls thought the baby suffered and was miserable (Kreitler).
babies are born . . .	through the navel (belly button) through the mouth (or nose or ears) through the anus (many 5–7 year olds) by the belly being cut open (many 5–7 year olds) As the vaginal opening cannot be seen, again children have no clue as to what exit could be used.

It is easy to see how children can become confused if they believe such things from an early age. The Kreitlers suggest these ideas are often not corrected by later knowledge but are merely 'covered up', which may partly explain neurotic anxieties about pregnancy, or lack of understanding of the full role of fatherhood. The Goldmans conclude children are able to understand even quite complex biological ideas much earlier than was first thought, so sex education can, and should, begin early. It is very important to find out what young children *are* thinking about sexual matters during this time, so if questions are not asked spontaneously then opportunities should be taken to open up the subject. A little new insight will be gained each time.

Pre-school sex education: important points

i)   Non-verbal communication is part of education.
ii)   Non-verbal questions from children, pointing, looking, staring, should be answered in the same way as verbal ones.
iii)   The same questions may be asked many times.
iv)   Correct words should be introduced as soon as possible.
v)   Opportunities should be taken to reinforce information whenever relevant situations arise.
vi)   The truth is protective:
from wrong concepts developing
from believing wrong stories
from not being able to talk about sex
from getting sex out of perspective
vii)   If a child finds an adult has not told them the truth, they may lose a little bit of trust.
viii)   To a child *anything* is possible, truth, fantasy and fiction fuse, help is needed to distinguish between these or confusion results.
ix)   Background talk by adults conveys information.
x)   Sex education is only a small part of a child's learning and will not seem more important to them than any other.
Young children are curious about *all* things. They accept the true facts of life with equanimity, if these are presented to them sensitively and lovingly. It is *adults* who can make life so complicated by adding innuendoes and their own hang ups, to the simple story of human love and reproduction perceived by this age group of children.

Books suitable for pre-school and first-school children 2–8 years
Books for young children arranged in a possible sequence of simplicity and acceptability, are:

i)   *How you began*, Hilary Spiers. 1971 Dent & Sons Ltd. Told in attractive colourful pictures and a simple story text.
ii)   *Peter and Caroline*, Sten Hegeler. 1957 Tavistock. A classic book with charming line drawings and a storyline text.
iii)   *A New Baby*, Terry Berger. 1974 Macdonald Raintree. A superb book (one of a series) ideal for promoting discussion of the *emotions* a child may feel when a new baby is expected in the family, including anxiety about parental love, jealousy, and so on.
iv)   *'Where do babies come from?'*, Margaret Sheffield. 1973 Jonathon Cape. This features pictures in a 'soft' flowery format, to aid acceptability.
v)   *A baby in the family*, Althea. 1975 Dinosaur Publications Ltd. Clear simple pictures, and a text which stresses love and commitment. Specially useful is the acknowledgement that parents may argue with each other sometimes, and, conversely, that making love is a pleasurable event.
vi)   *David and his sister Carol*, Althea. 1976 Dinosaur Publications Ltd.

David's viewpoint when his parents adopt a Jamaican baby girl, and sensitively involve him in all the events.

vii) *Emma's baby brother*, Gunilla Wolde. 1974 Hodder & Stoughton. Emma helps to care for her baby brother, with mixed emotions. Charmingly illustrated.

viii) *My new sister*, Bo Jarner. 1977 Adam and Charles Black. A delightful book with black and white photographs of a family eagerly anticipating a new baby. A four year old girl is very involved in the waiting process. Warmth and love abound in a more working class situation than shown in the previous books. Father is present at the birth, which can be explained as a personal choice both parents must feel happy about.

Books for older children, 6 or 7 onwards

ix) *'How you began'*, Lennart Nilsson. 1975 Kestrel Books has a more advanced text, introducing the concept of cells. Twelve pages detail growth in the womb, and the *behaviour* of the baby, kicking, thumb-sucking etc. Photographs of happy naked groups of females aged 4, 8, 14, and 24 and of similarly aged males are reassuring for comparison of stages of growth. Intercourse is described in the text, and by 'section' diagram.

Parents of pre-school children will also find the two BBC publications *How did I grow* useful, see page 34.

5–6 year old children

Sex education for this age should be incidental, but positive, in an atmosphere conducive to raising and answering questions. Children will already have gained knowledge and attitudes about sex, from home and outside. They may have wrong concepts (see previous section) and will need to ask many of the early questions again. Opportunities should be created for finding out their beliefs, so these may be reinforced or modified. Reception class infants will be meeting a wider range of other children and hearing new things, and need a trusted adult to give guidelines. The class teacher is ideal for this role unless prevented by strong personal reasons when someone else well known to the children could assist.

Parents should be involved from the beginning, and help provided for answering questions raised at home. This could start with discussions with pre-school parent and toddler groups or with members of the British Assocation for early Childhood Education, BAECE. The overall feeling should be of curiosity and interest in all living things and a sensible acceptance of human sexuality as part of the pattern of life.

7–8 year old children

By this stage a slightly more formal approach can be taken to draw together the incidental knowledge of the class and present it in more definite patterns. These children still tend to identify with the baby, so the emphasis can be on the need to care for young animals and plants of all kinds, and on a study of their growth. Life cycles, including some discussion of death, can be studied in a practical way, so sexual reproduction is put in perspective. Relationships and the interdependence of human and other animal families can be considered. Again the class teacher is the most suitable person to do this work. Parents can be involved, as before, so they too are ready for this stage.

The aims of sex education for 5–8 year olds
Children in their first years at school need to standardise the mixed bag of information and develop an acceptable base for future learning.

i)   They need to have access to correct information about their bodies and those of the opposite sex.
ii) They should develop an acceptable vocabulary for communication about them, in class.
iii) Sensible attitudes to body functions of elimination of waste should be developed.
iv) They should be made aware of different types of caring home backgrounds so no one pattern is seen as the only feasible model.
v)   They must be reassured they are still loved as much as younger brothers and sisters still with Mum and Dad 'all day long' while they are at school.
vi) They need an atmosphere conducive to asking such key questions as:
   a) Where do babies come from?
   b) How do they get out?
   c) How do they get in?
vii) Children at this age should develop ideas of non-stereotyped gender role, adapted to help individuals maximise their talents.
viii) They should begin a study of growth and reproduction in animals and plants.
ix) They need to become familiar with health care systems.

Access to correct information
Children with younger brothers and sisters will probably be aware of the differences between the sexes, although this cannot automatically be assumed. What is thought to be 'modest' behaviour varies very much between different cultures, generations, social classes and individuals. Some children from single sex families, or certain ethnic backgrounds, may not have had the opportunity to learn about the differences by seeing babies or toddlers being bathed, having nappies changed, or playing naked in the tub or paddling pool. If such occasions can be engineered, so small groups of children can observe infant anatomy, this would be a very appropriate learning occasion. A nearby nursery school or child clinic might help here. Babies are gloriously unselfconscious about their bodies, they do not 'mind' being viewed, so spectator embarrassment is minimal.

Follow up work could include putting names for all parts of the body onto pictures of male and female babies and toddlers. Suitable ones can be found in:
i)   Any of the books listed on page 55.
ii) PTM. Talking points Set 2. Life. Section 2. Our bodies (page 73).

iii)   Fit for life, see page 72.

iv)   BBC Radio vision film strips *'Where do babies come from?'* and *'Growing Up'* (page 73).

The words penis, testicles, vulva and anus, could be attached to pictures appropriately. As for pre-school children an explanation is needed that the vulva (or labia) cover the little girl's 'hole for wee or urine', and her vagina and clitoris. A penis after all, is triple purpose; for urine, for sperm (when grown up) and for pleasure. There are three separate parts to learn about the female genital anatomy.

If the naming game is played from time to time children will understand how boys and girls differ (nothing to do with length of hair or wearing trousers) that it is acceptable to talk about these parts and there is nothing furtive or naughty about doing so.

Developing an acceptable vocabulary for communication

Children arrive at school with their own words for sexual parts and body functions, so a class language which everyone can understand must be established. At the same time it is helpful to acknowledge families do have their own way of describing many things, and a child should not be ridiculed for using such a term. One chap, for example, referred to his 'peanuts'. His parents had told him the correct name for his penis, but he had changed it to a more familiar word, as children tend to do. One teacher [62] wrote 'after we had all the Willies, Georges and "Elephant Man" out of the way, the real body part names became the norm in class conversation.' She had also explained ladies had breasts 'which you won't have yet, because they only grow when a girl is older, and they are to make milk *after* the lady has had a baby.' The concept they are also deemed attractive to look at, is a later one, but may need some mention if newspaper on the painting table is turned over and reveals voluptuous frontages in page 3 presentations. Children are surrounded by sexual sign stimulae from the media and may already have some idea that grown ups find such things interesting. A check list of vocabulary for this age group is given on page 71.

Elimination of waste

Quite a proportion of an infant teacher's time is spent enabling children to get themselves to the lavatory in time to cope with their new school clothes, zips and all, as well as possible reluctance to use 'new' lavatories, or be near other children or 'strangers'. In this way the child can perform with dignity and efficiency and return to the class with no mishaps.

The realisation that this is a normal function for *every* person, and the calls of bladder and rectum must be responded to, no matter how fascinating the new school activities, is an important one for every child. It is part of developing responsible behaviour for your own body actions. Because the elimination of waste, and sexual functions are so closely linked anatomically, a feeling that one is somehow 'dirty' or 'messy' and not to be talked about can reflect on the other.

To become aware of different kinds of home backgrounds

Many story books are based on two-parent families, and these will be the norm in many areas. However, the increasing number of one-parent families, and of divorces and re-marriages means it can be very helpful for all children to hear cheerful, happy stories about a variety of home backgrounds. Young children do worry sometimes about what would happen to them if their parents died or went away, so learning about alternative caring systems is comforting for all. A teacher can select stories or invent others to provide the right balance for the backgrounds of the children in the class.

Reassurance that they are still loved

There should be constant emphasis on 'enough love for all', and good links between home and school, to help the child establish a secure image of a new 'school self', yet still within the supportive family context.

Creating an atmosphere conducive to asking questions

Questions about sex can be asked in almost any context. Some come in the form of statements, the child waiting to hear them confirmed or commented on. If they are answered at the time they will continue to arise and can be taken naturally in sequence with other work. Questions are most likely to be generated in the areas discussed below.

Ourselves

Discuss all about our bodies, what they are like now, how they have changed, and the idea that they will change again in the future. *Proof* of change can be brought in, such as baby clothes, equipment and toys which the children used to use. Direct comparisons can be made e.g. measure the length of arm of a baby jacket, then measure the length of arm of the child's present cardigan. Pin up both as a display and explain 'Alison's arm has grown x cm in y years.'

Each child makes a book 'When I was a baby' and so on. Time concepts are slow in developing, one 6 year old explained 'When my mum had me it was in the olden days!' Self concept is enhanced by comparison with younger children, and parents can be very involved in providing the items and anecdotes. Pre-warn them about this, and give a list of possible requests. Children can act out the baby stages in drama or PE and this can be developed into a sequence suitable for presentation at assembly, or a parents' evening.

Getting on with people

Work on relationships of all kinds with particular emphasis on promoting self esteem. Gender identity and roles will be implicit in this work. Perhaps use peel off sticky labels when appropriate, with 'Gary has been very kind today' or 'Amanda was brave when she hurt her knee.' These can be commented on by other children and adults, and give each child a chance to recall and retell a positive experience. At the end of each day a few words of *praise* for the class, can create a good feeling about school and a desire to return!

Develop non-stereotyped ideas of gender role

A distinction must be made for them between the concept of gender identity, i.e. I am a girl, I am female, or I am a boy, I am male, and gender role, i.e. I am a girl so I must always be (for example) helpful, good, quiet, pretty, kind (!), or I am a boy, so I must always be noisy, rough, untidy, clever, forceful (!).

It should surely not be necessary for society to require females and males to behave in certain ways only, or have certain temperaments to enable them to feel secure in their gender identity. If we enhance the conditioning for girls and boys to behave in the very fixed patterns suggested in the previous paragraph, and to develop limited expectations of their personal future potential, we perpetuate a divisive system where members of either sex who show characteristics supposedly of the other can be ridiculed and victimised from an early age.

Comments such as 'But girls don't like trains!' 'Boys aren't interested in babies!', 'You don't really want to play with dolls (cars) do you?!' have just such rigid conditioning effects when repeatedly heard by children.

All the talents of every individual need to be developed to the full. The community as a whole can then benefit from the total skills available in the population, regardless of which sex they appear in.

Most of us have been so conditioned to accepting unequal treatment for females and males, it takes a conscious effort to focus on the subtleties of behaviour training and expectations of performance around us.

A primary school teacher taking one class everyday for a whole school year has a vital part to play in combating entrenched classroom rituals which can otherwise be powerful reinforcements of damaging and restricting sex stereotyped behaviour.

Check points

i)   Dual standards should not be operating, for example boys being allowed to be more 'pushy' and physical, or girls placid non-contributors to the lesson.

ii)   Punishment and praise should be equal for girls and boys.

iii)   Equal listening to, and acceptance of, boys' and girls' ideas should be encouraged.

iv)   Tasks must be shared equally, e.g. moving things, making things, washing up, clearing up etc.

v)   'Cross sex role' activities and behaviour should be encouraged by giving praise to

girls using computers, constructional materials, for doing science and maths, and for being resourceful, adventurous, interesting;

boys for 'home care' activities, reading and language development and for being gentle, thoughtful, still.

vi)   Making general statements such as 'the girls' work is *always* neater, than the boys'' should be curtailed.

vii)   Avoid sexist material portraying girls only in subordinate, passive or decorative roles, whether in books, work cards, posters, displays, discussions etc.

viii)   *Collect* material (advertisements, books, etc) showing:

active, technological (etc.) girls; girls and women problem solving i.e. fixing a bike, car or tape recorder; women in leisure situations; and artistic, caring boys and men in parenting and home care roles, and families with both parents *sharing* activities whatever these are.

ix)   Do not separate boys and girls for *any* activity, nor for 'lines' in and out of the classroom.

x)   The register should be alphabetical (Sometimes take it from the bottom up. Self esteem can suffer if you're always last!) Why do we think we need to separate the sexes if they are not going to be treated differently?

xi)   Do not talk about home as if only the mother was the caring parent 'Take this home to show ...'

It takes a surprising amount of energy and concentration to make sure all these conditions are fulfilled (actually only in accordance with the Sex Discrimination Act 1975!).

Visitors, may need an explanation of this non-sexist work as road safety officers, police etc. often make such assumptions when talking to children.

Parents may also benefit from a discussion about the approach and the rationale behind it. This will hopefully raise awareness of sex stereotyping and its disadvantages.

With older children discussion of the concept of 'gender role' is possible and they could look for evidence of sex stereotyping, or of restrictions on activities. To be 'fair' to everyone is a sound moral principle.

Animals and plants
Begin a study of growth and reproduction in animals and plants. Visits to zoos and farms should be arranged. Keeping pets provides excellent stimulus for work on young animals. Projects on 'milk', or 'eggs' can be cross curricular and involve many skills. Follow up work on animal families can include

i)   matching pictures of father, mother and offspring
ii)   matching words and pictures of the above
iii)   'set' work, e.g. mapping between sets to show the adult and the baby.

Keeping pets
Arrange a pet show where children can draw, feel, stroke, hug, lift, weigh, measure, compare and survey the ones kept by all the children in the school. Emphasize the *care* of pets, responsibility, things they need, kindness to animals. Discuss the reasons for being responsible and *not* having a pet if you can't look after it properly.

Nature study
Animals and plants can be investigated in their 'natural' environment: school grounds, local park, or countryside. Small invertebrates may be brought in, temporarily, for further viewing, before being carefully put back where they came from. Some, such as water snails, are suitable for keeping longer in vivaria or aquaria, and may even be persuaded to lay eggs so natural life cycles can be observed and recorded.

Seed Growing
Seeds and plants of all kinds can be grown, their growth recorded, and their flowers and seeds investigated. See the *Teaching Primary Science* series (page 72).

Use large seed for small fingers and avoid chemically treated or 'pelleted' ones, as they cannot be directly related to natural seed, and the former may be poisonous.

Peas, broad beans and french beans will grow full cycle in a classroom within the summer term. All need extra heat, i.e. being near a radiator, for the first

6 May	Bean planted			18 June	Next layer of leaves, yellow.
11 "	Seedling visible				
12 "	First leaf unfolded			22 "	Petals from lower flowers have fallen off
13 "	Leaf 1·5 cm long, 1 cm wide				
14 "	" 2·0 " " 1·5 " "				
17 "	" 5·0 " " 4·5 " "			24 "	Pods forming
18 "	" 5·5 " " 5·0 " "				
20 "	" 8·0 " " 6·25 " "				
24 "	" 8·5 " " 8·0 " "				
25 "	Plant re-potted and mounted on a string				
27 "	Height 30 cm				
31 "	" 60 "				
4th June	" 120 "				
10 "	170 " 10 leaves on				
11 "	Bottom leaf starting to die				
14 "	Flowers appearing. Bottom leaf dead				
15 "	Reached the ceiling! 230 cm.				
16 "	Flowers turning red.				

Figure 2   Runner beans table of events and an open bean flower. Bean flowers are self-pollinating.

month. Start them in jam jars with blotting paper, so early growth can be recorded, 'plant on' into large pots, several in each. Some will require strings. 'Feeding' weekly later encourages good pod formation. Grow enough initially to 'sacrifice' one each week. Dig up, weigh, press, label and mount to form a visual record of growth. End with the open pod and 'seeds', so the cycle is complete.

Other work on seeds

Have a seed race. Start growing sunflower seeds in yoghurt pots to take home over the summer holidays to plant out and measure and keep a diary. Bring in the flower heads plus *seeds* in the Autumn term, *Count* the seeds, observe the pattern and stripes, note *variations*. Are they all the same?

Questions to be asked during this work

Do all the seeds *start* to grow at exactly the same time?

Do *all* the seeds grow quickly?

Do some grow more slowly than others?

These questions begin the concept of different *rates* of growth.

Are all the plants the same height by the end?

Are all the leaves exactly the same? (Measure leaf area on squared paper.)

Do all the plants have the same number of flowers?

Are all seeds from one sort of plant *exactly* the same?

These observations lay the foundation for the concept of *variation.*

What parts make up the flower?

What part grows to become the pod?

What is *in* the pod?

Have *all* the seeds in the pod grown?

The concept developed here is that flowers have sexual parts. Flower parts are best investigated earlier, using large simple ones such as tulips or cacti, when discoveries such as that anthers make pollen (male part) and the ovary makes ovules (female part) can be made. Lead on to the significance of pollen on the stigma i.e. pollination.

Open the ovaries of various flowers to show ovules inside.

Later ideas: Not all the seeds in the pod grow. New information can be given that this may be to do with pollination, and its success or otherwise.

Experiment: Cut off the *anthers* of *some* bean flowers, and cover these flowers with small polythene bags, so pollen cannot get to the stigma. Do the pods grow? Do they contain seeds? Compare with untreated 'controls'.

The idea that flowers need to be pollinated before they can make seeds, is the basis for later distinguishing pollination and fertilisation processes.

Concepts to be developed

In all this work, incidental or planned, the concepts to be developed over the four years, explained in the simplest way, are:

i) Like comes from like, earwigs from earwigs, oaks from oaks.

ii) All animals have a father and a mother in the beginning (asexual reproduction can be explained later).

iii) Some parents stay together to look after the young (most birds, some mammals).

iv) Sometimes only one parent looks after the young, for example the mother (most mammals) or the father (stickleback and seahorse fish!)

v) Sometimes the young can look after themselves, as can the young of most invertebrates, most amphibians and fish.

vi) Special names are given to the young of some animals (cubs caterpillars, cygnets).

vii) All animals (well nearly all!) are either male or female when they are young, and will grow up to be mothers and fathers when adult.

Confusing exceptions which teachers will need knowledge of are hermaphrodites such as earthworms, snails and slugs and of parthenogenetic aphid and stick insect stages.

viii) Humans can *choose* whether to become mothers and fathers (talk about famous non parents, as well as parents)

ix) Some male and female adults look different and some have different names: drakes and ducks, ewes and rams etc.

x)   Some male and female adults look exactly the same
a)   all the time, ladybird beetles, robins
b)   most of the time, frogs, newts, stickleback fish, these animals only look different in the breeding season.

xi)   Even if the male and female look the same outside they are different inside. Males have testes, which make sperm. Females have ovaries which make ova (single ovum) sometimes called eggs.

xii)   To produce young, the ova and the sperm must meet and join together which is called fertilisation – this process needs a lot of explanation (see page 66).

xiii)   For the ova and sperm to meet, the male and female animals must come close together.
a)   *In water* the ova and sperm can join outside the animal's body, as happens in most fish and amphibians such as frogs.
b)   *On land*, the sperm must join the ova *inside* the mother's body, or they would dry up. For this to happen the male and female must help each other, so *courtship* or mating behaviour can be seen (for example in birds in spring). The male must have a special part of his body to use for putting the sperm inside the female. In mammals this is called a penis. The female must have a special part of her body to collect the sperm. In mammals this is called a vagina. When the male and female come together so the sperm and the ovum can join, this is called mating.
Hens' eggs will not all grow into chicks. If a hen has not had sperm from the cockerel, the ovum has not been 'fertilised' and the 'egg' will not grow into a chick. An ovum cannot grow on its own. A sperm cannot grow on its own. Humans can choose whether they mate, or not.

Become familiar with health care systems
Visits by small groups of children to clinics or maternity units build the idea that regular help is available for families at all stages. Familiarity with the school health visitor, nurse and doctor means they can be seen as friends, rather than omnipotent beings who descend occasionally to cast a critical eye over our bodies, and may find us wanting! Many are willing to meet a class (out of uniform), and explain the work they do. The feelings generated by their official visits should be discussed and fear and apprehension allayed. It is also very helpful to build the concept of what a hospital is and does, as 50% of children go to one for some reason, before they are 8 years old.
Confidence and knowledge can be gained by:

i)   meeting local staff, a porter, ambulance driver, nurse, radiographer, teacher visitor etc. who could explain their work
ii)   a guided tour – by photographs – of the entrance, reception, childrens ward, X-ray department, etc.
iii)   making puppets, of the range of staff, in correct uniform for the local hospital, (ask for material from the sewing room) and using them in stories about their roles
iv)   writing to children in the hospital, sending pictures to decorate the ward

v)   reading of other children's experiences:
   A trip to hospital Anne Webb 1972 Young World Production
   Paul in Hospital J. C. Jessell 1972 Methuen
   Come inside the hospital Julie Simpson 1973 Studio Vista

vi)   *Children in hospital* packs for 5–11 years. ILEA Video cassettes, and 3 books of photo sequences of individual needs. Hospital ward, and teachers books.

vii)   ITV *My World* Programme 4, *My mum's a Nurse* (see page 72)
   ITV *Good Health,* Programme 13, 'Nurse!' (see page 72)

Children's questions. Concepts needed to answer them
The questions asked by this age group are many and varied, and often about the feeding, breathing and excreting of the baby in utero. Young children have difficulty understanding these processes as they require the concepts of liquids and the solubility of solids and gases. To build up these ideas do 'experiments' finding out how sugar, salt etc. 'disappear' i.e. 'dissolve' when stirred into water. We can't see them in the water, but we know they're there. Teacher demonstration dissolving a coloured crystal to make a coloured solution could help this idea in a more 'concrete'way. (Older children could 'recover' solids by evaporating the solution). Keep working on this 'dissolving' idea, (it also is the basis for understanding digestion).
   Then lead on to specific explanations.

Food
When we eat, the food our bodies need is turned into things which can dissolve and go into the blood. In a pregnant woman, blood takes them to the placenta, where they go into the baby's blood. The baby can then use this food, to grow, just like we do. In the placenta the blood of the mother and baby come very close (but *do not mix*) so dissolved things can go from the mother to the baby, and from the baby to the mother.

Waste
The waste from the baby is not solid, but again is dissolved, so it goes back into the mother through the placenta, and she gets rid of it. The baby does later make some very watery 'urine', which goes into the liquid surrounding it.

Breathing
The gas in the air that we need in order to breathe (oxygen) can also dissolve in water. Rather like the gases in fizzy drinks. You can't see them till you take the top off the bottle and they come out as bubbles. (The concept of a gas is difficult for young children, to them 'air' is 'nothing' and it is not usually practical to demonstrate a coloured gas such as bromine. Science schemes build up the concept by showing what 'air' can do). The mother breathes enough oxygen for both the baby and herself, the gas dissolves in the 'film' of water in her lungs, goes into her blood, is taken to the placenta and passes in to the baby. Carbon dioxide elimination can be similarly explained at a later stage. The baby does not need air in its lungs until after it is born, because it gets all the gas (oxygen) it needs from its mother in this way.
   Not all the children will understand these concepts, but they do provide an

accurate scientific basis for future learning and will anyway perhaps, help to counteract the idea of chunks of fish and chips making their way down the umbilical cord!

Fertilisation process

This requires an understanding of 'cells', and that there are some things so small our eyes cannot see them. Compare the sizes of 'very small' things. What's the smallest thing we can see? A speck of dust? Build up the idea that by using lenses or magnifying glasses we can make things look bigger or magnified. Osmiroid produce a wide variety specifically for primary schools. In some cases we can use two lenses at once to make things look even bigger – these lenses can be put together in a microscope. Then explain all parts of animals and plants are made of microscopic 'units' called cells, which are different shapes for different jobs. A human ovum is a cell smaller than a full stop – even people with good eyesight could not see one. It is a colourless, jelly-like, speck. We *can* see the ova of fish (in hard roe and caviare!) and frogs, as these are much bigger, and provide food for the young. Human sperm are much, much smaller cells than an ovum, so we can't see them either. They are colourless, jelly-like, specks, with 'tails', and can move by swimming. (All sperm cells are too small to be seen without a microscope but soft roe contains millions of them.) The ovum and sperm both need to be in liquid, as they quickly dry up and die if they are not. When the ovum and sperm meet, they join together completely (like two drops of water joining) This makes one new cell, which can grow into a new baby animal. The joining up of the ovum and sperm is called fertilisation.

Test tube babies

This does not mean that babies can be grown in test tubes! It means the baby is started outside the mother's body (fertilisation) then put into the womb to grow as usual. This is only done when the tubes from the ovary to the womb (Fallopian tubes) have both become blocked. The ovum, (or several ova), are taken straight from the mother's ovaries, by an operation, and put in some very special warm liquid in a little glass dish. The father collects some of his sperm to be added to the ovum, so it can be fertilised.

A later idea to be developed is that 'growth' of this cell first consists of dividing into lots of new cells, first two then four, and so on. This concept is needed for the understanding of identical twins, triplets etc., which children often ask about. Non-identical twins, are separate ova, and separate sperm. Twins occur at a rate of 1 in 80 births, so 1 in 40 people is a twin!

Multiple births resulting from the use of fertility drugs have made such questions even more likely. The implantation of the 'test tube babies' is after several cell divisions have taken place.

Umbilical cord

There are lots of questions about this, usually about the possibility of it being twisted round the baby. It helps to understand while still inside the womb the cord is filled with the baby's blood, so is quite stiff, and not likely to wrap round the child. Fill a long polythene bag with water, and show this stiffness perhaps.

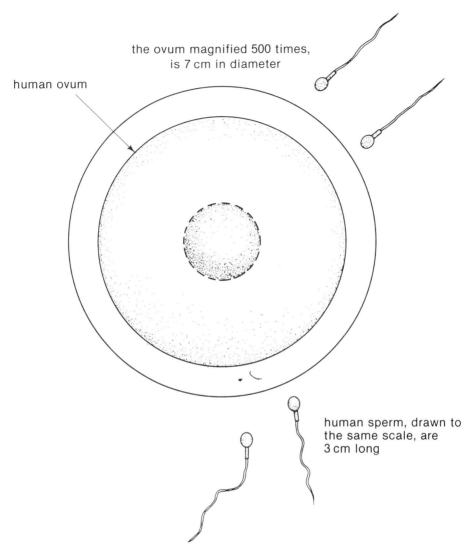

the ovum magnified 500 times,
is 7 cm in diameter

human ovum

human sperm, drawn to
the same scale, are
3 cm long

Actual size of ovum 0.14 mm diameter. Make plasticine models of ovum and sperm 1,000 times life size to demonstrate vast size difference. The ovum will be round like a ball not flat like a plate with a 14 cm diameter. The sperm will be 6 cm long. *Then cut each model ovum and sperm, into 10 equal pieces, and remould into shape. This will show a 100 times magnification of their actual size. Repeat from * to show a 10 times magnification of the real sizes. The sperm will nearly disappear! This process demonstrates the reverse of magnification.

Figure 3   Spot the difference: an ovum and sperm cells.

1. Three ova and three sperm result in non identical triplets.

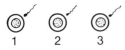

2. Two ova and two sperm result in identical twins plus one.

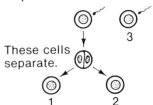

3. One ovum and one sperm result in identical triplets.

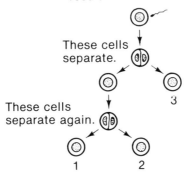

Each of the cells 1, 2, and 3, divides millions of times, and grows into a baby.

Figure 4   How triplets are formed.

After the birth, the blood has gone back into the baby, the cord is now soft and floppy and is cut near the baby (there are no nerves in the cord so there is no pain). The small piece left on the baby's tummy grows a skin underneath and after a few days comes off, like a leaf coming off a tree in Autumn, leaving the navel, or belly button. No blood escapes as the body is all healed up underneath. There is *no* further use for the navel, except perhaps for wearing jewels!

Conception

Questions such as 'do you have to have a baby?' are asked at this stage. It is important to explain this is not so. 'I shall just ask my husband not to put his penis into me', said one 7 year old. She had not developed the concept that sexual intercourse is pleasurable, and hence grown ups may want to do it more times than they want to make babies. ('Once for me and once for my brother?') As soon as this idea is established explain it is possible to stop the ovum and the sperm meeting. Children have usually heard of 'pills', and some, of sheaths, so this knowledge is most probably already in the class.

It is also very important to explain you don't have to be fully 'grown up' or married to be able to have a baby, but that any girl who's body can make an ovum (as soon as she's had her first period at say 12 or 13) could have a baby if the ovum was fertilised. Similarly any boy who was old enough to make sperm (at about 13 or 14) could become a father if his sperm joined an ovum. Discuss

Common frog tadpoles

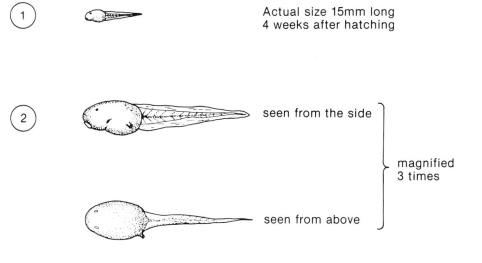

① Actual size 15mm long
4 weeks after hatching

② seen from the side ⎫
⎬ magnified
seen from above ⎭ 3 times

Human sperm
cells

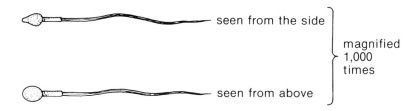

seen from the side ⎫
⎬ magnified
⎬ 1,000
seen from above ⎭ times

Human sperm average between 55 – 65 micron, in length.

1 micron = $\frac{1}{1,000}$ mm, so each is about $\frac{1}{20}$mm long.

Figure 5   Spot the difference: tadpoles and sperm cells.

the best conditions for looking after babies, and if it would be a good idea to have one so young. Children are extremely sensible about this and readily accept the 'preparation for having a baby' idea, and the beginnings of responsibility for behaviour.

Sperm

One other point to particularly emphasise is the small amount of liquid that the sperm are in (about a teaspoonful) and that sperm and urine are never produced at the same time. Otherwise 'concrete' knowledge of the volume of urine possible, could be anxiety promoting. Enlarged pictures of sperm cells also give the impression that they must be quite bulky. Keep emphasising the microscopic size, or 'tadpoles' may become a fixed image. The shape of sperm and frog tadpoles is also quite different. Look at the length of the tails!

Background information

Exhibitionism

This is the most common of all sexual offences [38]. One of the benefits of good communication on sexual matters is that children may be able to talk more easily about any sexual approaches made to them. It could be explained, 'There are a very few grown up men who find they like to show their sexual parts to other people. As everyone in this class knows all men and boys have a penis and testicles, this is not going to be such amazing news. However, because it is not polite behaviour, and some people might be very surprised, it is important to tell your parents, teacher or any grown up at once, if such a thing happens. Someone will then be able to talk to the man and help him, so he won't want to do it anymore, and you will have been a very useful person for being able to explain what happened.'

A child who has seen an exhibitionist may well need to talk about the experience for a while, to lessen any feeling of shock. Adult reaction is best kept calm, matter of fact and reassuring. Discuss the situation with the parents if possible, so they can express their feelings, possibly including those of shock and anger, and co-operate in this approach. Exhibitionists do not usually molest the children or women they expose themselves to, but seem to wish for some sort of alarm reaction.

Paedophilia

This of course is potentially much more serious as besides exposing himself, a paedophile may desire active participation, either by touching the child's genitals, or asking them to touch his, or masturbate him, or he may even attempt penetration. A paedophile, usually heterosexual, prefers to approach pre-pubertal children, boys or girls between the age of about 6 and 11, so it is important children are aware of such possibilities. Many schools have asked the local police to show the film 'Never go with strangers' to children and their parents, to highlight the dangers of going with *any* adult they don't know, whatever the bribe or story they are told. The social skills needed to cope with such an approach can then be discussed and practised. As the majority of paedophiles are known to the child [38], during the follow up work it must be explained that the person who likes children so much may in fact be someone they've met before, and not a complete stranger. However nice the person is, or however much they ask the child not to speak to anyone, it is not right for any grown up person to behave in that way, so it is very sensible and correct to tell some other adult at once. This subject does need a sensitive approach to seek a balance between not frightening or worrying the children unduly, but enabling them to recognise and respond to potentially damaging situations. Parents need to play their part by insisting that they know where their children are going and with whom, and in being suspicious if an adult male seems to frequently want to be alone with a child. Much harm might be prevented if children were able to talk about any fondling, caressing etc, so the situation could be identified early. The child may be under threat, or have feelings of guilt or fear, so *any* change in behaviour after being with a male adult should be followed up tactfully. Dr Christopher [38] gives advice on what to do when a child has been sexually abused, and also discusses incest, which typically involves rather older girls, of 10 or 11.

Evaluation

At primary level the evaluation of sex education could include assessment of:
i) the children's concepts (list on page 63), correct understanding of basic facts of human reproduction and early science concepts
ii) willingness to ask and answer questions, identify pictures eg. of males and females of all kinds, without embarrassment
iii) knowledge of names and use of basic parts, and sensible attitudes to them.
iv) boys and girls co-operating together, little or no inter-sex rivalry or aggression
v) broad ideas of gender roles
vi) caring attitudes to others, particularly those younger than themselves
vii) ability to communicate with parents and teachers on sexual matters
viii) viewing the medical profession as helpful and non frightening
ix) good self image.

A health education officer might be able to help teachers devise evaluation schemes covering these areas.

Vocabulary check list of words in sex education for 5–8 year olds

birth	navel	sperm
bladder	nipples	testicles (testes)
breasts	ovaries	tube from ovaries to womb
cell	ovum	tube from testicles to penis
clitoris	penis	umbilical cord
female	placenta	urine
fertilisation	pregnant	vagina
hole for urine (urethra)	scrotum	vulva
male	sexual intercourse (making love)	womb (uterus)

Resources for infant/junior classes
1.   School's Council Health Education Project 5–13 (SCHEP 5–13) *All about Me* (5–8 years), Nelson.
1)   Teacher's Guide.
   This discusses sex education in the wider context of health education. The emotional side of growth and development, and of relationships between family members and pupils are considered fully at every stage. The sections are *Finding out about myself, How did I begin?, What is growing?, What helps me grow?, Looking after myself.*
ii)   *All about me,* 16 copyright-free spirit masters, of associated pictures, to use in classwork.
2.   Schools Council and Health Education Council project for slow learners. *Fit for life,* Level 1 (5–8 years) 1983 Macmillan.
i)   Teacher's Guide
   The guide explains that this project was developed from the original SCHEP 5–13, but includes much new material specifically designed to help slow learners. It is extremely flexible in its use, however, and the attractive, high quality illustrations in the guide (which may be reproduced for class use), and the carefully planned sequences, mean it could be used most effectively with children of all abilities.
ii)   Visual material
   18 colour cards, to be cut up for class use, and 24 pressurefax masters, of pictures illustrating the work outlined in the Teacher's Guide, are available.
3.   Schools Council, Nuffield Foundation, and Scottish Education Department. *Science 5–13 Project,* Macdonald.
   This excellent series of books for teachers, explains how to introduce science through broad-based curriculum activities. Particularly relevant are the books *Ourselves,* which enables children to make comparisons of height, growth, and so on, and *Minibeasts,* which has practical advice on finding, keeping, investigating and recording details of all kinds of invertebrate animals.
4.   Chelsea College Project, Teaching Primary Science, Macdonald.
   Most helpful in this series is the *Introduction and Guide to Teaching Primary Science* which gives advice on keeping animals and plants in the classroom, and on using museums and zoos, and *Seeds and Seedlings,* with full details of a wide range of activities with plants, including ways of measuring growth.

Television series
1.   *ITV My World* For children of 4 to 6. A series of 28 15-minute programmes. Particularly relevant in the *Caring* theme,
i)   *My baby brother*
ii)   *Families*
iii)   *My Mum's a nurse*
iv)   *Dad looks after us*
v)   *Buying a pet.* The teacher's booklet gives many suggestions for integrated work.
2.   The revised version of the ITV *Alive and Kicking* (1982–3) is for 6 to 8 year olds. The series is child centred, multicultural and realistic. There are 9 15-minute programmes in the main series.
i)   *Growing*
ii)   *Looking after Young,*
iii)   *Homes and Families,*
iv)   *His and Hers?,* being particularly relevant. Teacher's notes available.
3.   *ITV 'Good Health'*
For children between 8 and 12 this series of 14 programmes is very relevant for building background concepts for sex education. Lively, child orientated with full teacher's notes providing excellent follow up ideas.
i)   Programme 1: *Everybody's different,* the foundation to the series, shows the

unique nature of each individual,
ii)   Programme 7: *Fit and healthy*. The need for exercise, hygiene and rest. Introduces various body systems.
iii) Programme 10: *What next?* About physical and emotional changes at puberty. A good basis for a lead in to more detailed discussion of physical changes.
iv)   Programme 13: *Nurse!* The work of a student nurse.
For more details of any of the ITV programmes, contact your local ITV Education Officer, list in appendix.

Film strips
BBC Radio Vision series 1970, *Nature.*

i)   *Where do babies come from?* Film strip and tape commentary. For 7 and 8 year old children. The basic 'facts of life' are explained simply, using painted pictures of children and adults. Conception and birth are dealt with in a sensitive and truthful way, and the teacher is able to set the context of a loving relationship.
ii)   *Growing Up* This follows on and explains pubertal changes, brief details of menstruation, and emphasises these processes take some time to be completed.
These film strips, sound tape, and teacher's notes can probably be obtained from the local Health Education Officer, or Teacher's Centre. The BBC no longer supplies them alas.

HEC Source lists
from the Health Education Council, or the local HEO.
1.   *Books for children 5–8* an annotated bibliography. Sections include, adoption, concept of self, death, divorce, home and family, relationships and communications, basic anatomy and sex education.
2.   *Teaching aids for children 5–8* list of selected audio-visual aids for similar areas.
3.   *Health Education Material for Ethnic Minorities* Details of material for promoting greater understanding of the needs of immigrant families, and leaflets and posters produced in several languages,

Photographic teaching materials.
Visual aids for use in language development.
1.   *Talking points Set. 2 Life.* 1980
   A set of black and white photographs on cards 25 × 20cm, designed for use at primary level.
i)   Love and affection in human relationships
ii)   Physical differences between females and males
iii) Intercourse, pregnancy, birth and the care of babies.
Each card has a 'teacher's statement', and suggestions for discussion. Teacher's notes included.
2.   *Conversation Aids I. The Family* 1980
   Similar in format, 36 photographs illustrate family situations. Both sets are extremely useful and sensitively presented. Each card could lead to a further collection of pictures on the same theme.
   Available from : Photographic Teaching Materials, 23, Horn Street, Winslow, Buckingham. MK18 3AP.

Books
1.   Books for Teachers
i)   *Learning about life.* A child-centred approach to sex education Mary Lane. 1973. Evans.
   This is most valuable and details work for children from 5 to 12 years old. Chapter 6 is devoted to children's questions.
ii)   *School broadcasting and sex education in the primary school* BBC Publications 1971.

This report explains the development and rationale behind the BBC sex education programmes and the reactions of pupils, teachers and parents to them.
Also see list of books for teachers and parents, pages 34, 35.
2.   Books for children
i)   *Health and Growth* 1973. Scott Foresman and Company. This series of books from the USA, has excellent coloured photographs illustrating a text building up health care ideas. The first 3 are for 6–8 year olds, the 'teacher's editions' have added notes. Most inspiring.
ii)   *How did I grow?* 1977. BBC Publication See page 34
iii) Knowing about sex. *A baby arrives* Hemming and Maxwell Editors
      Knowing about sex. *Growing up* Macmillan See page 35

See page 55 for details of a book sequence suitable for children from 2–8.

Body functions

The Body book, Claire Rayner 1979 Piccolo. This gives a down to earth approach to *all* functions, with a simple text, and coloured pictures.
How you are made, Christina Palmgren. 1972 Dent. Adapted by Hilary Spiers. A delightfully illustrated book suitable for 7 and 8 year olds.

Family life resource list

TV: *ITV My World* series (see above) for 4–6 year olds. Programme 6 of *Caring, Dad looks after us.*

ITV *Alive and Kicking* series: for 6–8 (see below). Programme 3, *Looking after young*, excellent portrayal of a family who share in the care of the baby, with Dad changing and bathing him. Programme 6 *Homes and families* shows a variety of cultures and home circumstances.
SCHEP 5–8 Teachers' Guide, *Homes and Families* has many imaginative suggestions.
BOOKS In addition to those on page 55:
I am adopted Susan Lapsley. 1974. Bodley Head; For very young children.
Suzanne's Parents Get Divorced Birgit Erup.
A & C Black *Big Sister, Little Brother* is one of an excellent series for exploring emotions, all by Terry Berger, illustrated with coloured photographs and with a simple text published by MacDonald Raintree in 1979, about a West Indian family. Others in the series are:
Being Alone, Being Together about a boy's activities with and without his friend.
A friend Can Help a girl's feelings after her parents have separated.
Dad Doesn't Live With Us Anymore
'Olly sees it through' is a splendid series by M. Gydal and T. Danniclsson (1976 Hodder & Stoughton).
i)   When Olly went to hospital
ii)   When Olly had a little brother
iii) When Gemma's parents got divorced
iv)   When Olly's Grandad died
These sensitive texts are illustrated with colour drawings.

Sexism and gender role.

TV: ITV 'Alive and Kicking', programme 7 *'His and Hers'* explores this theme in detail.
BOOKS: *Sexism in Schools* Sheffield Women & Education Group. From Jenny Kavanagh, 29 Parkes Road, Sheffield S1D 1BN. Analyses sexism in reading schemes, and has a list of recommended books. The group has produced a series of adventure stories in 4 non-sexist and non-racist supplementary readers, the *'Space Seven Series'* from Sheffield Women & Education Collective, Bridge Cottage, Edale Road, Hope, Sheffield S3D 2RF
Do you provide equal educational opportunities? a valuable guide from the Equal

Opportunities Commission (and see page 84).

White J. *Beyond the Wendy House*. Sex role stereotyping in primary schools. Most useful suggestions. 1984. Schools Council.

Animal care

Most useful: *RSPCA catalogue of educational material*, which includes colourful wall charts on how to look after all usual pets. *ITV 'My World'* Programmes 10, Buying a pet, 21, The Shepherd, and 24, The Country Vet.

Nature study

i)   *Science 5/13* Schools Council. *Minibeasts*. MacDonald Educational
ii) The *School Natural Science Society* has a helpful journal 'Natural Science in Schools' and an extensive series of very useful publications.

Table 3   Summary of suggestions for curriculum and resources for use with five to eight year olds.

Summary sheet. Curriculum and resource suggestions 5–8

Reception class 5 year olds	6 year olds

SCHEP 5–8 *All about me*
Assembly: My family
My home: My family, sisters, brothers.
All about me: names for all external parts of the body, and understanding of functions. Differences between boys and girls, and women and men, girls and women, boys and men.
Me: feelings, likes, dislikes, my school self, my home self.
Animal families: males and females, matching family groups.
Pets: caring and loving, the needs of living things.
Our friends: the school health visitor, nurse and doctor.
Being nice to people: getting on together, right and wrong behaviour.
(ITV *My World*,
   "My baby brother"
   "Families"
   "Dad looks after us"
   "Buying a pet")
See also book list pages **55 and 74**
	SCHEP 5–8 *All about me*
	Assembly: me as a baby, me now.
	Mothers and fathers: young grown inside, young grown outside.
	Caring for the young: ITV *Alive and kicking*
	Growing things: all sorts of plants and seeds.
	Seasons: young in the Spring (Science 5–13 *Ourselves*)
	People who help us: nurses, doctors, health visitors, our clinic.
	Range of homes and families (ITV *Alive and kicking* "Homes and families").
	Emotions: love and caring, anger, sorrow (PTM Talking points Set 2 "Life")
	See also book list page **74**.

7 year olds	**8 year olds**
SCHEP *All about me* Assembly: girls and boys are equal Growing: growing before birth, gestation, periods, birth, milk, egg incubation, hatching, all about eggs. Life cycles: length, death. Measure: self, plants, pets, keep records. (ITV *Alive and kicking*: "Growing" and Science 5–13 *Minibeasts*). People who help us: ambulance drivers, "Our hospital" project. Gender roles: can we all do everything? (ITV *Alive and kicking*: "His and hers" PTM *Conversation aids 1:* "The family") Revise: outside body parts, lead on to inside body parts.	Assembly: Responsibility (*How did I grow?* BBC) Revise: life cycles. Human cycle: conception, fertilisation, process. Begin idea of cells (BBC Radio Vision *Where do babies come from?*) Courtship: setting up a home. Growth and variation: experimental work with plants. (ITV *Good health*: "Everybody's different") Feelings: friendships, responsibilities (Film *Never go with strangers*, ITV *Good health* "Fit and healthy")

Chapter 5

THE SCHOOL CURRICULUM 9–13

Preparation for future changes

Points to keep in mind when planning the sex education curriculum for this age group are the changes involved in puberty, the necessity to involve parents, and the need to consider the sexism inherent in the present system.

Pubertal changes

Knowledge of pubertal changes before the event is essential, to allay anxieties. The earlier maturation of children over the last 20 years, the 'secular trend', has meant a few girls will have their first period when 9 years old.

As the ages at which boys and girls enter puberty vary so much, from 9–15 for girls, and in boys up to two years later, information has to be repeated every year, from 9 till 13. The materials therefore need to be different at each stage, and increase in sophistication with the age of the pupils.

Pubertal changes take from two to five years to complete, so the work will be relevant to a high proportion of the class. The implications of puberty, particularly the potential child-bearing role for girls, can cause anxiety (see page 26) so time should be allowed for feelings about changing relationships and body growth to be expressed.

Involvement of parents

Relationships within families can be altering rapidly during these years, and parents often welcome an opportunity to discuss adolescence and gain support from the school (see page 29 and 103). There is very little other help for them at this time, and, unlike teachers, most will not have had any special training about the needs of pubertal children.

Consideration of sexism

There is evidence [60, 172] that at puberty the expectations of the potential of girls, by pupils, parents and teachers, change, and they are perceived to be less able and have more limited career prospects than boys. Research also suggests teachers give more attention, time, courtesy and marks to the boys in a mixed class than the girls, regardless of their true ability. There is therefore a need to be immensely self-critical about one's own attitudes as a teacher, and analyse carefully exactly what is happening in the classroom. Subject choices begin to be made at this level, often with far reaching consequences. It is important to check there are genuinely equal opportunities for boys and girls to take, and succeed in, all subjects. See page 84 onwards.

Teachers
Children of this age are used to having a range of teachers for different subjects, so although the class teacher would ideally do some of the work, one or two other teachers could become particularly involved.

It is extremely beneficial if teachers of feeder schools can liaise with those of the next level, so they each know the approach and materials used. A planned sex education programme can then be maintained across the change of schools.

Some schools make use of trained speakers from commercial firms to talk about menstruation, usually to the girls only. This can be helpful especially if the class teacher is male, and at that stage feels himself unable to talk about the subject. However, it should not be the only way in which the sex education programme is covered, as a common core of knowledge needs to be built up for all children and teachers, including males. In lower secondary classes the work is often covered in biology, as in many schools all children take this subject for the first few years.

If sex education is spread over several subjects it becomes essential to co-ordinate the work so all children have the opportunity to partake in it.

The aims of sex education for 9–13 year olds

i)   To assess concepts of human reproduction, reinforce and develop these where necessary, and determine the children's needs.

ii)   To pre-prepare for pubertal changes, physical, emotional and social.

iii) To increase awareness of the range of human sexuality, and of 'hidden messages' about it.

iv)   To increase consideration for others by moral and relationship education, and the development of social skills.

v)   To further consideration of gender roles and dual standards.

vi)   To begin an understanding of contraception.

vii) To increase knowledge of health care services.

viii) To begin knowledge of sexually transmitted diseases.

ix)   To increase biological knowledge of reproduction.

x)   To maintain communication on sexual matters.

xi)   To liaise with parents.

Concepts of human reproduction

Similar questions to those used by the Goldmans [53] in their survey, could be tried here e.g. 'Do the bodies of boys and girls grow any differently as they grow older?' etc. etc.

Details of how to analyse the answers are given in their work, but shortcomings in understanding will be very apparent. The children's needs will become clear from such testing if done regularly, and can be amplified by using the anonymous question box or questionnaire, asking what subjects they would like to know more about. Parents can also be asked what they would consider appropriate for sex education at this stage. (See page 20 for source of survey sheet.)

The curriculum can then be planned in response to the information obtained, making sure all the aims as given are achieved, but with priority on those perceived as most important to the children and parents, as well as the teachers.

Preparation for pubertal changes

These changes are physical, emotional and social. A sequence of visual aids for each year group is given in the summary chart, pages 107. Adolescent changes are considered in detail in Chapter 6, but how will you know it's happening?

Girls have their 'growth spurt' fairly early on in the sequence of changes, so growing out of shoes and cardigans rapidly, will be an early indication of puberty. The growth spurt for boys occurs later in their sequence, so early signs here are likely to be the more personal ones of enlargement of the penis, scrotum and testes. Actual growth in height may be very slow at this stage and cause some anxiety.

Early developers: girls

Early developing girls can be under stress in several ways. They may rapidly become the tallest in the class. Girls are not 'supposed' to be taller than boys, so this can cause embarrassment. In assembly, it is kind to organise things so they may stand at the end of the row.

New curves attract attention, boys, men (even Dad?) look at them differently. Some girls can cope with this, and may enjoy it, to others it is unwanted and embarrassing and they may curve over, hide behind long hair, or become somewhat withdrawn. Early developers can feel extremely self-conscious, so suitable arrangements are needed for changing for swimming and PE, for the full kit to be worn (more than just a vest and tight pants?) to allow for privacy and dignity.

Such girls may sometimes be taken to be much older than they really are, and can be 'chatted up' or 'bumped into'. Help in developing the social skills needed to cope with such events is therefore very valuable. Some such girls are vulnerable because they do not realise what effect they are actually having on males. They need help in understanding the responsibility attached to having a grown-up body.

Parents and teachers may expect a sudden onset of sensible adult behaviour from early developers, whereas contemporaries will still be allowed to be 'childish'.

If a girl is the first in the class to have periods, she may have no one at school to confide in, and feel a bit weird or freakish.

Girls like this do need extra sympathy, help and reassurance that

i) once periods have started their growth rate will have slowed down considerably,
ii) the rest of the girls will soon catch up, and will welcome their advice and expertise!

iii) adults do understand the situation, have experienced it many times before, and are willing to be specially friendly to ease the seemingly premature transition into the grown-up world.

Early developers: boys
Early developing boys, by contrast, can be at an advantage. Their extra height and strength helps in image-raising sports activities, and they may become gang leaders. Their sexuality tends to be more approved of, and they may even be encouraged to have girlfriends, (perhaps to confirm that they're not homosexual?) 'Quite a lad is our Peter!' They, also, need help in understanding the responsibility attached to sexual maturity, and in how to cope with dares and challenges. 'Did you score with her?'

Late developing girls and boys are often at a disadvantage, perhaps boys even more than girls (see page 114).

The range of human sexuality
Up to this age human sexuality has probably only been discussed in the context of 'baby making', and love, with or without the element of pleasure. At this stage it is necessary to increase awareness of the range of human sexuality and hidden messages about it.

Pubertal children are on the verge of the great commercial market aimed at 'sex for fun', and it is hypocritical to pretend this does not exist. Advertising is directly aimed at young teenagers. 'Wear this, puff on ...', and you will increase your (sexual) attractiveness'. TV comedy programmes, wife swapping sagas (why not husband swapping?) stories in the daily press, show children that adults are extremely interested in sexual sign stimuli which are powerful attractants used in virtually every way for commercial gain. If children have had education enabling them to talk about sex sensibly, this process can be continued by examining the forces at work.

The facts:
    many people like to be sexual,
    many people like to see sexual things,
    sex is used widely in advertising,
can be acknowledged and discussed.

Project work: hidden messages
Children of 12 or 13 could do a general survey of advertising in the usual national and local press using the following framework.

i) What attracts you to an advertisement? Colour? Action? Layout? Children, babies, young animals portrayed? Punch lines? Humour?

ii) What other means are used to attract attention to advertisements? Men's bodies? Women's bodies? Clothed or unclothed?

iii) Make a collection of advertisements using all the attractants already mentioned. List the products using each method e.g. puppies and toilet paper! A collection could show women's bodies used to advertise yoghurt, alcohol of all sorts, microelectronics, cars, chair coverings, paint, pastry, sportswear, gas cookers, duvets, electric fires, holidays, mustard, watches, cough medicine and breakfast cereals.

The situation when analysed in this way is seen to be quite ludicrous, and children readily learn to identify the 'sex sell' approach. Also the types of people shown appear to be nearly all young women (men are rare!) with one particular body type i.e. slim, long legs, full frontage etc.

iv)   Consider the 'hidden message' thus spread into our daily lives:

women/men are valued for their shape, which enhances any product,

you won't be valued unless you can approximate that particular shape (which only a small fraction of the population possess!) and remain young for ever,

this makes many of us feel dissatisfied with what we've got!

v)   What shape do you think you'll grow into? Collect pictures of ordinary people (not glamorous film stars or sports people, already a 'selected' group) showing the wide range of shapes and sizes. This is real life.

vi)   Relate these pictures to the statistical survey of heights of women and men in Britain (see page 116).

vii)   Lead on to consider what other characteristics attract us to people for instance personality, cheerfulness, kindness or interest in us? etc, etc. Which of these is to be valued the most?

Children of this age can begin to appreciate more abstract qualities such as loyalty, thoughtfulness, consideration, reliability, patience etc.

Homosexuality

This should be spoken of openly and sensibly as it is relevant to children beginning to choose special relationships. It could be led into from the consideration above. Conclusions drawn from the survey of advertisements could include that nearly everyone is attracted to babies and young animals and that men are attracted to women, and women to men, then discuss whether there are any other sorts of attractions.

Do some women like seeing pictures of women and some men, of men? Indeed, we are nearly all a mixture of feelings, and find things in both sexes to attract us [52]. Some will always find people of their own sex more attractive than those of the opposite sex, and are called homosexual or gay (from the Greek *homos* meaning 'the same', not *homo* Latin for 'man') Homosexuals can be either male or female. Women homosexuals are sometimes called lesbians.

There are so many negative jokes and presentations of homosexuality: 'Here comes a poof!', 'You great pansy', 'She's a lesie' etc, that children have sometimes developed a fear of physical contact with their own sex. If a teacher puts a hand on a child's shoulder 'Ere get off Sir! What d'you think I am!', 'Miss! I'm not like that!.' (Smirks all round.) This can spoil the 'best friend same sex' relationships so common in early adolescence. For the approximately 1 in 20 boys and 1 in 40 girls who are truly homosexually orientated it can be a time of great personal turmoil and identity crisis. Homosexuality is considered in more detail on page 185 but at this age the subject does need to be raised, myths explored and questions answered. The following points are likely to be useful:

i)   it is not possible to tell just by looking at someone, whether they are homosexual or not (some famous 'Butch' filmstars were homosexual);

ii)   the homosexual 'types' portrayed on TV comedy programmes are no more representative than beauty queens are of women;

iii)   homosexuality is not caused by any physical, hormonal or genetic condition, and seems to be a normal variation of human sexuality;

iv)   homosexuality is not 'catching', and talking about it, or experience of it will not cause 'conversions';

v)   homosexuals do not have any more interest in young boys or girls than heterosexuals do (there is often much confusion with paedophilia);

vi)   there are equally nice, reliable, hardworking, thoughtful, talented people among homosexuals as heterosexuals;

vii)   if 'approached' by a member of your own sex who you don't want to begin a relationship with, treat the matter exactly as for the opposite sex i.e. you are 'too busy, got too much homework, already going out with ———, thanks', Don't be afraid or upset, but flattered someone finds you attractive and wants to get to know you better. Persistent unwanted advances from anyone, of either sex and whatever age, do not have to be tolerated. Get help at once from parents or teachers. No-one has to make a relationship if they don't want to.

This introduction may enable questions on relationships to be asked from time to time, help sought if necessary, and it may pave the way for a fuller discussion of the subject with older children.

Masturbation

At puberty, with increasing sensitivity of the genital organs a proportion of children may begin to masturbate for the first time, though many may already have experimented when younger, so it is helpful to discuss this phenomenon again. It used to be thought such activity would cause blindness, growth of hair on the palms of hands, or madness, but explain we now know that masturbation (rubbing the penis, or rubbing or squeezing the area around or on the clitoris leading usually to a climax of pleasure) is part of finding out how one's body responds, and begins as a learning process. It is thought proper in our society to keep sexual activities private, so the same applies to masturbation. This practice is not weakening, degrading or perverted, and no-one should feel guilty about doing it. As it is not necessarily totally superseded by heterosexual or homosexual activity later, many men and women, with or without partners, find pleasure in masturbating throughout their lives.

People in some religions still feel it is not an allowable activity and will teach accordingly.

Wet dreams

These may begin in boys of about 14 years, or earlier and are another normal part of growing up. The body practices the sperm/semen release system, often while a boy is asleep. He may have sexual dreams at the same time, linked with a pleasurable sensation, and again this is absolutely normal. At puberty the fine coiled tubes in the testes become hollow for the first time, and begin to produce sperm. Other glands also become active and make the liquids that go together to make semen. The whole system then 'rehearses' so all parts are in working order. In some cultures it is felt the release of 'too much' semen must be weakening. This has been shown not to be the case, the fluid lost is replaced in the same way as any other body fluid. The numbers of sperm cells in the semen will go down after repeated ejaculations, but these are subsequently replaced by more from the tubes in the testes.

Both boys and girls will find it helpful to know:

i)   the normality of 'wet dreams', sometimes called 'nocturnal emissions';
ii)   that parents will be understanding when they occur (and hopefully hosts and hostesses too, as there can be anxiety in not knowing how to cope in a strange place);
iii)   only a small amount of fluid is involved, about a teaspoonful or so, which can be very easily washed off pyjamas or sheets;
iv)   it is possible to minimise their event by masturbating, using a handkerchief to collect the semen, but not everybody would consider this the right thing to do.

Anti-social sexual behaviour

Children should be reminded of how they should behave if they see an exhibitionist, or are approached by a possible paedophile (see page 70). The words themselves can be explained to older children, and also that among the laws made to safeguard children there are ones to protect them from sexual advances. It might also be wise to explain that a very few males like watching girls getting undressed, so it is a good idea to make a habit of pulling curtains while changing.

Naivety can cause problems. It should be stressed that *nobody* has to be sexual unless they want to be, and it is important to get help if *anyone* ever tries to make you do something sexual you don't want to.

The question of incest is a complicated one, but it seems to arise most often in families where relationships between husband and wife, and wife and daughter, are unsatisfactory [38] Incestuous advances are often begun at puberty, and most often involve girls. About half the girls apparently initially acquiesce to the relationship and may gain extra 'love' attention, or temporary power out of the situation. The rest are deeply disturbed and distressed from the beginning. Incest has been show to be psychosexually damaging in many cases, and is almost universally condemned. The longer the relationship continues the more serious the consequences are likely to be.

If a teacher suspected a child was being involved in such a way, with her brother, father, stepfather or uncle, it would be advisable to discuss the matter as an anonymous case with a senior colleague, and seek advice on the 'hypothetical' situation from the social services. They may well have drawn up guidelines for procedure, or be able to refer the teacher to an expert in such cases. The whole family is put at risk when incest occurs, so there is a great need for help from trained counsellors, as well as the medical profession and the police.

Consideration for others

This can be increased by moral and relationship education, and by the development of social skills. The increasing ability of children in this age range to think in an abstract way, means they can develop understanding of moral principles, such as consideration for others, responsibility for one's own actions etc. However, there is a huge gulf between knowing how you ought to behave, and actually behaving in that way so it is helpful to develop social skills facilitating the bridging of the gap.

The 'skills' to be practised could include:

i) how to be a good friend (develop the idea that this requires effort and thought);
ii) how to encourage other people, rather than criticise all the time;
iii) how to end a relationship kindly, and remain friends;
iv) how to react to praise ('How kind of you to say so');
v) how to say thank you, and show appreciation (including to the family!);
vi) how to say you're sorry (not allowed in some cultures as it is an admission of failure);
vii) how to ask for help (for any worry or anxiety);
viii) how to admit to a failing, and learn how to redeem it;
ix) how best to react if someone's being cross with you

... and so on.

Children often anticipate far worse reactions from adults for misdemeanors than in fact actually happens, so learning to face a small bit of perceived 'unpleasantness' early on, to save having to deal with a much greater one later, is a very useful skill, and praise should always be given for doing this.

Resources

Two sets of material particularly useful for class discussion of moral values and consideration for others are:

i) TACADE 1981. *Understanding Others*, for 12–16 years. This pack of 20 situation cards is of material originally from the magazine *Jackie*. The teacher's guide analyses approaches to discussion and role play exercises, and has suggestions for extending the work. Each card has a list of questions on the back, and topics include jealousy, family tension, lies, stealing, platonic friendships, trust, moodiness and shyness.
ii) Health Education Council 1977. Cambridge University Press. *Living Well*, for 12–18 year olds. (see page 174) Particularly relevant are the cards and teacher's guide *And how are we feeling today?*, where humour introduces family relationship situations.

All this material will only be effective if the scenes depicted are perceived as being realistic. The *only* arbiters of this are the pupils! They could be invited to

make suggestions on how materials could be modified, to make them more life
like. 'Realism' varies according to your own background and social class so
viewpoints sometimes differ. Groups could produce a pack of 'situation' cards,
illustrated with their own photographs or drawings, to try out with a parallel
class.

Other useful resources can be found in the Schools Council Project
curriculum material, detailed on page 108.

Gender roles and dual standards

The hidden curriculum aspects have already been mentioned (page 76) The
following two books should be read by every teacher, and could form the basis
for staff discussion on equal opportunities.

i) *Sex discrimination in school. How to fight it.* Harman H. 1978. National
council for Civil Liberties. This summarises statistical evidence of sex
differences in curriculum options and careers guidance, and gives a detailed
explanation of the working of the Sex Discrimination Act 1975.

ii) *Do You Provide Equal Educational Opportunities?* Equal Opportunities
Commission. This has clear guidelines for schools on the implementation of
the same law and the offer of more specific advice and guidance on request.

Project work with children

This area lends itself to project work, collecting and analysing the messages
given about the roles of men and women by everyday comments in the press,
radio, TV, conversations, discussions etc.

Theme 1: women and men at work

Mixed groups of boys and girls could investigate:

comics and children's magazines

advertisements in the press and on television

school text books

children's television programmes, etc.

Each group could prepare an illustrated report or display eg.

i) the jobs men and women are shown doing,

ii) the way they are portrayed, i.e. as active, directing, organising, in control,
independent etc, or passive, supportive, dependent etc, a 'Chiefs and Indians'
approach;

iii) the value attached to the work. This is a more subjective quality but the
discussion may promote thought about what would happen if certain jobs
were *not* done.

Continue the analysis. Did all the groups have the same findings or did one
particular medium show 'stereotyped' roles more than another? Were some
jobs e.g. secretary, nurse, telephonist, housewife (househusband?) shown as
being done only by women? Is there any real reason for this? Are all men
unable to learn to type, do shorthand, run messages, care for ill people etc?
Why are some jobs thought of as being exclusively male or female? Historical
reasons? Do these still apply? Is housework really 'work'? (Try it and see!) Who

would do it if all the family were 'out' at work? What would this cost?

Collect careers information booklets and analyse them in a similar way. Note what subjects are needed for entry into each career. Send back any sexist material to the organisation concerned, with class comments attached. Do they really recruit from only half the population? Use EOC 1980 career information guidelines also reproduced in *Class, gender and education* [172].

Invite people doing jobs usually associated with the other sex, to talk about their experiences, the reasons for their choice, and the attitudes of others to them.

Theme 2: women and men at home

Consider a young couple both working full time, or sadly, more realistic, both unemployed and at home. In small groups list all the jobs to be done using separate pieces of paper for:

i)   daily jobs e.g. making beds, getting meals, washing up, drying up, putting things away, clearing up rubbish, etc;
ii)   weekly jobs e.g. shopping, washing, drying, ironing clothes and sheets, cleaning floors, baths, lavatories, sinks ... etc. writing letters, having friends in, gardening, etc;
iii) monthly jobs e.g. remembering birthdays, visiting relatives, paying bills, cleaning windows ...

Compare the lists from the groups, and make a combined one for each section. Each child copies this down or it could be reproduced for class use. Now ask each individual to tick or underline in green the jobs that women do, and in brown the jobs that men do. The lists are now handed in anonymously. Discuss, 'Is there any reason why any of these jobs could only be done by a man or a woman?' 'Which would be the fairest way of sharing them?' 'Equally!' 'In that case there should be an even number of green and brown colours on the sheets. Hold up the lists so the class can see the distribution of colours. Are they equal? If not, why not? Discuss possible reasons, such as:

'What will the neighbours think!' Are some men only willing to help with housework 'emergencies'? Are there any other examples of restrictive practices in the home? Do some women never 'mend' anything mechanical?

Pin up all the lists, and find out:

Does everyone agree on the division of jobs?

Which ones are listed by some as men's jobs and some as women's jobs?

Why do people have different ideas on this? Is it because their own parents always do these, i.e. father always ... mother always ...?

Discuss one-parent families. These parents have to do everything themselves. What might happen to a partnership if a man and woman made different assumptions about who was going to do the jobs (or were not even aware there were jobs to be done!) before they lived together? Key words here are resentment, disillusionment, tiredness, exhaustion etc. What would happen if one was ill, or had to go away for a while? What conclusions might we draw from this study? List them.

A survey in *Woman* magazine, 30.10.82, on how much help women got from their male partners, revealed in one in ten homes he does not help at all, in one in four he will help if asked, and in about one in three he is very good at housework. This was regardless of whether the woman worked outside the home or not. Children however *are* being brought up to help more, so there is hope for the future!

This project could be followed up by interviewing other pupils and staff to find out which jobs on the lists *they* thought of as male or female ones. The data could be collated into bar charts and used as discussion material or displayed at PTA meetings, even the local radio might be interested in the project.

Theme 3: women and men at leisure

The class could collect information on the chosen leisure activities of

i)   boys and girls
ii)   young women and men
iii)   middle aged women and men
iv)   older women and men

Make a table:

> *type* of leisure activity, sport, indoor, outdoor, craft work, at home, at classes etc. voluntary work etc. ...

versus

> *time* spent on it per week

versus

> *cost* per week etc.

Are there any differences between male and female pursuits? Do they vary with age? Is there any evidence to explain why the children in the Goldman [53] survey did not think women *had* any leisure? Is this because women may spend their leisure time making things rather than in visible active sport? If there *are* any differences in leisure time, what could be the reasons for this?

Encourage class leisure activities of all sorts, have a 'hobbies' display, or talks from children with specialist interests. It is increasingly important to help self-image with absorbing, creative or active leisure pursuits, as in the future most people will have more 'free' time than ever before. Again encourage 'cross gender' hobbies whenever possible.

Theme 4: helping at home

As children grow older they are more able to help in the home, and this is vital training both for looking after themselves later, and for harmony in personal relationships!

Discuss the situation with parents. Do they encourage boys and girls to help equally at home? Or are the boys 'excused' because of:

i)   cultural reasons ('men don't help in the house')
ii)   they are 'too busy' with homework, football practice, meeting friends ... 'I *must* just ...'
iii)   family sanity, as they make such a fuss or a fantastic mess (suds and water

all over the place) it's much easier to do the job yourself? This is the 'make trouble – get results' principle as explained by Dale Spender [60].

It is very important that boys develop basic skills, e.g. ironing a shirt, as well as their jeans! Are girls expected to help more, and be more thorough when doing tasks in the home? Explain that abundant praise should be given, again, equally, for jobs done satisfactorily and all children should have genuine leisure time of their own.

The following class investigations could be carried out.

i) Small groups can investigate one 'job' in detail, and suggest improved ways of doing it. Devise a sort of consumer test and link this with work in home economics.

ii) Find out about the 'housework' i.e. 'bull' done in the services, where every member is expected to spend time keeping self, kit, bed, hut etc. organised and immaculate as a matter of course.

iii) What 'housework' is needed in the classroom? Draw up a rota of jobs, to be done in boy/girl pairs? Girls, boys alternately? Discuss the advantages of everyone increasing these skills, and of working with each other. Try to reduce antagonism between the sexes during these activities.

As with all project work, the subjects should not be considered 'done' once investigations are finished, but the knowledge applied to other situations so more insight can be gained into the changing roles of men and women. There may be in the future many more families where the male chooses to remain at home, and the female works outside the house.

The following books may be useful (and see pages 244 and 249).

Spender D. and Sarah E. (Eds) *Learning to lose, sexism and education* 1980. The Women's Press Ltd.

Hannon V. *Ending Sex-Stereotyping in Schools* A sourcebook for school-based teacher workshops. Equal Opportunities Commission.

Tiedt I. M. *Sexism in Education* 1976. Silver Burdett Company.

Sharpe S. '*Just Like a Girl*': How Girls Learn to be Women. 1976 Pelican.

Contraception

The aims are to allay children's anxieties about the implications of puberty by their understanding:

i) nobody has to become a parent if they do not want to;

ii) some couples may not wish to have a family at all, as not everybody likes children;

iii) for those that do, it is now possible for them to plan when to have their babies, so they can look after them in the best possible circumstances;

iv) free help and advice is available, for planning a family, and for care before and during pregnancy and birth;

v) deciding to have a child is a very important stage in anyone's life, and should be taken seriously and after much thought;

vi) any act of intercourse between a fertile couple could lead to parenthood.

It is advisable for the teacher to read all the latest leaflets on family planning methods from the FPIS as well-informed children of this age can ask quite detailed questions.

Children will need pre-knowledge of:

i)   the pleasure aspect of sex;
ii) the process of intercourse, fertilisation and implantation;
iii) the normal female cycle, including changes in cervical mucus production.

Happy families

During work on families, the question can be raised 'Is there a best time to have a baby?'

It can be suggested that though different couples may wish to have their babies at different times, many are taking advice from doctors that one of the best times for a first baby might be when the mother is in her mid-twenties, as more healthy babies are born then, and the mother's body is fully grown.

They may also want to consider that a woman's fertility slowly decreases between the age of 25 and 35, and sharply after this [78]. Approximately 10% of couples find they are infertile, but many can now be helped. It is important to include some mention of this, as family planning does involve help to *have* babies, as well as *not* to have them. This can lead on to a discussion of family planning methods, see page 91.

The numbers game

Animal	Mouse	Rat	Syrian Hamster	Mongolian Gerbil	Guinea Pig	Rabbit
Age *in weeks* when can reproduce						
Male	6	4-5	8	9-12	10	16-24
Female	6	4-5	6	9-12	4-5	16-24
Gestation period, in *days*	19-21	20-23	15-17	25-28	59-71 Average 63	30-32
Number in litter (average)	8-11	9-11	5-7	4-6	3-5	4-6
Litters per year	8-12	7-9	3-4	8-12	3	7-9

Figure 6   Mammal reproduction, adapted from J. D. Wray and J. F. Gaitens *Small Mammals* (1974) Schools Council.

House mice - breed all year round
from 2 mice, there
could be
2,500 by the end
of the year!

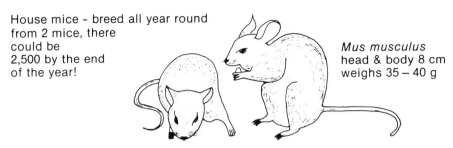

Mus musculus
head & body 8 cm
weighs 35 – 40 g

Harvest mice - are so small that
many do not survive the winter
only 20% may live till the next spring

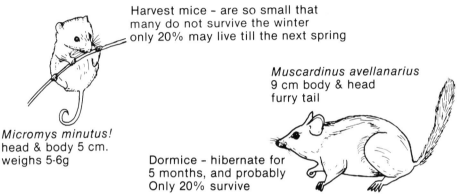

Muscardinus avellanarius
9 cm body & head
furry tail

Micromys minutus!
head & body 5 cm.
weighs 5-6g

Dormice - hibernate for
5 months, and probably
Only 20% survive

Figure 7 Animal numbers.

Consider the number of young which could be produced by various different animals in 3 years. In groups calculate the maximum reproductive rate for a chosen species. Information will be required on:

i) the age at which the animals become sexually mature (the 'generation time');
ii) the possible number of breeding cycles per year;
iii) number of young in each litter;
iv) the gestation period (or time from mating to birth);
v) the fertility span of the female, how long can she go on producing young?

Assume an equal number of males and females are produced each time, maximum fertility etc. The information can be displayed in chart form.

It will soon be appreciated that if maximum breeding rate was achieved, and all the young survived to maturity, the numbers of cats, dogs, rabbits, flies, spiders, birds etc. would be absolutely astronomic!

This does not happen because animals in the wild are 'in balance' with the other animals and plants around them in their environment. Wildlife television programmes often show the hazards young animals have to face: predation, starvation, cold etc. Some animals also have inbuilt ways of controlling their numbers; for example in good conditions, white-tailed deer breed when one year old, and many twins are born. In poor conditions females do not breed until they are three, and then often only have one fawn. For other examples see *Animal Reproduction* [110].

Now let's consider whether humans have the same sort of controls. How many children would it be possible for a couple to have in their life time? We need to know several things to find this out.

i)   When does fertility start?
As soon as a girl has had her first period (menarche) *average* age 13, she is fertile. (It could even be before this, if ovulation had occurred in the first cycle though this is unlikely.) So it is possible for a girl as young as this to become a mother. A girl would not be married at this age in this country and in these times but it used to be the custom for girls to marry before puberty. In some countries today such arrangements are still made.

Discuss changes in age and patterns of marriage over the years, and differences between cultures and races (see page 236). Revise the understanding that it *is* possible to conceive a child without being married. It is the act of intercourse, not the ceremony which is the critical factor, but in many cultures these are meant to be linked. In some, though, the girl is expected to 'prove' her fertility by having a baby before marriage.

ii)   How long can a woman go on having babies?
A woman is fertile till the age when her ovaries stop releasing ova, usually about two years after her last period, the time called menopause. The most usual age for this to happen is between 45 and 50, say an average of 47.

iii)   What about fertility in the man? Does this end at the same time as periods do in a woman?
A boy can become fertile as soon as he has ejaculations of sperm, at about the age of 14. Once started, a man can go on producing sperm even when he is 70 or 80 years old. (Young boys may have lower sperm numbers than later, but this can vary.)

iv)   How long is the human gestation period?
Pregnancy lasts about nine months or 40 weeks, but it might be more reasonable to allow a short recovery time for the mother (!) and consider one baby a year as possible (though not advisable, see page 223).

v)   Considering all these factors then, pupils can work out that, theoretically, about 34 children could be produced! A classful indeed. Whew! Has anyone ever had this number?!

Some incredible feats are described in the Guinness Book of Records 1978. So unless a couple is aiming to beat these records (!) they may want to consider carefully how many children they would like, and when they would like to have them.

But how can a couple choose when to have their family? In order not to have a baby before they're ready, they can use various things to stop the sperm joining the ovum. Remember that conception (fertilisation and implantation but see page 257) is meant to happen after intercourse, and that 300 to 500 million sperm are striving to this end! To thwart the process then, positive action is needed. Ask the class if they've heard of any methods and explain the basic facts about each as simply as possible.

Table 4   Family size records taken from the Guinness Book of Records, 1978.

Family size records	
All time record: 69 children	A Moscow peasant, Fyodor Vassilet (1816–1872) and his *first* wife(!) 27 confinements: 16 pairs of twins 7 sets of triplets 4 sets of quads
Modern world record: 32 children	In 1972 a Brazilian couple had 24 sons and 8 daughters.
UK Record: 22 children	Margaret McNaught of Birmingham (1923) had 12 boys and 10 girls, all singletons. Mabel Constable of Warwickshire (1920) had 22 children including 1 set of triplets and 2 sets of twins.

Barrier methods

These involve putting a 'barrier' between the sperm and ovum.

The sheath

This is a very thin, soft rubber tube, with one closed end. It is rolled on over the erect penis and catches the sperm so they can't swim into the vagina. It is necessary for the woman to put some special sperm-killing cream (spermicide) in her vagina as well, so any particularly adventurous members of the 500 million are rendered extinct!

The cap

In this case the soft rubber is made into a cap which the woman is taught how to slip inside her vagina so it fits neatly over the neck of the womb. Again she should use the special spermicide. The woman cannot feel the cap at all, if it is the correct size, and this must be decided by a doctor. It is left in for at least six hours to stop the sperm from getting into the womb. Afterwards it is easily taken out, washed and dried, ready for use next time.

Chemical barriers

Spermicidal creams, foams or pessaries are best not used on their own, but always with a rubber barrier as well.

Chemical control

'The pill'

There are now many different kinds of contraceptive pills to suit all sorts of women and they work in different ways. They can only be obtained on (free) prescription from a doctor, as it is necessary to decide which is the right sort for each person. The woman is taught how to use them, what time of day to take them, and so on. Just like any other drug, they must only be taken according to instructions. Discuss the 'Medicine Code' here, and test class ability to follow any series of instructions in sequence; a very useful skill to develop.

The shot

This is also called the jab, injectable or Depo-provera. If a woman has one injection of this single hormone, it prevents her becoming pregnant for up to three months, and it acts in a similar way to some types of 'the pill'. In this country it is not used as a regular method very often but is suitable after a man has been sterilised, while the couple are waiting for the sperm in the top part of the tubes to be all used up, or after the woman has had an injection against *Rubella* or if other contraceptive methods are not suitable.

The coil, loop or IUD (Intra Uterine Device)
It was discovered a long time ago in Africa, that a few pebbles put into the womb of a camel would prevent her becoming pregnant during the long months of trekking across the desert. An 'expectant camel' or a baby would have slowed the caravan down too much. The same sort of idea works when specially made plastic shapes (*not* pebbles!), some with fine copper wire bound round them, are placed by a doctor into the womb of a woman. How they work is still not exactly known, but they may speed up the ovum as it travels down the tube from the ovary to the womb, or they may prevent the fertilised egg from 'implanting' in the lining of the womb.
'Morning after' pill or coil
These are methods of post-coital contraception which are available only at some clinics. They are for use within 72 hours of a single 'accident' during intercourse, such as a hole in the sheath or cap, which the sperm may have swum through. (The coil can be used slightly longer after the event.) A doctor gives the woman special pills, or puts in a coil to stop the possibly fertilised ovum implanting in the womb. This cannot be used as a regular method, but is for emergencies only.

Self-control or 'natural' methods
The safe period
(This is also called the rhythm, natural, calendar, mucus, Billings, muco-thermal, or symptothermal double check, methods.) The man and woman agree not to have intercourse on days when it would be possible for an ovum to be fertilised. This means they must find out exactly when the ovum comes out of the ovary each month. This is probably about half-way between periods, about day 14 of a 28 day cycle, but it could be earlier or later. There are several 'clues' to when the ovum might be ready, which the woman notes carefully.

i) She keeps a detailed record of all her periods for six months or a year, to find how they vary, and the shortest and longest time between them. (Discuss here perhaps the technique of recording periods, see page 156).
ii) She takes her temperature first thing every morning to see if it has gone up a little and stayed up, which it does after the ovum has come out of the ovary.
iii) She examines the mucus from the neck of the womb, to see if it has changed, as it often does a few days before the ovum is released.

Some couples use all these ways to try and get the best idea of when the ovum has been produced. Sperm can stay alive inside the woman for up to 5 days and the ovum can be fertilised for 2–3 days, so calculations have to be made about which are the 'safe' days to have intercourse, i.e. those days when the sperm are *not* likely to fertilise the ovum. This can be quite complicated, so training is available for couples wishing to use this method.

If a couple want to have a child, and have tried for a while without success, they can use this method to find out the most likely time to make a baby.

Note to teachers

Discussion of this method is useful because it implies:

i)   that cervical mucus and vaginal secretions are normal;
ii) that it is acceptable for a woman to examine herself to investigate this;
iii) that the couple are thoughtfully co-operating for a shared aim;
iv) that self-control is possible in sexual relationships.

For more details contact the FPA, or the Catholic Marriage Advisory Council.

One of the skills needed for this method, and for child care in general is in reading a thermometer. This can be developed whenever they are used in class experiments. Older pupils might at some stage take each other's temperatures with clinical thermometers, but stress not everyone will be at exactly 37°C (or 98.4°F) as it is normal for the temperature of individuals in a group to vary, and for any one person's to vary a little during the day. Ask the class why the woman's temperature must be taken first thing in the morning, if she's using the rhythm method?

Link this with work on how the human body keeps a more or less steady temperature, and with what is the best temperature for sperm production, which explains why not all body parts are at exactly the same temperature. Use a 'thermograph' picture to show the variation displayed as a difference in colour.

Withdrawal or 'being careful'

This is not considered a very good method as it relies on the man being able to take his penis out of the vagina before ejaculation. Unfortunately a few drops of semen often come out before this happens, so several million sperm may already have been released. (See page 206 for more details.)

Sterilisation

If a couple decide they have had all the children they wish for, they may consider either one of them having a sterilisation operation. The tubes either from the testicles to the penis, or the ovaries to the womb are cut, and the ends tied or clipped so no ova or sperm can pass. Nothing is taken away (other than a very small piece of the tubes sometimes) so all other parts of the body work just as before, so periods still occur. The ova or sperm just dissolve and disappear. Semen is made, but does not contain any sperm, though after a vasectomy it takes between ten and twenty ejaculations to clear the sperm already present. The man is asked to provide samples of semen, for checking, a few months after the operation.

Children often confuse sterilisation with a hysterectomy operation where the whole of the womb is removed. This will also sterilise the woman of course, but she will not have any more periods.

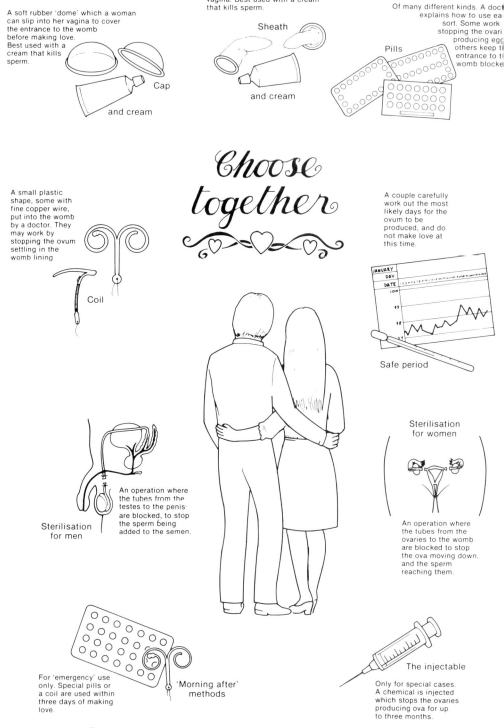

A soft rubber 'dome' which a woman can slip into her vagina to cover the entrance to the womb before making love. Best used with a cream that kills sperm.

Cap

and cream

Made of soft, thin rubber, and put over the penis before making love, to stop the sperm getting into the vagina. Best used with a cream that kills sperm.

Sheath

and cream

Of many different kinds. A doctor explains how to use each sort. Some work stopping the ovaries producing eggs, others keep the entrance to the womb blocked.

Pills

Choose together

A small plastic shape, some with fine copper wire, put into the womb by a doctor. They may work by stopping the ovum settling in the womb lining

Coil

A couple carefully work out the most likely days for the ovum to be produced, and do not make love at this time.

Safe period

Sterilisation for men

An operation where the tubes from the testes to the penis are blocked, to stop the sperm being added to the semen.

Sterilisation for women

An operation where the tubes from the ovaries to the womb are blocked to stop the ova moving down, and the sperm reaching them.

For 'emergency' use only. Special pills or a coil are used within three days of making love.

'Morning after' methods

The injectable

Only for special cases. A chemical is injected which stops the ovaries producing ova for up to three months.

Figure 8   Choose together: different types of contraceptive.

General points

The family planning methods have been described so far in the simplest way, avoiding technical jargon (barriers to understanding?) where possible, and without listing advantages or disadvantages, or relative efficiencies.

To the question 'Which is the *best* method?' explain although 'the pill' is the most efficient it may not be suitable for all women at all stages of their lives, so other methods may sometimes be best, and can also be efficient if used properly, as taught by a doctor or nurse.

It is never safe to have intercourse without using a contraceptive unless the couple wish to have a baby, or the woman has had 'menopause' and two years without periods. More details of each method can be given if asked (see page 205), but if disadvantages alone are raised, they should be countered with equal advantages, and a reminder of the alternatives, abstinence or children.

The overall message could be:

i)   there are a large number of family planning options available;
ii) it is up to each couple, with advice from a doctor, to decide which method they would be happiest with, in accordance with their religion, culture and values;
iii) all the methods are reversible, except for the sterilisation operations which must be considered final (though with new techniques some have been successfully reversed);
iv) all couples who care for each other, and for children, will want to talk about their parenthood potential (which is real from the very first sexual occasion, even if full intercourse does not take place);
v)   contraception won't cost them anything, as advice and all supplies are free at Family Planning Clinics and from their own, or any other doctor (but GPs do not give free prescriptions for sheaths);
vi) if a couple wish to have a baby and find after some time they do not, they can get advice from their doctor or clinic. If they find it is probably not going to be possible for them, they might like to think about adopting a child, so they can give their love and care to this very specially chosen person.

Sensitivity is needed to the 'hidden agenda' in all this discussion. The suggestion that some children are not planned might infer that they are not 'wanted'. It should be made clear if this idea does arise, that even if a pregnancy came as a 'surprise', the baby from it could be very much wanted and loved.

In the case of adopted or fostered children, it is important they feel it was lack of accommodation, or money, which forced their parents, reluctantly, to come to the decision to give them a chance of a better life than they could provide themselves. It should be stressed that it is not easy to allow one's child to be adopted or fostered.

The age of consent
If questions are asked about the age at which family planning advice can be obtained, it should be explained that doctors will help anyone of any age, in absolute confidence. The BAC publications *Under sixteens* and *Sex and the law* explain the legal position and how doctors always try usually successfully to get young patients to confide in their parents, and will not prescribe contraceptives without carefully assessing the background and medical risks involved. This can lead in to a wider discussion of confidentiality in all medical matters.

Consider the law in this country (1956 Sexual Offences Act) which means it is illegal for a man (or boy over 14) to have intercourse with a girl under 16 [64]. The girl is not acting illegally, but of course may be emotionally and physically at risk.

Discuss the reasons for this law. The following points might be raised.

i)   The protection of a girl from being pressurised into having sex. What is meant by 'pressure' to behave in certain ways? What are the 'pressures' on all of us? Are some pressures good? How could someone avoid pressure to act in a way they didn't really want to? Could they ask for help from a friend, teacher, parent, doctor or nurse? How would they go about asking for this?

ii)   Girls under 16 are unlikely to have grown inside enough to have healthy babies, [65] even though they may have had periods for years.

iii)   Some young teenagers might not be good parents? Why not? What does it take to be a good parent? Time? Patience? Love? Money? Accommodation?

iv)   People change a lot as they grow up, especially between mid and late teens, so their feelings and ideas change too? Might they prefer not to have too much responsibility at this stage? Early marriages are particularly 'at risk' but teenagers often feel 'fully mature', of course, even at 14. (The Age of Marriage Act, 1929 means that 16 is the minimum age for marriage with parental consent, and 18 (16 in Scotland) without parental consent, for both sexes).

v)   What advantages and disadvantages would there be in waiting until the girl or boy was older?

Pupils particularly at risk
Analysis of the backgrounds to teenage pregnancies has indicated those particularly at risk are often from deprived inner urban areas, large families (4.5 children, or more), lower socio-economic groups, daughters of previous teenage mothers, low achievers with no employment prospects, or, because of cultural and religious attitudes, West Indians and Rastafarians.

It may also be wise to remember that some emotionally deprived children come from very sumptuous surroundings.

Teachers might find helpful reading for this section in:

i)   The Pregnant at School report [7]
ii)   Simms, M. & Smith, C. 1983 *Teenage Mothers and their Partners* [177]
iii)   Reid [17] who suggests children need not only information, but help in developing the skills necessary to resist social pressures and increase communication with their parents.

Knowledge of health care services

Leading on from previous work on the local clinic or hospital, the class could find out how many different kinds of clinic there are. Did everyone go to the baby clinic? Do they remember what it was like? What other clinics do children in the class go to, eye, child, teeth (or ophthalmic, orthopaedic, orthodontic)? The names can be confusing, so 'crack the code' and begin a list explaining the meanings. Ask children to describe what happens at their clinic (restraining overdramatic presentations!), explain how they have been helped, and give them a mandate to find out more next time they go. The class could make a short list of questions for them to take. This will help increase the 'status' of clinics and clinic patients within the class, and create a positive view of attending one. Most of us will do so at some time in our lives.

The class might design and make appropriate badges for each type of clinic, or create decorated appointment card holders, for young patients to use. Lead on to pre-natal or ante-natal clinics; the Latin *ante*, 'before birth' as in *ante meridian*, a.m., should not be confused with the Greek *anti*, 'against', as in 'antiseptic'.

It is crucial that both boys and girls understand how vitally necessary it is for expectant mothers to go to a doctor or a clinic from the very beginning of their pregnancy. Stress how the parents-to-be are taught about the woman's body gradually changing to help the growing baby, what to expect during the birth, when there will be lots of help, and how to look after new born babies, so both parents feel they can cope.

Use ITV *Living and Growing* programmes, *5: Pregnancy, ante-natal care, and labour*, and *6: Birth and the new baby*. Allow plenty of discussion time after the programmes, so the subject is fully explored, and accepted. Discuss the HEC poster, *'If you're pregnant, don't wait for your baby to prod you into going to the Doctor.'*

Pre-conception clinics

These are sometimes called 'Preparation for Pregnancy' clinics. They are relatively new, and are aimed at helping couples become as fit as possible before conceiving and:
i)   to space pregnancies adequately, to give the mother's body time to recover (unlike the one baby a year for 34 years previously discussed!);
ii) to test for immunity to Rubella, and for any other infections which could affect the baby;
iii) to stop oral contraception and introduce another method of birth control for a few months before conceiving, so the natural cycle can be re-established;
iv) to give help for decreasing, or stopping, smoking, drinking alcohol, and taking unnecessary medicines;
v)   to encourage eating sensibly, so the mother in particular is not too thin;
vi) to test for high blood pressure, diabetes, blood Rhesus factors etc. as these may call for special care during pregnancy;
vii) to find out if there are likely to be any unusual problems.

There is so much that can be done now, in preventive medicine, stress that if couples used all the pre-conception, ante-natal, birth and post-natal care available it would give them the very best chance of having a healthy baby.

Getting to know how to use the national health service is an important step in this chain, as is a positive view of the services, so they are not seen just as curative i.e. you only go if you're ill. Understanding of the concept of 'immunity' is important here too. Teachers have a vital part to play in fostering this 'good' image of NHS facilities, and liaising with local health services.

Health programmes in school

There is an ongoing campaign to try and reduce the number of Rubella-damaged babies. Rubella can cause serious malformations of brain, eyes, ears and heart, and is most dangerous during the first month of pregnancy (50% risk of damage), the second month (20% risk) and the eight weeks following (7–8% risk) [65]. The District Health Authorities and Education Authorities can co-operate to arrange for an immunisation programme for girls between 10 and 14, which can be done in school. Only one injection is involved and side effects are uncommon and mild. See the HEC leaflets on Rubella.

The reasons behind the campaign should be explained to the class and the following points discussed. Rubella or german measles (but avoid confusion with measles) is a virus which can cause a mild disease in young children, though adults may suffer painful joints. The greatest damage is to unborn children, who may be affected if their mothers catch it while they are pregnant.

The number of babies damaged could be very reduced if certain precautionary measures were adopted.

Firstly everyone who had the disease could avoid all contact with adults while they were infectious. Women in the first months of pregnancy are not obviously bulging of course, so cannot be specifically avoided.

Secondly all girls betweeen 10 and 14 could be immunised against Rubella whether or not they think they've had it before. They would then not catch the disease later, which would be important if they ever wanted to have a baby.

Finally any woman able to have a baby could have a simple blood test to see if she was immune to Rubella. If not, she would then have the single protective injection, and would avoid conceiving for at least three months after this.

This provides an excellent opportunity to discuss what is meant by a community health programme and of people co-operating, not just for their own health, but for the sake of others, and future generations.

Abortion

Questions such as this one may arise.

'What happens if the mother knows she *has* caught Rubella and is in the first months of pregnancy, so the baby might have been badly damaged?'

This could be answered as follows.

'The couple will probably want to go to their doctor, or a clinic, and discuss the situation. The woman's body itself may decide not to continue with the pregnancy, and she may have what seems like a very heavy period, during which the minute foetus is passed out. This is called having a miscarriage or a spontaneous abortion, and it is the body's way of dealing with an unhealthy beginning, so giving itself a chance to start again. If this doesn't happen the couple and the doctor might think it wise for the woman to have an abortion. During this operation the very tiny damaged foetus can be removed. Then, after waiting for a few months, and having checks to see if the woman's body is healthy again, and free of the Rubella, the couple may decide they would like to begin another baby, which would not be "at risk" of being damaged.' It can be explained that not everyone would think this was the right path to take, as some people feel an abortion is never justified.

Suggest it is sensible for couples to discuss their feelings about this, and decide what is right for them, according to their circumstances and beliefs. Children of this age have often heard of miscarriages and abortions, but are not very clear exactly what is meant by these terms.

Note to Teachers

Rubella itself increases the likelihood of a miscarriage [65]. It has been estimated that 75% of all fertilised human ova spontaneously abort [71]. Many of these will not be recognised as they happen so early, but the figure includes the 15% of established pregnancies which miscarry. A detailed analysis of foetuses lost in this way has shown up to 60% of those from the first three months of pregnancy have chromosome damage, and would not have developed normally. It would be appropriate at this stage to talk about the care of handicapped children, as in spite of all precautions, some will be born every year, and this is not the fault of the parents. Many children will have handicapped brothers, sisters or parents, and it is helpful if teachers are aware of this, and are always sensitive to the needs of their families.

The ITV *Good Health* programme *One of the family*, shows a family with a handicapped child, encouraged to do as much as possible for himself.

Going to the doctor

To build up confidence in patient/doctor relationships, it is helpful to role play a visit to the doctor. Many children have played 'Doctors and Nurses' games when younger but probably to give 'permission' to touch and look at another person's body (which we give the medical profession the 'right' to do) rather than building knowledge of the health system!

Explain a doctor needs to find out what is wrong, and will need information from the patient in order to do so. Perhaps a local doctor would spend a little time with a class to explain what sort of 'clues' are needed and show the most often used instruments, stethoscopes, ophthalmoscope (eyes) otoscope (ears) etc.

It should be made clear the patient can ask the doctor questions, and is not wasting valuable time by doing so. Children of this age will probably always see a doctor with an adult, but should still be encouraged to speak for themselves, so they can develop this art.

The class could make a display on 'Having a health check', or 'Happy to be Healthy', using all the information they have collected with the emphasis on positive health and preventive measures: 'Good! You're fine … next one please!'

Sexually transmitted diseases STD

This subject can be introduced in the context of personal hygiene (see page 127). Explain our bodies normally have some microbes living, for example, in

Table 5   Sexually transmitted diseases.

Sexually Transmitted Diseases	
How many are there?	There is a wide range of sexually transmitted diseases, only a few actually called venereal diseases. Some of the others are caused by viruses, fungi or single celled animals.
How do you catch them?	By very close contact of bodies, as happens during sexual intercourse. Much reassurance is needed that very few can be caught by normal use of lavatories, door knobs, cups, towels etc, by being breathed or coughed on, or from food or water, or by rubbing against people in a crowd. "Can you catch VD at a bus stop?"
How can they be cured?	The diseases can be cured fairly easily in their early stages, so people are asked to go at once for free treatment and expert advice, to their own Doctor, or straight to a 'Special Clinic,' probably held in a hospital.
Can you only get them once?	Unfortunately unlike measles, Rubella or mumps, the body does not become 'immune' to the sexually transmitted diseases, (possible exception Herpes p.268) and it is possible to be cured, infected, cured, infected, indefinitely, if people choose a life style which means they go on catching them. They can also catch several at once.
Are they serious?	If left untreated they can be very damaging and cause long term illness, or mean a woman is unable to have a baby (it has been estimated that 1,500 people become infertile each year because of gonorrhoea for example), but when treated early, most can be completely cured, and then have no lasting effects.
What clues are there for someone who's infected?	The symptoms vary, there could be 'painful piddling', smelly, frothy or yellow discharge from penis or vagina, a rash, sores, or itching, but sometimes there may not be any symptoms, especially for women. Because of this, anyone going for treatment is asked to say who they might have caught it from, or who they might have given it to, so these people can be contacted (very discreetly) and offered help. All treatment is absolutely confidential – a clinic will not tell *anyone* about it.
Are special clinics only for STD?	No, people with other diseases not sexually transmitted can also get treatment, because of the expert advice there. About one quarter of all the patients attending for a check up are actually found not to be infected, (70) but then feel reassured and can stop worrying that they might be.

the rectum, or vagina. Some of these are useful e.g. in keeping the vagina slightly acid, so other harmful organisms cannot grow there. It is only when the balance of this 'human zoo' is upset (by long term use of some antibiotics for example) or when certain organisms get into parts of the body they do not usually live in, e.g. the urethra, that they can cause trouble. Some of the other micro-organisms always cause disease if they are present. The aim is to keep the useful ones in the right place and keep the others away by correct washing and wiping.

The SCHEP 5–13 *Think Well* Unit 3, *From Sickness to Health*, lists venereal diseases in the chart of infectious organisms. Talking about them necessitates acknowledgement of the wider implications in terms of human behaviour i.e. that some people do have sex with more than one person. It should be made clear that anyone can choose whether or not they wish to run the risk of catching these diseases, and that if they only have sex with one non-infected partner, or do not have sex at all, they will not become diseased themselves. (NB. There are possible exceptions to this rule, see page 265.)

Questions to be answered
Great tact is needed during this discussion, for example if a child comments 'Dad got VD from the dirty loos at work', the answer is just 'Mmmmm, really?'. The truth is required, but clothed in diplomacy, as relationships can be at stake.

Develop understanding of the meaning of 'completely confidential'. Do some 'professionals' e.g. teachers, doctors, nurses, need to keep some information they have, very private? If someone tells you something 'in confidence', what does that mean? Would you have to ask their permission if you wanted to tell someone else about it?

The overall approach should be matter of fact and sensible. A balance must be kept between giving adequate knowledge of the risks involved, and not over dramatising the 'dire consequences', so possibly arousing a counterproductive fear, which might prevent those at risk later, from seeking help. It should be made quite clear again that nobody has to include these risks in their life style. The majority do not.

Biological knowledge of reproduction
Some of the previous work could well be done in biology, but more specifically biological areas are:

i)   reproduction in a variety of plants and animals
ii)   the nature of various ova and sperm
iii) non-sexual reproduction
iv)   increasing knowledge of patterns of inheritance
v)   sex determination.

Reproduction of 'the birds and the bees', has to be taught, in the same way as for other animals!

It is useful at this stage to put human reproduction in perspective, by an 'overview' of reproduction in a variety of animals and plants, in water and on land. Practical first-hand observations of ova and sperm can be made by viewing the fertilisation of the ova of the tube worm, *Pomatoceros triqueter* under a microscope. Children find this a fascinating experience. Questions on human reproduction can arise at any time during this work, and should be answered in context. Make clear it is to be considered in more detail later in the course, and emotional and social factors can be emphasised then.

Inheritance
During biology work over several years, children can continue to collect information to add to 'data banks', on plant and animal variation. General information based on direct observation, and discussions with animal breeders, pet fanciers or farmers, will enable thought processes about the nature of inheritance to develop, and pave the way for an understanding of the mechanics of genetics later.

The only 'fun' thing about them is drawing their shapes!
This is what they look like in the blood and cells of an infected person:-

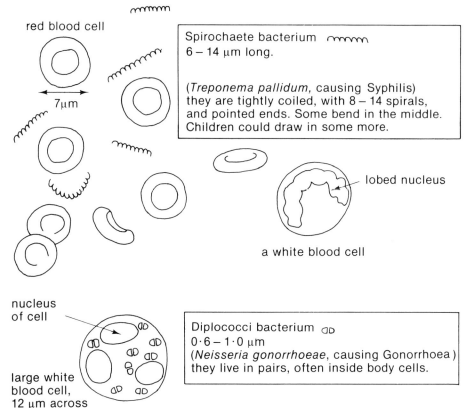

red blood cell

Spirochaete bacterium
6 – 14 μm long.

(*Treponema pallidum,* causing Syphilis)
they are tightly coiled, with 8 – 14 spirals,
and pointed ends. Some bend in the middle.
Children could draw in some more.

7μm

lobed nucleus

a white blood cell

nucleus
of cell

Diplococci bacterium
0·6 – 1·0 μm
(*Neisseria gonorrhoeae,* causing Gonorrhoea)
they live in pairs, often inside body cells.

large white
blood cell,
12 μm across

This is an idealised picture, as the techniques for staining and viewing
these two types of bacteria are quite different. It would not be possible to
view both on one slide, but someone could have both infections at the
same time.

NB.

$$u = 1 \text{ micron} = \frac{1}{1,000} \text{ mm} = \frac{1}{1,000,000} \text{ m} = \mu m \text{ (micrometre)}$$

mm = millimetre   milli = one thousanth   micro = one millionth

Figure 9   Bacteria which cause sexually transmitted diseases.

Sex determination

The sex of any individual can be decided in different ways in different kinds of animals and plants.

i)   One sort of alligator lays her fertilised eggs in a nest on the river bank. If the nest is warm, about 30°C, the eggs all develop into females, if it is warmer still, about 34°C, they all develop into males. So in this case the temperature at which the eggs develop decides which sex they will be.

ii)   In bees, fertilised eggs from the queen grow into females (either worker bees or queens depending on how the larvae are fed) but, unlike most animals, the unfertilised eggs she lays can also grow and in this case become male bees, called drones. In this example it is whether the egg is fertilised or not which makes the difference between male and female.

iii)   In mammals, including humans, it is the sperm that decide the sex of the offspring. Some sperm carry instructions to be male, and some, to be female. So the sex of the young animal depends on which sort actually fertilise the ova. So it is the father who is responsible for the sex of his children. (The ova are all alike as far as the sex of the young is concerned, but may be quite different for all the other features of course.)

There are other factors involved, including the conditions in the female reproductive system, which will determine the chances of a male or female sperm reaching the ovum first. It is very important to be extremely careful when discussing human genetics with children, even in the simplest terms, because of possible implications for the family. This is particularly so in these days of artificial insemination by donor, or of adopted children, where this fact is not necessarily known to the child. It is wiser to use well documented case histories of Royal families or film stars, and never make categorical statements about the likelihood of such and such a character being passed on in humans. It takes skilled genetic counsellors with extensive expert knowledge and much statistical evidence to make any valid predictions, as so many factors can be involved.

Communication

If the suggested previous work has been done, and full discussion time allowed, children will have accepted the idea that the questions they raise about human sexuality will be taken seriously, and answered honestly. If several members of staff have been involved there will be a choice of adults to ask, and pupils will be able to select the person they feel most easy with.

Liaison with Parents

The benefits of PTA meetings have already been discussed (page 29) but parents of this age group may find it helpful to have one specifically on 'Adolescent Growth and Development' when the importance of explaining to children in advance what pubertal changes are going to occur can be stressed.

Because of the nature of adolescence, there will be endless opportunities during it, for criticising 'Why are you so untidy, late, noisy, uncouth, unappreciative, selfish, thoughtless, clumsy, careless, forgetful and childish?'! Even buoyant children have self-doubts when the only communications are negative ones. Explain the school will try and give praise, encouragement, status (and house points?) to a wide range of activities and qualities, so every child has some chance of a positive experience. Such rewards will not just be reserved mainly for sports activities, where late developers and non-athletic types are penalised so much.

There could be an explanation of the school's pastoral care system, and of the opportunity for children from one parent families to be in a tutor group with a teacher of the opposite sex from the parent, as this could be particularly helpful during the adolescent years. Stress the importance of equal 'expectations' and subject choices for boys and girls. Finally discuss the school curriculum in sex education, and the tasks the children will be asked to do during it, which will give parents a chance to raise these subjects with their children if they wish.

The school could prepare a 'Parent pack' on adolescence, with relevant leaflets, a booklist, and a summary of the evening's discussion. Many children will have no particular problems during puberty, but if those that have can be helped early on, the consequences and worries can be minimised.

Table 6   The changes which take place at adolescence.

Changes at Puberty	
Physical changes	These can happen fairly quickly or be more spread out (see chapter 6, on adolescence) nearly *everybody* has been self-conscious or awkward at *some* stage during these changes – even if they seemed fine to everyone else.
Emotional changes	For example feeling excited at new prospects and opportunities, but not being sure if you can cope or not (feelings of self-doubt) again, *everyone* has these feelings. Rapid changes in emotions, feeling elated one minute, and depressed the next, are also common at this time.
Communication changes	It is important children are able to *keep talking* about how they feel about what is happening to them. Stress that it can be very helpful if parents find time to talk to each child, alone, during the week, just to keep in touch "How do you feel about . . . ?" This will reinforce the child's feeling of being considered and loved as an individual, as well as a member of a family or school. If the child is away from home, teachers, counsellors or house tutors take on this role. It *does* matter to children what their parents and other adults think of them, however blasé and unconcerned they sometimes seem, and attitudes are conveyed to them non-verbally, as well as verbally, of course.
Social changes	Making friends, being in the gang and 'conforming', are all very important to children. Being isolated and friendless lowers self image drastically. Explain the school will help here by discussing such matters in class (see SCHEP, 'Think Well') by developing friendship skills and keeping a close watch for teasing or bullying, which will be dealt with immediately.

Children's questions

The questions on sex from this age group can be very wide ranging, so parents and teachers have to be prepared for almost anything. Here are some examples of questions asked by boys and girls of 12 and 13.

i)   Why do we have pubic hairs?
ii)   What does it feel like to have a baby?
iii)   What's a 'Caesarian'?
iv)   What's an 'induced birth' and why is it done?
v)   Why are some girls' breasts big and others' little?
vi)   When boys get an erection, what do girls get?
vii)   Why is it dangerous to use a tampon when just starting periods?
viii) If you don't use tampons during a period, how can you have a bath?
ix)   Can you have sexual intercourse while you have a period?
x)   Is it dangerous to have sex when you have not yet started periods?
xi)   How do you get VD?
xii)   How do you get rid of VD?
xiii) What's inside the testicles?
xiv)   What is foreskin?
xv)   What is an abortion?
xvi)   How do you get triplets and twins?
xvii) Why have some people got white skins and some dark?
xviii) Is it right to live with someone without being married?
ixx)   What's a vibrator?
xx)   Is it safe to have a bath after my brother?

Answers to most of these questions are given in context in this book, for the others, here are some possible approaches.

Answers

i)   Nobody really knows. One idea is they might protect bodies rubbing together during sex or that they look or smell attractive.

ii) Do you mean during the pregnancy or the actual birth? See page 230, for explanations, but the answer should deliberately interpret 'feelings' as emotional and physical and include those of the father.

iii), iv)   Pages 232, 233. v) Page 163, body images, vi) Page 135. vii) Page 150.

viii) The blood flow is not (usually) so great it will affect the bath water. It can be relaxing to have a nice warm bath at this time.

ix) Yes, it is possible, though it could be a bit messy if the flow was greatest, but some people do not mind this. Some cultures and religions however, do not allow sex at this time.

x)   It really would be very unwise as the girl's body would not be ready for sex, and she might find it very uncomfortable. It would be much better for her to wait for a few years, even after her periods had started, when her body would be more likely to be ready, and she would be more able to cope with her feelings and emotions about the relationship as well.

xi), xii)   Pages 99, 100. xiii) Page 139. xiv) Page 141, xv) Pages 98 and 256.

xvi) For twins see page 66. Triplets could be from three separate ova and sperm, twins plus one, or, for identical triplets: the fertilised ovum divides once, and the two cells separate. They then each divide again and one of the two pairs of cells formed separate yet again (page 68).

xvii)   People living in very hot countries need protection from the sun so their skins (and eyes) are dark. In cooler countries there is not such a need, so skins (and eyes) are often lighter. In fact this helps their bodies make Vitamin D when the skins are in weak sun. People with dark skins may need extra vitamin D when they live in this country, people with light skins have to be careful not to get sunburnt when they live in hot countries. A long time ago people did not travel so much from country to country, so their bodies became 'adapted' to suit the conditions they lived in. Each particular skin colour is inherited by the children from the parents.

xviii)   Teachers will need to be sensitive to the varying pupil families here: 'Opinions differ on this. Some people's cultures and religions think it is not right, ever, other people feel if a couple care for each other and agree to stay together, it does not matter if they are not actually married. Legal points need to be considered though, particularly if they have children, so these should be discussed before they finally decide what is right for them.'

ixx)   A small battery driven object which when held on the skin gives it lots of little taps or 'vibrations'. Some people enjoy this feeling, and may use it on all parts of the body, including the clitoris, because it gives them pleasure.

xx)   Sperm do not 'leak' out into the bathwater. They are only produced after an ejaculation, so it would be quite safe. (NB. Getting pregnant from bathwater is a fairly common myth or excuse!)

Evaluation

As the aims for each section have been specified, the evaluation can be structured to find out if these have been achieved. In some cases this will be of factual recall and understanding, for example of the vocabulary, in others it will be evaluation of skills such as:

i)   reading a thermometer,

ii)   perceiving 'hidden messages' in advertising etc;

iii)   a change in attitude towards male/female roles, so these are not seen as tightly stereotyped;

iv)   increased willingness to help at home (ask parents at the end of term);

v)   ability to communicate with nurses and doctors,

vi)   friendship skills;

vii)   ability to ask questions about sexual matters without embarrassment.

Resources

Curriculum Projects 9–13

1.   *Schools Council Health Education Project (SCHEP 5–13) 1977 Nelson. Think Well 9–13.* Teacher's Guides, Resource sheets, Spirit masters. Of the 8 teachers books in this project, the two key ones for sex education are units 1 and 2.

Unit 1. Myself, for children of 9–11 Sex education is put in the context of family relationships. The material covers: *Awareness of myself,* feelings, values, self image, *Myself and others,* on relationships, *The same but different,* showing variation is

Table 7 Summary of suggestions for curriculum and resources for use with nine to thirteen year olds.

Summary sheet. Curriculum and resource suggestions. Years 9–13.					
	9 year olds	10 year olds (2.2% of girls begin menstruating by the age of 10 [58])	11 year olds (15.2% of girls begin menstruating by 11 [58])	12 year olds (39.2% of girls begin menstruating by 12 [58])	13 year olds (Over 73% of girls begin menstruating by 13 [58])
Schools Council projects	Moral education: *Startline* Home economics: *Home and family*.	Moral education: *Startline* Home economics: *Home and family* Health education: *Think well* Unit 1. *Myself*, on relationships and growth	Moral education: *Startline* Home economics: *Home and family*. Book 5 *Interdependence* Health education: *Think well* Unit 2 *One of many*, on pubertal changes and relationships; Unit 3 *From sickness to health*, on transmittable diseases including STD.	Moral education: *Startline*	Moral education: *Lifeline*
	Health education for slow learners: *Fit for life*, Level 2.	Health education for slow learners *Fit for life*, level 2	Health education for slow learners: *Fit for life*, level 2.		Health education for slow learners: *Fit for life* Level 3
Film strips and slides	BBC Radio Vision. *Growing up*.	Camera talks, *Primary health and sex education 1 & 2*. BBC Radio Vision. *Life cycle. Into the wide world*.			Camera talks, *Adolescence* 1, 2, 3
Television	BBC Sex education. 3 programmes.		ITV *Good health*. Programme 5 *Germs, germs, germs*. Programme 10. *What next? Living and growing*. All 8 programmes are relevant, but some could be used with 13 year olds.		ITV *Living and growing*
Other material, curriculum suggestions & books				Nuffield Combined Science. Sections 3, 8, and 9, for work on animal life cycles. Menstruation in detail. Gender roles. HEC booklet *How we grow up*.	Nuffield Combined Science Sections 3, 8, and 9 Film *Then one year* summarises pubertal changes Health Education Council project *Living well*, on relationships. TACADE pack, *Understanding others*.
	Book list on pages 55 and 74.	Book list on page 34.	Book list on page 110.	Book list on page 110.	Book list on page 110.

normal, *Myself as a changing person,* looking at physical and emotional growth, *The sex education component,* where the teacher's notes discuss the approach to this subject.

Unit 2. One of many, for 11–13. Very good coverage of relationships, in *Myself and others, Making up our minds,* on choices made in social situations. *People that matter,* relationships with groups and family, *Beautiful friendships,* about being a friend, *The other sex,* physical and emotional changes at puberty and the need for responsibility. These two units form a sound basis for Middle School sex education. The unit 3. *From Sickness to Health?* begins a study of transmissable diseases, and 7. *Get Clean!* includes hygiene, so these are also helpful.

2. *Schools' Council Project, Home Economics in the Middle Years. 1979* Forbes. *Home and Family 8–13.* The pack consists of 6 books.

   i) *Planning for home and family education.*

This introduces the rationale behind the project, indentifies the 5 key concepts and surveys development in children of 8–13, with helpful tables of the characteristics of children in this age group.

   ii) *Five Teacher's Guides*

Development suggests activities suitable for middle school pupils to assess the physical development of children younger than themselves; and *Interdependence,* this is about relationships and personal responsibilities within the family, at school and outside.

3. *Schools Council Moral Education 8–13* 1978 Longman *Startline*

   i) Teacher's book *Moral Education in the Middle Years.*

   ii) Series of 6 *Choosing Books* for children, coloured illustrations of scenarios depicting realistic 'choice' situations. Attractive presentation.

   iii) *Photoplay 1* and *2* large black and white photographs of faces and people to use as stimulus material.

   iv) *Growing. How it happens, making it happen.* Setting the scene. A series of cards to use with or without the photoplay material.

   Extremely useful for relationship and moral education, as a very flexible approach is possible.

4. Schools Council and Health Education Council project for slow learners.

   i) *Fit for life,* level 2 (for 9–12 years) 1983 Macmillan.

The teacher's guide comprising the material at this level, has good suggestions about teaching the sex education component, which comes in the section called Growing Up. The photocopy masters in the guide include excellent work sheets on pubertal changes, and the emotions they involve.

   ii) Level 3 (for 13 + years) This teacher's guide and photocopy masters, continue the explanations of pubertal changes, and have a sensitive treatment of the fertilization process, and of how a baby grows. Also included are most effective sequences about personal appearance and hygiene and the social pressures involved. (See page 72 for details of level 1.)

5. *Nuffield Combined Science* 1970 Longman/Penguin

   Relevant Sections:

   Section 3 *How living things begin.* Activities book 3 A brief introduction to human reproduction in the context of animal and plant reproduction.

   Section 8, Subsection 3. *Cells, eggs and seeds.*

   Section 9 The life cycle and reproduction of locusts, butterflies and aphids (parthenogenesis). In all sections the work is based on experiments and full details given on organising these.

6. Health Education Council Project *My Body* (10–12 years) 1983 Heinemann. These lively packs of classroom materials, divided into 6 main units, include information and discussion on the reproductive system. The work is practically based throughout, and develops early science concepts, including that of cells and the size, shape, and orientation of body parts.

Television Programmes

1. BBC *Sex Education. 1984 Series, for 8–10+* years.
Three 20 minute programmes, *Growing, Someone New,* and *Life Begins,* cover pregnancy, birth, pubertal changes, including menstruation, and conception. Comprehensive teacher's notes are available.
Two background books *How did I grow?* are detailed on page 34.
2. ITV *Good health* series. 14 programmes over 3 terms. (See page 72) most relevant No. 10 *What Next.*
3. ITV *Living and Growing* A new series for 1983. Eight 15 minute programmes for 10 to 13 year olds explain the biology of human reproduction, while emphasising human relationships. The topics covered are, social and emotional development, individual differences, physical growth, erection and ejaculation, menstruation (in some detail) masturbation, loving relationships, intercourse and conception, pregnancy and birth, the need for ante and post natal care, details of a pelvic examination, family planning is mentioned, and how families adapt to the new baby. A teacher's booklet has background information, drawings, and suggestions for follow up work.

Film strips and slides.

1. BBC *Nature.* Radio Vision. *Where do babies come from?* and *Growing up* (see page 73).
2. BBC *Life Cycle,* Radio Vision. 1972 Filmstrip BBC Publications *Into the wide world.* Age 11–13. 33 frames of coloured pictures and photographs explaining reproductive organs, conception, fertilisation (good photos of ova and sperm) implantation, gestation and birth, new-born baby girl and boy, and stages of growth to adolescence. Menstruation is mentioned briefly at the end. A most useful programme which emphasises loving relationships. Background information in the teacher's notes. The commentary tape is no longer available.
3. BBC *My Body.* Film strip associated with five radio 4 programmes.
4. *Camera talks.* Film strips or slides.
    i) Primary Health and sex education; *Let's talk about ourselves.* 10–15 year. *Part 1.* 24 frames. Tape commentary 18 mins. Survey of all parts of the body including sensory organs, clear diagrams of reproductive organs and a good description of their use and of circumcision. A long description of endocrine glands follows, more suitable for older children.
        The commentary by a male voice is rather solemn.
    ii) *Part 2.* 29 frames. Tape commentary 26 mins. Pubertal changes are shown by diagram and photographs, menstruation and wet dreams are mentioned (but semen is equated with 'seed') Animal reproduction leads into consideration of human conception, gestation and birth.
        These could be usefully used with the younger age group by selecting frames from the whole series, and adding a commentary from the teacher, adapted to the needs of the class.

Films

Then One Year
British version. 16mm 21 minutes; colour, sound. Boulton-Hawker. An excellent summary of pubertal changes, and the wide range of times, rates and final shapes. Illustrated by photographs of British school children, and good diagrams. Skin changes and the need for hygiene and sleep are mentioned. Masturbation, erections and wet dreams, the structure and function of the sex organs are all clearly explained. The film notes give the full commentary, and extra information. This could be used as a lead in, or summary of a sex education programme, and would be very suitable for showing at parents meetings. Available for purchase or hire from Concord Films Council, or National Audio-Visual Aids library.
Human heredity 16mm sound colour 14 mins. A most useful introduction to human

genetics for 12 and 13 year olds. Details of availability as above.

Books

(see list on page 34). Hemming J and Maxwell Z. Ed. *Knowing about sex* series. 1975 Macmillan:

1. i) *A Baby arrives!* Text suitable for 8–10 year olds, coloured line drawings of human reproduction in a family context.

   ii) *Growing up* (see page 35)
2. Lance J and Went D. *Animal Reproduction.* 1974 Evans. Sexual and asexual reproduction, courtship, mating, birth and parental care in all vertebrate groups in the context of animal population numbers. Illustrated with photographs and diagrams. Suitable for 11–13 year olds.
3. Barnard, C (ed.) *Body Machine.* 1983 Kestrel.
4. HEC Booklet *How we grow up* A most useful resource with a series of questions about young children. Pubertal changes are illustrated with cheerful pictures and diagrams in colour. Erections, wet dreams, menstruation, intercourse, pregnancy, ante natal care, birth and care of a new baby are all clearly explained. These booklets are free, and can be obtained from the HEC in quantity. They would be very suitable for class use, for group work or cutting up to make files and notes, or to take home to discuss with parents.
5. *Understanding. Conception and Contraception.* 1971 Ortho-pharmaceutical This extremely useful book is available free to teachers. The illustrations are simple, accurate, and most acceptably presented. Details of the female reproductive system (but not the male) are given, organ by organ, each with scale, orientation and texture carefully explained in the context of the whole pelvis. Most helpful is the very clear picture of female genital openings, including the hymen (no pubic hair, and vagina shown open for clarity). There is a detailed explanation of the menstrual cycle, and conception and pregnancy are illustrated with life sized drawings of the developing baby. Finally there is a summary of contraceptive methods.

HEC Resource list

i) *Books for children 9–13*
ii) *Teaching Aids for children 9–13*

Both include details of material on body care and cleanliness, human biology, sex education, adoption, death, divorce, child development, concept of self, home, family and friends, health workers and hospital visits.

For parents and teachers of less able and mentally handicapped children

1) Shennan V. 1982. *Help your child to understand sex.* MENCAP
2) HEC Source List. *Health, hygiene and sex education, for mentally handicapped children and adults.*
3) *Fit for Life* See pages 72 and 108.

Teaching about family planning

1. Specimens of contraceptives can be obtained from the FPA or BAC, or may be on loan from the local Health Education Resource Centre.
2. Kit. The FPA produce a series of colourful cards, *All about Contraception* one for each of the nine methods.
3. Flip chart. Understanding Family Planning. Ortho Pharmaceutical. This large, free standing chart, includes excellent drawings of the womb in situ, an enlarged picture of an isolated womb, with a circular disc rotated to show menstruation, conception and the use of cap and foam. Others are included and there are teacher's notes on the back of each sheet,
4. Slide set. *Adolescence 3. Contraception.* Camera talks. A selection from the 33 slides could be used, emphasising the positive value of planning a family.
5. Poster. *His and Hers* Scottish Health Education Unit. Good coloured photographs of all contraceptives, useful for cutting up to make individual cards.

6.   Television. ITV *Living and Growing* series, programme 7 introduces the idea of family planning and the need to discuss it.

Going to the doctor

1.   TACADE *Free to Choose* Unit 1 *Images*, for children 11 and over investigates the influence of 'images' on the promotion and use of socially acceptable drugs.
Unit 2. *A pill for every ill*, encourages children to think about the correct use of drugs.
2.   *Health and Growth series* (see page 74)   Books, 4, 5, and 6 have excellent pictures for increasing understanding of all body parts. Book 6, *Why have a health examination?*, is particularly relevant.

Animal and plant reproduction

A.   Most attractive series of books by Jill Bailey called *Nature in Action,* 1979 Purnell, is lavishly illustrated with superb colour photographs from Oxford Scientific films. The lively text would be very suitable for 12 and 13 year olds. Most relevant:
   1) *'How Creatures Multiply'*, reviews reproduction in plants and animals, and has a section on non sexual reproduction, and 2) *'Growing Up'*, the development of plants and animals, with details of larvae, embryos etc, and examples of metamorphosis.
B.   Revised Nuffield Biology Text I, *Introducing Living Things.* 1974 Longman, has good coverage of all the areas mentioned, and excellent drawings, diagrams and photographs, some in colour. The Teacher's Guide I, gives background information and details of practical organisation, including the technique for keeping *Pomatoceros*.

Vocabulary

abortion	gender	nucleus
cervix	gestation	orgasm
circumcision	homosexual	paedophile
climax	hormones	periods
conception	hymen	population
contraception	implantation	puberty
chromosomes	labia	pubic hair
embryo	labour	sanitary towel
erection	lesbian	semen
ejaculation	lining of the womb	sexually transmitted diseases
exhibitionist	lubrication	smegma
Fallopian tube	masturbation	tampon
foetus	membranes	urethra
foreskin	menstruation	uterus
genetics	menopause	virgin
		wet dreams

Chapter 6

THE SCHOOL
CURRICULUM 14–18

Developing adulthood

This is the age of increasing sexual awareness and, for some, of sexual relationships.

By 14 a high proportion of girls will have almost completed puberty, and about half the boys will have begun their changes. The majority of children may have no difficulties, for others the combination of a sexually mature body and an emotionally and socially immature being, means they can be very vulnerable to pressures to be sexual. 'Are you *still* a virgin?!' These pressures are also perceived by pre-pubertal teenagers, so ongoing reassurance must be given to 'late' developers whose behaviour characteristics are discussed later (page 114). Many 14 year olds will still be in gangs of same sex groups, and reassurance is needed that interest in the opposite sex is not obligatory, and conversely, being 'best friends' with a member of the same sex does not indicate a necessary predilection towards homosexuality. This subject itself needs further discussion in a sensitive way (see page 185).

Moral education, though essentially programmed in from the beginning of school education, becomes increasingly relevant as children develop more independence and the potential for abstract thinking. So it is important to allocate time in the curriculum for discussion, reasoning and value clarification processes.

The curriculum

Helping agencies

Examples of these are school counselling facilities, tutor group support system and the work of the NMGC, FPA, PAS, BPAS, BAC, HEC, NHS family planning, relationship and child care services etc.

Teachers will again know that parts of the discussion will be more relevant to some pupils than others. However, if children have followed a sex education programme as outlined earlier, many of the concepts will be familiar to them, and the syllabus can build on previous understanding.

A detailed curriculum is given in following chapters.

Several teachers will be involved for any one age group and the subject can be interdisciplinary, or taken as a separate strand under one title such as 'personal development' for a whole year group throughout the year.

Table 8 Suggestions for the curriculum for fourteen to sixteen year olds.

The Curriculum for 14 – 16 Year Olds	
Families	Changing relationships. Is there a 'generation gap?' The needs of teenagers and parents. Independence and responsibility. Consideration of others.
Body images	Media presentations. Gender identity and role. Mass persuasion techniques. Biological sign stimuli.
Human sexuality	Variations. Homosexuality. Positive views, tolerance. 'Rules' of behaviour, morality. Considerate life styles. Exploitation. Sex and the law.
Social Pressures	Behaviour at discos and parties. Alcohol and sex. Casual relationships and possible consequences. STDs and their cure. Abortion and alternatives. Learning from mistakes. Redeeming self-image. The right *not* to be sexual.
Personal relationships	Making and keeping friends. Finding a partner. Ending a relationship. Marriage and alternatives. Changes in the expectations of marriage. Marriage guidance. Separation, divorce, re-marriage. Bereavement.
Education for parenthood	Choosing to become a parent. Conception, gestation, birth, childcare. Single parent families. Practical involvement with pre-school children. Parents as sex educators.
Helping agencies	School counselling facilities, tutor group support system etc. The work of the NMGC, FPA, PAS, BPAS, BAC, HEC, NHS family planning, relationship and child care services etc.

Parental involvement can be continued through the PTA, and by asking parents regularly about their concerns, and offering to arrange talks or courses on specific areas of interest.

Higher education 16–18 age group

Sixth forms, sixth form colleges and colleges of further education have an important role to play in on-going sex education programmes. The scope is wide for discussion groups, seminars, group work, research projects, visiting speakers, and so on. The topics are perhaps best chosen by the students themselves at this stage. As by no means all will have been involved in sex education previously many may wish to include some of the areas already mentioned. Other subjects of interest might be ethical issues raised by any of the following:

sex education in schools
'test tube' babies
genetic engineering
'surrogate' mothers
sperm banks
artificial insemination by donor
pro-and anti-abortion groups
choice of sex of the unborn child
the women's liberation movement
sexism and society, sexual harassment, and so on.

Many colleges and schools have been able to provide opportunities for students to work in the community during this time which can act as an introduction to a wide variety of life styles, and give opportunities for further education in the social aspects of sex education.

The secular trend

Over the last century, records show children have been entering puberty earlier, by about 0.3 years per decade, and growing to larger final adult sizes, an increase of about 1cm per decade [51] These changes together constitute the 'secular trend'. In some industrialised countries this tendency now seems to have levelled out, in others, and in most developing countries, it is still continuing.

It is thought to be due to such factors as:

i)   improved nutrition, particularly in early infancy;
ii)   the lessening of diseases which retard growth;
iii)   the hybrid vigour, or heterosis effect, which occurs if inherited characters for tallness dominate in a population, thus increasing the height of individuals by more than might be expected by a simple 'average' amount. This happens particularly with a greater genetic mix of people, as happens when a wider choice of partners is available, through more travel and emigration and immigration.

Consequences

Manufacturers of children's equipment and clothes have had to take these changes into account. For teachers and parents it has meant there is a need to talk about pubertal changes earlier, and provide help during the lengthening gap (for some) between apparent physical sexual maturity and socially and medically acceptable sexual activity.

Physical changes at adolescence

At puberty, changes in body shape and proportions have the effect of strongly differentiating between males and females, a condition known as sexual dimorphism (from the Greek *di* meaning two, and *morphos* meaning form or shape). Each sex is therefore easily recognisable to the other, which has great social implications and to be mistaken for the opposite sex during this time can be felt to be very humiliating!

The timing of pubertal changes cover so many years it is possible for teachers to meet some girls only after their puberty, as they have completed these changes before arriving in the first year at secondary school, whereas some boys may leave at 16, still only beginning the metamorphosis. Mixed ability teaching it seems is therefore very necessary, as there is a link between mental ability and maturity. When children of the same chronological age are given intelligence tests, there is a definite tendency for the more physically mature children, and the actually physically large children, to score higher than their contemporaries, from about the age of six onwards [73].

The emotional and social effects of an early maturation have already been referred to (page 78). Research on late developers [74], has shown such boys to be at a disadvantage socially and psychologically. They often show more attention seeking behaviour, are less able to concentrate and are more talkative than their peers; facts many teachers will be able to substantiate. The analysis also identified deep feelings of anxiety and inadequacy in late developing boys and a fear of being rejected by their group where they tended to be less popular and had a lower social status.

The majority of girls will have had some degree of pubertal change by the age of 16, but late developers may well crave for curves and periods, and the trappings of 'sophisticated' mature classmates.

Both teachers and parents can but try to keep these findings in mind, and be particularly patient and supportive to late developing children. In all cases, both for the timing of puberty, and final shapes and sizes, a constant reminder is needed: *'average' is normal but normal is not just 'average'!*

Conviction on this point may be increased by the following studies, though teachers will need to develop convincing sales techniques to combat powerful media messages to the contrary!

Height changes

History

Consider historical records of average heights using evidence from clothes, suits of armour, doorways, beds, chairs etc. A report on skeletons of Romans, found at Cirencester, suggests the average height of men to have been 168cm, ($5'6\frac{1}{2}''$), and women 158cm ($5'2''$).

Geography

Survey the average heights of different races. What is happening to the heights of these populations, are they changing? Tanner [51] and [75] discusses the interaction of heredity and environment on the control of growth, and the genetic differences between the races.

Sociology

Does height make any difference to success or esteem? Make a montage: John Cleese, Dudley Moore, Diana Rigg, Lulu, Napoleon, Churchill, Mountbatten, Mother Theresa, Ghandi, politicians, musicians, sports personalities. Note the range of shapes and sizes. Think of boys and girls at school and locally who are well liked and respected, and note their heights. Do these cover the whole range?

Biology

Remind the class of previous work measuring growth in plants and animals. Even within one species they did not all grow at exactly the same rate, nor end up exactly the same size or shape at the end.

Mathematics

Persuade a female 163cm ($5'4''$) in height and a male, 174cm ($5'8\frac{1}{2}''$) (average heights) to stand in front of the class. Ask the children to write down on paper, and in their books,

i) an estimate of their heights
ii) whether they are, 'average', below 'average' or above 'average', for the men and women in this country.

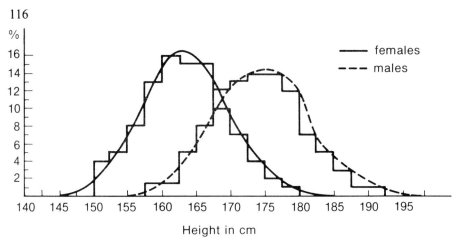

Figure 10   Percentage distribution of heights of males and females in Great Britain. 10,000 adults aged 16–64 were measured in their own homes (from OPCS Monitor data SS81/1 J. Mills).

Collect in the papers, and consider the statistics presented in the OPCS Monitor *Adult heights and weights survey* Ref. SS81/1 27, Oct. 1982. (Fig. 10)
What do these curves show?

i)   There are more women than men in Great Britain?   (No)
ii)   Women are taller than men?   (No)
iii)   The spread of heights among men is greater than among women?   (Yes)
iv)   The most frequent height of women in great Britain is 163cm? (approx. 5′4″)   (Yes)
v)   As the curves are approximately symmetrical, about how many women have heights greater than this?   (Half)
vi)   About how many women have heights less than this?   (Half)
vii)   What is the most frequent height of men in Great Britain?
(174cm approx. 5′8½″)
viii)   How many men have heights greater than this?   (about half)
ix)   How many men have heights less than this?   (about half)
x)   Are some women and men the same height?   (Yes, see overlap of curves)

The horizontal gap between the two curves shows there is a steady 10cm (4″) difference in height over most of the range. However, the difference increases with height, the top 20% of men being 12cm (4¾″) taller than the top 20% of women.

This work may demonstrate:

i)   Actual heights are not easy to assess without practice. Give the spread of the class guesses. How good a witness would you be? Did the answers vary very much?
ii)   The two chosen individuals may well have been estimated to be below the average height. What might be the reasons for this? Does the media present above average heights as 'the norm' e.g. model girls? Does television distort perception of height? Does posture and confidence have anything to do with perceived height?

iii)   The calculations from the graphs, will show about half the population will be 'below average', and about half 'above average' height. Convinced?

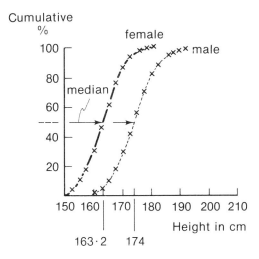

Figure 11   Cumulative frequency curves of heights of males and females in Great Britain (from OPCS Monitor SS81/1 J. Mills).

The OPCS Monitor gives details of how these statistics were collected and the variables considered. It has information on association of height with age (it declines, slightly, with age, after the mid-twenties) and social class. 'Average' height for women and men in social classes I, II and III non-manual, is higher than those in social classes III manual, and IV and V.

(Also the more children in the family the lower is their growth, and the less their final height [51].) OPCS Charts are included for weights, in relation to heights. The 'average' weight for males in 73.6kg (11st 8lbs) and for females 62.0kg (9st 11lbs). The complex factors involved here are also discussed.

Comparative rates and timing of growth in height again can be most clearly appreciated in graph form

Actual height changes After Tanner

(Tanner defines 'typical' as children with mean birth length, growing at mean velocity, and having their peak spurt at mean age.) Parents might be interested to know (see FIG 12 overleaf):

a–b)   that typical girls are slightly shorter than typical boys until puberty. (They are, however, actually 20% more 'mature' than boys, from birth, as measured by skeletal growth, and this is reflected in their abilities [51].)

b–c)   from 11 to 14, girls, on average, will be taller than their male contemporaries, as demonstrated in school assemblies.

c–d)   from 14 onwards typical boys will be about 13cm (5.1 inches) taller than typical girls. Social difficulties may be experienced by 'short' boys and 'tall' girls.

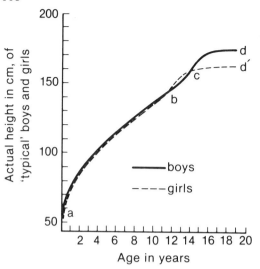

Figure 12 Actual height changes, after Tanner.

Rates of change of height

Children find 'rates' much more difficult to interpret than actual heights, but understanding of the significance of the slopes of curves in graphs can be developed.

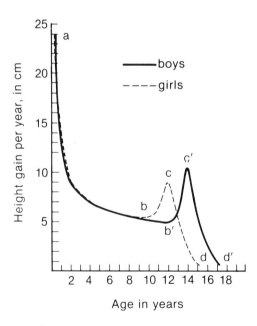

Figure 13 Rate of change of height, after Tanner.

a–b, a–b¹) Shows the dramatic drop in the rate of growth after birth, and the steady fall in rate (growing less every year) until the sudden 'growth spurt' at puberty b–c, b¹–c¹. The rate of growth just before this spurt is minimal, particularly for boys (at b¹ the line is very nearly horizontal and growth can be as little as 3.5cm), which can cause despair in late developers. It is some consolation to have this fact explained.

b–c) Girls on average reach puberty two years earlier than boys, and have their height spurt earlier in the sequence of changes (see Fig. 9) starting at about $10\frac{1}{2}$, and peaking at 12, adding 9cm in this year. They may begin to 'catch up' older brothers at this stage.

b¹–c¹) Boys on average reach puberty two years later, starting at $12\frac{1}{2}$ and peaking at 14 with 10.3cm of growth. Boys' growth spurt is later in their sequence of changes (FIG 10).

Measure out the actual average growth in height in the three years of growth spurt (Fig. 6): girls total 20cm (7.9 inches), Boys total 23cm (9 inches) Many families keep records of children's heights, on the back of doors or walls, these could be 'collected' as of historical value, and different ways of presenting growth discussed (FIG 7).

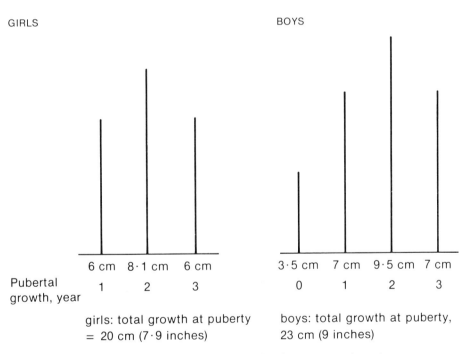

Figure 14   Growth in height during the three year pubertal spurt.

Seasonal changes in children's height

Growth in height in Europeans is greatest in the Spring and Summer, between March and July. This may be a response to increased day length, as blind children do not show this association, though their growth also varies during the year (Marshall). Growth in weight tends to increase in the Autumn(!).

120

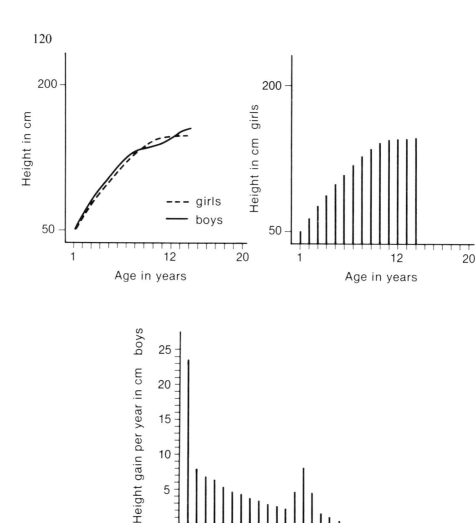

Figure 15   Comparison of ways of measuring growth.

Sequence of growth, all children

i)   Hands and feet grow first, peak growth rate 3 months after beginning of spurt, which may cause temporary clumsiness, and the 'clonking into everything' syndrome.

ii)   Legs grow next, some 6–9 months before the main pubertal spurt, so colt-like leginess may ensue, emphasised by mini skirts and high-rise shoes. Trousers recede up. Because boys enter puberty later than girls their legs grow proportionately longer, as they have more years to grow in. Chorus girls in high heels and costumes split to the hips attempt to redress the balance, but why should a woman want to be more like a man?!

iii)   Hips, then chest and shoulders increase in size about four months later.

iv) Trunk length increase is the main feature of the pubertal spurt, but happens last. It can be measured by sitting height.

Face changes

During puberty, forehead, jaws and noses all grow, altering facial proportions and effectively making the eyes seem smaller and move up the head! Fig. 8.

We are very sensitive to proportions and react strongly positively to 'baby faces', as advertisers and Walt Disney productions know well. Face changes in adolescents can disturb parents as they are visibly losing their 'little boy or girl', and a new person is emerging, whom they may react to crossly on occasions. 'Don't look so sullen!'

Eyeball changes

The eyeball may grow in length slightly from front to back during puberty, which can affect eyesight. Watch for children 'peering' at the blackboard or television, as the incidence of short-sightedness increases in girls of 11 and 12, and boys of 13 and 14. Conversely, previously long-sighted children may find their eyesight improving during puberty. Regular eye tests are advisable.

Teeth

These seem more vulnerable to decay during adolescence, so dental checks may pay off socially.

Skin changes: Acne

Increase in secretions of sweat, and from apocrine and sebaceous glands occur. Both the sex hormones affect the skin, sometimes causing closed pores, trapping sebaceous secretions, which can lead to an actual infection. The effect of spots, or in the extreme form acne, should never be underestimated. It can make a young person already very vulnerable to negative assessments of personal image, feel absolutely wretched. Doctors can give advice, and one particular antibiotic may help control the situation and prevent scarring.

The sequence of pubertal changes

These are less variable than the age at which puberty occurs, but the speed of each of the changes can vary.

Girls

i) Increase in growth rate begins, though may not be noticed at first.

ii) Breast development starts, and some girls find 'breast buds' tender, and they may be uneven. This is quite normal. Five stages are defined, stage one being before growth starts. Some girls complete all stages in $1\frac{1}{2}$ years, others take 4 to 5 years or more.

iii) Pubic hairs grow, in five definable stages. Stage one is before hairs appear. Again the speed of progression varies, and is not synchronised with any other feature.

iv) The first period occurs, known as menarche. This stage is closely linked with the rapid drop in the rate of growth in height, after the adolescent spurt. These changes can be shown diagramatically (FIG 17).

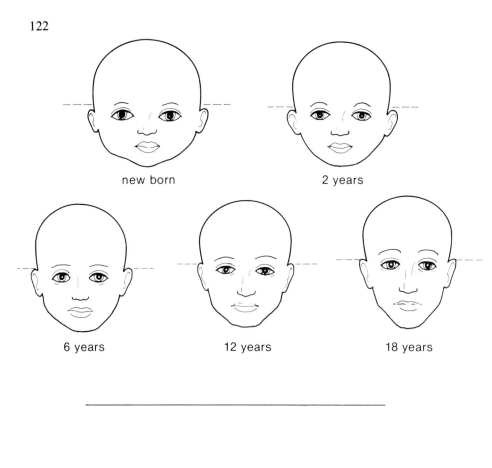

new born

2 years

6 years

12 years

18 years

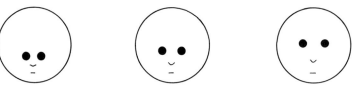

Try the effect of moving cut out features around, in a circle which looks the oldest?

Figure 16   Changing face proportions (from J. M. Tanner and Raltray Taylor, *Growth*, Time Life International).

Other physical changes in girls

i)   Hips widen more than the shoulders. The waist is more defined.

ii)   There is an increase in muscle and muscle power in the limbs, but not to such an extent as boys.

iii)   Hair grows under the arms, and increases on face, arms and legs. The amount and pattern of hair growth differs very much between individuals and races.

iv)   Fat layers do not increase much [51] (unless due to unwise eating) but become distributed in a feminine pattern of a more rounded-shaped body.

v)   The womb grows, the lining responds to the female hormones, progesterone and the oestrogens.

vi)   The vagina and its glands enlarge, vaginal secretions increase, and become more acid (about pH 4.5).

vii)   The genital organs grow:
the labia enlarge and darken, the outer ones grow hair;
the clitoris enlarges, becomes sensitive and erectile.

viii)   The sweat rate increases and glands in the arm pits become active.

ix)   Skin changes occur which may lead to spots or acne.

x)   The voice deepens slightly.

xi)   Face changes occur (see page 121).

Boys

i)   The testes enlarge, the scrotum changes in texture, and darkens.

ii)   The penis enlarges, darkens, and becomes more sensitive, erections increase, wet dreams may begin in about a year.

iii)   Pubic hair grows in five stages, stage one being no hair. Growth of hair up the abdomen in a line towards the navel is normal and used to be called stage six. It occurs in 80% of men and 10% of women [61].

iv)   Spurt in growth in height begins, and is thus later in the sequence than in girls.

Other physical changes in boys

i)   Growth in width of shoulders more than in the hips, giving a 'masculine' shape.

ii)   Changes to hair. Hair grows under the arms and also on the face where the sequence starts at the corners of the upper lip. Body hair increases, the amount and distribution being related to race and ancestry. Hairs on the chest are not a reliable indicator of virility! Hair begins to recede at the temples and on the scalp, the amount of eventual baldness determined by hereditary factors. Choose your parents carefully! It may be some consolation to know that eunuchs have low hair lines and thick hair.

iii)   Some breast development may occur. Up to 1/3 of boys experience this. Do not panic, it usually lasts only for a year!

iv)   The voice 'breaks', or deepens gradually, usually quite late in the sequence of changes.

v)   Fat layers actually get less, giving an angular appearance. This may affect buoyancy so some boys have difficulty learning to swim and may also get cold very quickly (but will *not* come out of the pool, though blue and with chattering teeth, as this is obviously unmanly).

vi)   Muscles increase in size and strength, greater proportionately than those of girls. Boys also have relatively larger hearts and lungs; a higher blood pressure; greater oxygen carrying capacity; lower heart beat at rest and more chemical resistance to fatigue. These are reasons why directly competitive sports are usually kept separate for men and women.

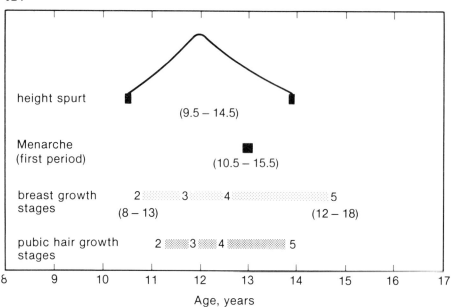

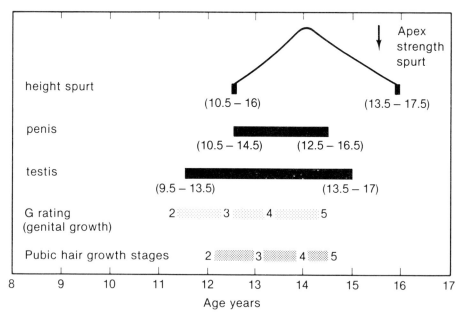

Figure 17 Sequence of pubertal events: above, girls; below, boys. From Marshall and Tanner. The spread of ages is shown in brackets.

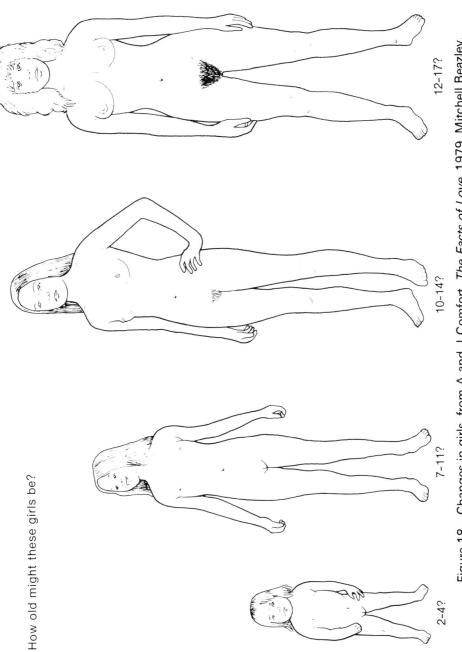

How might these girls be?

2–4? 7–11? 10–14? 12–17?

Figure 18 Changes in girls, from A and J Comfort, *The Facts of Love*, 1979, Mitchell Beazley.

126

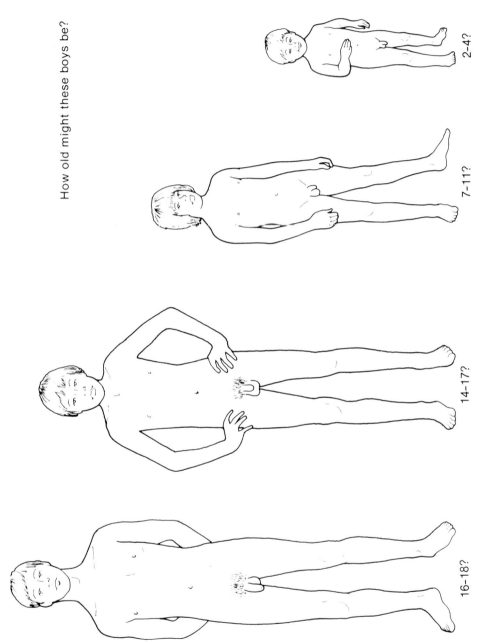

How old might these boys be?

16–18?   14–17?   7–11?   2–4?

Figure 19   Changes in boys, from A and J Comfort, *The Facts of Love*, 1979, Mitchell Beazley.

During adolescence many pre-pubertal boys will not have reached these stages, so are very much at a disadvantage. Great tact is needed in arranging for them to succeed at something during PE sessions.

vii)   Increased sweating occurs. Skin changes may lead to acne, as a boy's skin is particularly sensitive to the male hormone testosterone.

viii)   Face changes occur, proportionately greater than in girls (see page 121).

The hormonal control of growth

The brain controls the level of many hormones concerned with growth, by acting through the hypothalamus, which secretes chemicals stimulating or inhibiting hormone release from the closely associated pituitary gland.

Pituitary hormones

The interaction of these hormones with the parts of the body sensitive to them is complex, and can be influenced by stress, and intense emotions. Much can be done to help children who are not growing within accepted norms (see Tanner [151]). All can encourage communication about feelings, and try to ensure children have enough exercise and *sleep*, both of which seem necessary for the production of the growth hormone, GH [152]. Too much late night television watching during puberty may not be so advisable!

Hygiene

At puberty new glands become active, and the character of sweat and body secretions changes. Bacterial action on such natural effluents can lead to a socially unacceptable smell and certain infections have a better chance of developing on undisturbed areas of the body. Lessons on the washing of self and clothes therefore become particularly appropriate, and may ensure a reasonable working environment for the teacher!

Personal hygiene

An historical lead in, on fashions in washing or not washing e.g. only one bath a month was usual before the 18th century, can be a non-threatening approach. Then proceed to modern washing possibilities e.g. film star glamour baths, pictures of wild extravagance and the shapes of modern baths.

In science lessons construct a 'Which' survey of soaps and prices, advertising and packaging. Also try making soap.

Discuss the merits of baths versus showers, and the relaxing or invigorating effect of water on skin, a sensual occasion to be enjoyed. Religions such as Hindu, Muslim and Sikh, consider baths unclean, and always prefer running water.

Consider the problems of those who do not have baths or showers at home, or have to share them with a large number of others.

Washing clothes

Liaise with the home economics department, again using the historical approach e.g. massive 'wash days', etc. Contrast this with the ease of washing modern fibres, some of which dry more quickly. Survey advertising claims for new low temperature washing powders, and supposed effect on the family; is it only women who can wash clothes? (and only men who can offer advice!).

Table 9   Pituitary hormones influencing growth.

Pituitary Hormones	
Thyroid Stimulating Hormone	TSH, causes the thyroid gland to produce thyroxine necessary for normal growth.
Growth Hormone	GH acts on the liver, stimulating the production of somatomedin, which promotes the growth of cartilage and muscle.
Adrenocorticotrophic Hormone	ACTH acts on the adrenal cortex to produce i) Adrenal androgen, with a similar effect on growth to testosterone, but it is produced in girls as well as boys. ii) Cortisol (hydrocortisone), which has an anti-stress action, but also inhibits growth.
Follicle Stimulating Hormone	FSH in females stimulates the ovaries to produce oestrogens (see below) and in males the growth of the seminiferous tubules and the production of sperm.
Luteinizing or Leydig-cell Stimulating Hormone	In females LH is involved in the menstrual cycle, and the production of the corpus luteum and progesterone. In males it stimulates the Leydig cells in the testes to make testosterone. (See below)
Insulin	This comes from the pancreas and must be present in adequate amounts for normal growth. The treatment for diabetics allows for this.

Table 10   The sex hormones in girls and boys.

Hormones in girls		Hormones in boys	
Oestrogens control	The increase in growth of the vagina and its glands, the genital organs, the womb (and its lining, in the menstrual cycle), and growth of breasts and pelvis.	Testosterone	i) When present in the foetus it causes male genitals to form, and may also effect the hypothalamus causing it to be non-cyclic in response later, unlike the female. ii) At puberty the large increase causes the adolescent spurt in growth in bones and muscles, particularly of shoulders and spine. iii) Growth of the genitals (rated as the G factor!) iv) Growth of all hair (and thinning that on the head). v) Possible increase in aggressiveness. vi) Deepening of the voice. In old men with less testosterone the voice may become higher again.
Adrenal androgens control	i) Probably the adolescent spurt in height and strength. ii) The growth of body and facial hair. iii) The sex drive.		
Progesterone controls	The menstrual cycle (in conjunction with oestrogen) growth of breasts, and pregnancy.		

Give a class assignment e.g. find out how each item of school clothing (including sports wear) is washed and ironed. Make a chart of the findings. Presoak? Washing temperature? Soap or detergent used? Number of rinses? Drip dry? Spin or wring? Ironing temperature? Dry clean only? Find out the facilities provided at launderettes and other commercial laundries.

Bonus marks and praise must be given to those who show they can wash and iron some of their own clothes. Discuss techniques for the removal of stains: mud, grass, ink, body fluids, sweat, blood from nose bleeds, cut fingers, periods etc.

Smelly children

Most teachers have come across this problem, which raises issues of personal liberty and 'interventions' for the common good. It is always a delicate matter, but *does* need to be tackled.

i)   This must be done primarily for the good of the individual concerned. Personal relationships do not flourish if nobody wants to sit next to you. What does this do to your self-image? Disadvantaged children may have bladder control problems, which do not help; 1% of 16 year olds may still wet the bed [80].

ii)   If an individual has never been shown acceptable standards of hygiene, how can they teach their own children, if they have any, later? The vicious circle would continue.

iii)   It will benefit other members of the class or group.

Possible strategies

i)   Try a private chat during the lesson. How easy is it to wash self and clothes?

ii)   Enlist assistance from the health visitor attached to the school, who could liaise with the social services to find out whether help could be given for washing facilities at home. These may well be very inadequate, or lack privacy.

iii)   The parents could be contacted. Would it be possible for the teenager to join the 'Laundry Club' and learn how to use the school washing machine if there is one, and do ironing ... and so be more helpful at home?

iv)   Showers after games can be strategic, with privacy, and perhaps an extended time for one class which could report on new soaps donated by local chemists.

v)   Swimming: chlorine in the water may reach the parts ... Unfortunately children most in need of showers or a swim often contrive to miss them, of course.

vi)   Have a heart to heart talk with the child. Would they like to have help and make an effort to look and smell nicer and make the most of such lovely hair ... hands ... skin ... Practical help for the physical arrangements will have to be given, as well as moral support and encouragement. It is worth the effort, and facing possible accusations of 'interfering', for everyone's sake.

More specific matters
Feminine hygiene

Because of the moist nature of the mucus membrane of the inner labia, it may be preferable for girls to have pants or pant-linings of cotton as this absorbs the normal vaginal secretions, and sweat. Wiping and washing the vulva, should always be from front to back, to avoid transferring normal bacteria in faeces, into the vagina or urethra, where they could cause infection. Talk here of caring for baby girls, and how they should always be washed in this way. Toddlers too need help, their arms aren't long enough to cope!

Girls (and boys) of the Hindu, Muslim and Sikh religions are taught to wash themselves with water, rather than use paper, so they appreciate access to water in the same cubicle as the toilet.

Special care with hygiene is necessary during a period (see page 150).

Masculine hygiene

Because of the need to keep the testes cooler than the rest of the body, the scrotum and groin are liberally supplied with sweat glands. Evaporation of sweat lowers the temperature. This area therefore needs special care, particularly as one fungus specialises in living here, causing 'Dhoby's itch', (this is easily treated however). Uncircumcised boys are wise to pay attention to regular washing under the foreskin, as there are glands in this region which produce a waxy substance called smegma, which can become smelly or infected if allowed to accumulate, and could become a potential source of infection to a sexual partner.

Describing personal plumbing

The way you feel about the parts you are growing does matter. Psychosexual effects are very real. Too often the only information children are given is from poorly presented diagrams, where the relative sizes, positions and orientations of organs are not clear. Ovaries and womb are depicted far too large, with an open cervix inviting problems. Testes are apparently small, level, and stuck on the sides of the legs!

Female organs
The womb and vagina

Ask everyone, girls and boys, to put one hand on their womb, or where it would be if they had one. There will be some hesitation here, partly because it is rude to put your hand down low in public (this can be discussed later). Generally the consensus is that the womb is right in the middle of the abdomen, firmly across the navel (related to the pregnant condition possibly).

Now, produce a pear, approximately 8cm (3″) long. This is the actual size of the womb in a non-pregnant woman. Show it is three-dimensional, rotate it, stalk-end down to demonstrate the neck of the pear as the cervix. (Take the stalk out!)

It is possible for a woman to touch the cervix with her (clean) finger, and it feels like the end of a nose ... 'everyone feel the end of your nose ...' only it's silky smooth. (Some women have mistaken the cervix for a growth.) Hold the

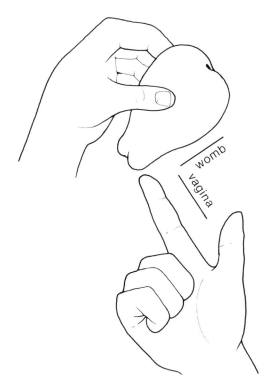

Figure 20   The pear-fect visual aid!

pear at right angles to the index finger to show the angle of the womb to the vagina, about 90° or rather less.

The vagina points backwards, towards the small of the back, and the womb tips forwards. Where must it be in the body then, if it can be felt with a finger? Correct ... right down low, close to the vulva, and certainly not half way up the body, with ovaries under the armpits!

Hold the pear at the side of the body, at the correct level and orientation, to demonstrate how relatively small it is. The womb is able to rotate slightly backwards, to accommodate a full bladder, and in some 10% of women it quite normally tilts backwards, called a retroversion [81]. If a human skeleton model is available, show the position of the womb inside the pelvis (and relate to the figure below).

The Ortho-Pelvic model

Confirm the position, size and angle of the womb and vagina, by using the ortho-pelvic model [76]. This is in two halves, of transparent and pink plastic, held in a frame and stand. Some practice in using it is advisable, the

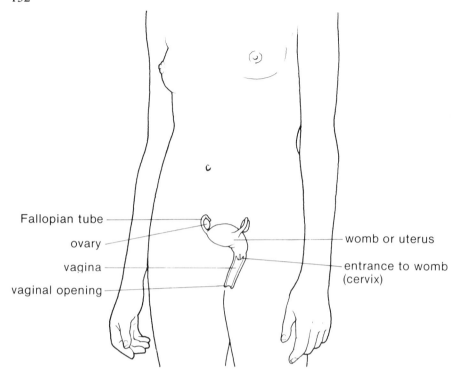

Figure 21 The position of a girl's reproductive organs (from A and J Comfort, *The Facts of Love*).

accompanying notes explain how to slot the sections in and out. It helps to reduce any tension if it is endowed with a name, e.g. 'Orthina'. The model is slightly less than full adult size, more like an adolescent. When in the stand, the organs are in the position of a person lying down (see the figure on page 133). so rotate the model to compare them with the pear, previously shown.

Work with small groups.

i)   The side view: demonstrate the angle of the womb and vagina again, the womb can be seen to be more horizontal than vertical.

ii) Show the front view, as if looking through a transparent abdomen wall (FIG 23). Note the *top* of the womb, with the two (fallopian) tubes leading from it (10cm, 4″, long in reality), ending in fringe-like structures near the ovaries. In an adult the ovaries would be about 3.5cm (1½″) long and have been variously likened to almonds, walnuts, grapes or pigeons' eggs!

iii) Next, turn the model as if Orthina were lying on her back. Put the two halves back in the stand if necessary. Show the transparent vulva, sadly lacking a clitoris, so indicate where this would be (and the interesting sociology of its omission), the outer and inner labia the opening of the bladder and the anus, a little misleadingly placed as it seems to be included in the vulva. Get each child to look down the vagina, (usually about 10cm, 4″

ORTHO PELVIC MODEL 1. SIDE VIEW

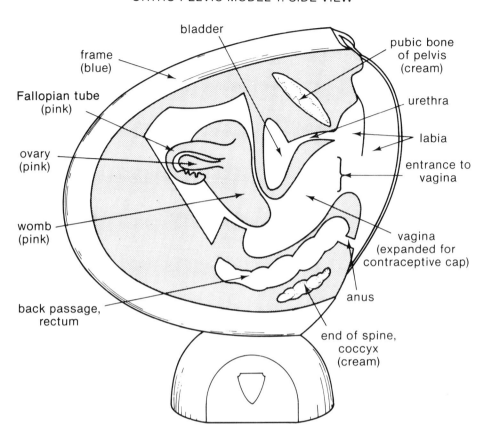

bladder

frame
(blue)

pubic bone
of pelvis
(cream)

Fallopian tube
(pink)

urethra

ovary
(pink)

labia

entrance to
vagina

womb
(pink)

vagina
(expanded for
contraceptive cap)

back passage,
rectum

anus

end of spine,
coccyx
(cream)

2. SIDE VIEW OF MODEL, ROTATED TO A 'STANDING PERSON' POSITION

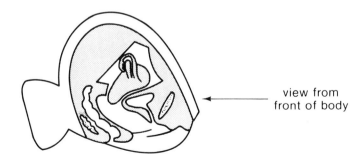

view from
front of body

Figure 22   A side view of the ortho-pelvic model, i)"lying down" and
ii)"standing".

3. 'FRONT' VIEW OF ORTHO MODEL

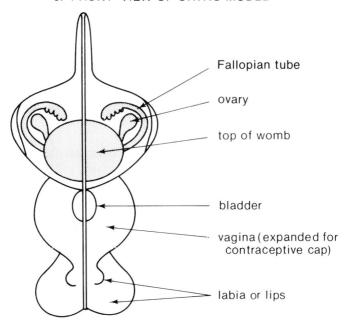

Fallopian tube

ovary

top of womb

bladder

vagina (expanded for
   contraceptive cap)

labia or lips

ORTHO MODEL, VIEW DOWN THE VAGINA

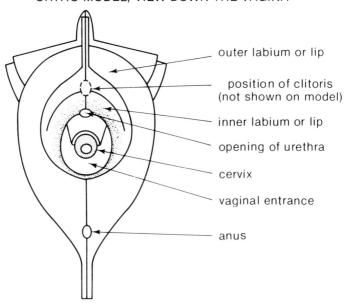

outer labium or lip

position of clitoris
(not shown on model)

inner labium or lip

opening of urethra

cervix

vaginal entrance

anus

Figure 23   Ortho-pelvic model, front view and view down the vagina.

long, when not sexually excited), to see the cervix, clearly protruding at the far end. (FIG 23) Note the *very* small opening in the cervix, no tampon could enter here. Explain the vagina does not really stand open like this – it would be very draughty if it did (!), nor has it usually got the sideways bulge which has been built in to the model to demonstrate the use of a contraceptive cap. The vagina is really soft and stretchy, with slightly folded walls, touching each other.

If doctors want to get this view show by the model, to take a cervical smear for example, they use an instrument called a speculum, to hold the vaginal walls open. An ordinary pelvic examination does not require this, a couple of fingers are used, sometimes with gentle pressure on the abdomen, to check all is well. The importance of relaxing during this event can be stressed, and how quick and painless it is.

iv) When everyone has appreciated the 'whole organ' orientation, slide out the right side of the model (as viewed from behind) to see the mid-line sectional view. This shows the thick muscular wall of the womb, in pale pink, and the darker pink lining, which would be shed during the next period (FIG 24). Rotate the model again, vulva downwards, so it can be related to diagrams of 'half women', which are so difficult to interpret otherwise. The relatively small cavity of the womb can be commented on. Again, it does not 'stand open', but the walls touch each other. Demonstrate the position of the bladder and how the womb would tip up when the bladder was full. The pear can now be cut both longitudinally and transversely, and have the core removed, to show the womb cavity, which is flattened from front to back (FIG 24).

The vulva

Having seen the plastic model it is much easier to relate to drawings and diagrams of the vulva. Explain the clitoris is the most sensitive part (very like the tip of the penis) and is linked with tissues under the labia and around the vagina about 30 times the size of the visible shaft and glans of the clitoris, which react to sexual excitement by becoming swollen, and filled with blood, in exactly the same way as a penis does [77]. There is no need for women to feel deprived of sexual equipment.

Labia differ in size and shape, in some women the inner labia normally protrude a little for example. Muscles of the 'pelvic floor' run under the labia. Pre- and post-natal classes include strengthening exercises for these, and similar ones could be done in routine PE lessons. It would help to make this part of the body as acceptable as any other, and might help prevent a prolapse developing in later life.

The hymen

Children find the concept of the hymen difficult. Explain it is a very thin skin, or membrane, partly covering the opening to the vagina. Again its exact nature varies and some girls have larger openings than others, or several smaller ones. Very often the opening enlarges, by the hymen becoming naturally stretched during sports activities, gymnastics or dancing, or by the insertion of tampons during a period.

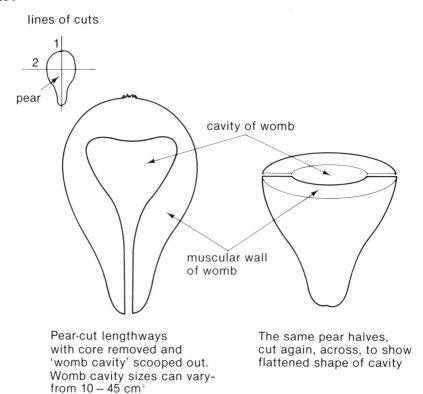

lines of cuts

pear

cavity of womb

muscular wall
of womb

Pear-cut lengthways
with core removed and
'womb cavity' scooped out.
Womb cavity sizes can vary–
from 10 – 45 cm³

The same pear halves,
cut again, across, to show
flattened shape of cavity

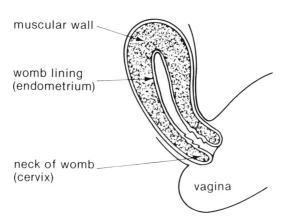

muscular wall

womb lining
(endometrium)

neck of womb
(cervix)

vagina

Figure 24   Top: cut pear to show shape of womb cavity. Bottom: lengthways
section of womb (shown in ortho-pelvic model).

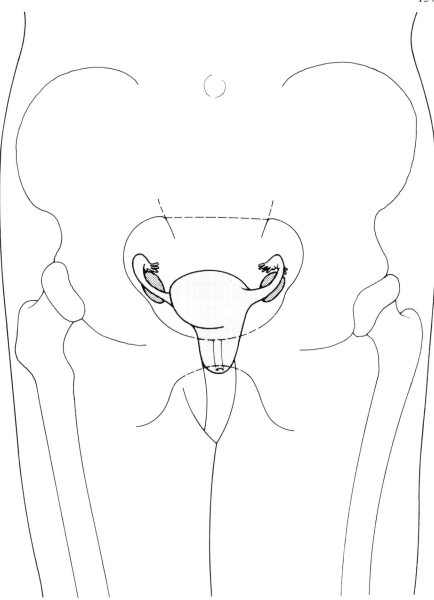

Get the class to find:

i) the navel   vi) the neck of the womb (cervix)
ii) the hip bones   vii) the vagina
iii) the womb (uterus)   viii) the pubic bones
iv) the two Fallopian tubes   ix) the pelvic girdle
v) the two ovaries   x) the bones of the leg

Relate the position of these organs to a model
skeleton wherever possible.

Figure 25   Female reproductive organs approximately $\frac{1}{4}$ size.

A useful aid to understanding is the inner tube of a toilet roll, covered with plain paper, and slightly squeezed into an oval shape, to represent the vagina, with a piece of cling film (about 15cm square) taped over one end, in which a small opening has been made with the little finger, to represent the hymen and its opening. Show how easily this opening can be stretched, using one finger, with a slight rotary action. The cling film is sufficiently elastic to let the opening expand in a natural looking way. Discussion of the hymen may well lead on to the nature of virginity.

Is it possible for a doctor (or sexual partner) to tell if the girl is a virgin? No, it is not always possible, for the reasons explained above. Natural openings vary very much in size.

Does the hymen always bleed on first intercourse, as folk-lore and novels about 'being broken into', would have it? No indeed it does not, some being more elastic than others.

So deep is the conviction that bleeding is 'proof of virginity' that some girls arrange their wedding nights to coincide with a period. If virginity is used as a highly prized commodity, proof of it is exacted ... from the girls.

How could boys prove their virginity? Discuss the dual standards which have arisen from the basic anatomical differences between men and women.

In a few cases a hymen may be resistant to stretching, necessitating a gradual dilation procedure, or a small operation. This condition is different from vaginismus, which is the contraction of the vaginal muscles on attempted examination or penetration, due to fear or pain. Treatment here is by psychotherapy, enabling the woman to understand and overcome her fears.

Male organs

As these are much more visible, understanding of them is usually better than for the female equivalents.

The scrotum and testes

The following teaching points could be included. The reason why the testes are suspended in such a vulnerable place is that sperm only develop at 35°C, at 2°C lower than the average body level. Temperature control involves sweat glands and the (reflex) capacity to lower the scrotum and testes slightly, when hot, or raise them tightly against the body, when cold. Boys will be aware of this phenomenon. School medical rooms are best kept warm, or the task of the doctor examining this region will be more difficult! Such a check is advisable as the testes usually descend from inside the body cavity, to the scrotum, about one month before the baby is born, as in 96% of mature baby boys at birth. Some do descend later but should be in position preferably before the boy is about 5 or 6 years old, or subsequent fertility could be affected [78].

The pathway of the testes out of the body cavity is over the top of the pelvic bone, through the inguinal canal, and this can be a point of weakness if it does not close properly and allows a bulge of the abdominal wall, or even the gut, to protrude into the scrotum. This then causes an inguinal hernia, which can be surgically corrected at any age.

Some young boys have discovered they can push their testes back up the canal. 'I do it while I'm watching boring TV', said one. This may not be such a good idea as it could encourage a later hernia, and consternation if they don't come down again easily!

The growth of the testes at puberty is great, from a volume of about 4cm³, to one of 12 to 20cm³ or more. They are oval, about 5cm (2″) long, and are worn asymmetrically, the left one usually being lower than the right, – despite evidence to the contrary from classical sculpture.

Inside the testes are a mass of very finely coiled tubes, about 0.25mm in diameter. Their total length is about 200m, and their function is to produce sperm. About 100 million of these are made every 24 hours, a rate of 1,000 per second, after maturity, the number gradually declining in old age.

As sperm are so miniscule, vast numbers, up to 500 million, are contained in the 0.5 – 10cm³ of semen produced at each ejaculation. Over 99% of semen is the fluid produced by glands; Cowper's glands, the prostate gland and the seminal vesicles. (These last do not actually store the sperm, as previously thought.)

As sperm are damaged by acid, a reflex system automatically closing the bladder on ejaculation means sperm and urine are never passed at the same time. This is why it is difficult for boys to urinate while they have an erection. Chemicals in the semen help to neutralise acid from the urine, or in the vagina.

Special cells between the fine tubes in the testes produce the male hormone testosterone, so the testes are in fact dual purpose.,

The names associated with the male system are nearly as long as the tubes! They can be simplified as much as possible, but it is useful to know about them.

i) The vas deferens is the tube leading from the testes to the penis, and is fundamental in male sterilisation operations (and can make a vas(t) difference!).

ii) The prostate gland is about the size of a golf ball. As it surrounds the urethra, should it enlarge in later life it can cause problems. Many children have heard of operations involving this gland, often misnamed the prostrate.

iii) The urethra is the dual purpose tube down the penis. Its relatively long length is somewhat protective, males having fewer bladder infections than females.

For those that enjoy words, 'epididymis', can be added, and is useful in spelling tests and crosswords, it is the tube from the testes where the sperm wait and mature.

The penis

There is probably more concern about the size of this organ, than almost any other part of the body!

Boys worry theirs is not 'big enough'!

Girls worry that 'it' will be 'too big'!

Big enough for what?!

i) For male pleasure? Any size of penis is able to erect and orgasm, so there is no problem here.

ii) For female pleasure? The areas of a woman's genital organs sensitive to pleasure are the clitoris, the labia and the outer region of the vagina. No

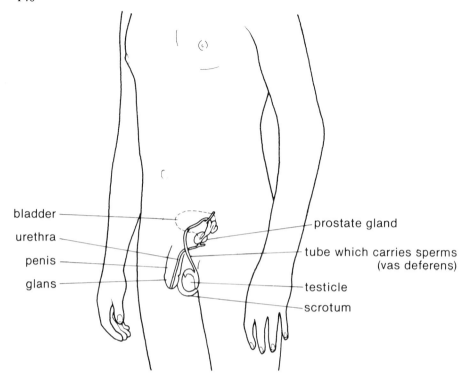

bladder
urethra
penis
glans

prostate gland
tube which carries sperms
(vas deferens)
testicle
scrotum

Figure 26 The position of a boy's reproductive organs (from A and J Comfort, *The Facts of Love*).

sensory cells (even of the much discussed 'G' spot) are buried down the far end of the vagina or on the cervix, (a contraceptive cap, or a tampon correctly placed cannot be felt at all).

iii) To be impressive? To whom? Anyone understanding the above facts will know there is no correlation between size and function. Smaller penises tend to increase proportionately more when erect anyway. Circumcised and uncircumcised penises function equally well.

Too big?

The size of a penis, which can vary from about 3.5 to 10cm ($1\frac{1}{2}$ to 4″) when limp (or less if it's cold!), and from about 9cm to 20cm ($3\frac{1}{2}$ to 8″) average 15cm (6″) when erect can be a shock factor, and a worry to females. They can be helped by reassurance that the vagina is extremely elastic and flexible enough for a baby to be born through remember, and during sexual excitement becomes wet and lubricated and increases in length and width, the inner third 'ballooning'.

The erection process

This hydraulic system is in full working order even before birth, being an involuntary action triggered by physical or mental stimulation. Erections do increase in frequency at puberty, and can cause embarrassment. Boys have to learn to cope with this situation, and girls should know that boys too can have

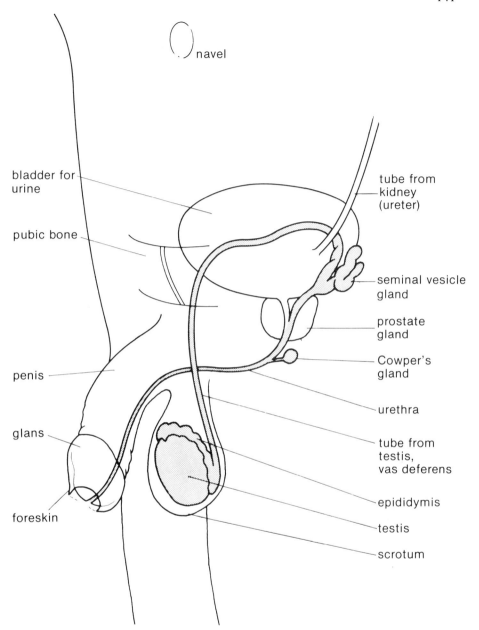

navel

bladder for urine

tube from kidney (ureter)

pubic bone

seminal vesicle gland

prostate gland

Cowper's gland

penis

urethra

glans

tube from testis, vas deferens

epididymis

foreskin

testis

scrotum

Figure 27   Male reproductive organs, side view, $\frac{1}{2}$ size, after R.J. Demarest.

problems while growing up.

Orgasms can occur from an infant age and are not necessarily linked with ejaculation, which can begin fairly early on in pubertal changes, and may occur at night, with or without an erection. The three processes, erection, orgasm and ejaculation are therefore not always linked.

Menstruation

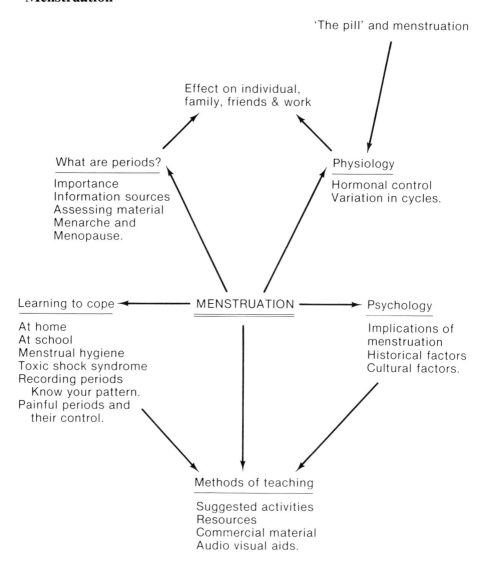

'The pill' and menstruation

Effect on individual,
family, friends & work

What are periods?

Importance
Information sources
Assessing material
Menarche and
Menopause.

Physiology

Hormonal control
Variation in cycles.

Learning to cope ← MENSTRUATION → Psychology

At home
At school
Menstrual hygiene
Toxic shock syndrome
Recording periods
  Know your pattern.
Painful periods and
  their control.

Implications of
menstruation
Historical factors
Cultural factors.

Methods of teaching

Suggested activities
Resources
Commercial material
Audio visual aids.

Why? No-one knows exactly why this process has evolved. It occurs only in apes, old world (African) monkeys, and humans. It appears to be a wasteful process, but until relatively recently women probably did not menstruate very often, because they were pregnant or breast-feeding for most of their lives. Only with family limitation and increased life expectancy has the situation arisen where a woman may have periods for 65 days or more per year for 30 years, and then possibly live another 20–30 years without them.

Effects

Menstruation affects everybody, directly or indirectly.

In any one month in the United Kingdom, up to 600,000 women and girls have to take time off work or school, because of menstrual problems [82] (see page 146). Apart from the personal misery involved, this means a loss to British industry of millions of working days per year.

Pre-menstrual and menstrual tension are probably experienced by about half the female population of childbearing age and for some this can influence performance [83]. Weekly grades of school girls can drop by 10%, and in 'O' and 'A' level examination results there are more failures and lower average marks. Factory workers become more accident prone at this time and are slower and less accurate. There are more cases of battered babies and accidents in the home increase. The likelihood of road accidents increases and the toxic effect of alcohol is greater. There is lowered resistance to infectious diseases from flu to meningitis. Epilepsy, asthma and migraine are more likely to occur. More criminal offences are committed: shoplifting is 30 times more likely in the second half of the menstrual cycle, as is the suicide rate, which increases sevenfold.

There are some sceptics who do not believe the syndrome exists, but it may be a majority of women at some stage in their lives know it as a very real phenomenon. The law now recognises PMT as constituting mitigating circumstances in some cases, when women have committed crimes. The syndrome does, however, put women in one of the greatest 'double bind' situations of all time. If they talk about their problems frankly and honestly, will they be seen as making excuses, or the facts used by some as justification for excluding all women from certain situations? Will men, and the women who do not have these difficulties, understand and be sympathetic, tolerant and helpful to those that do?

Should we warn girls of what might happen, or will this encourage psychosomatic symptoms and dread of the event? Indeed it is desirable to lift the secrecy from the very real problems experienced by so many, to enable them to seek help, relief and comfort. More research is needed into the exact nature of the physiological changes causing cyclical disturbances, so more specific treatments can be developed.

The good news

There has been progress in the understanding of the menstrual cycle and clinics for the treatment of pre-menstrual tension and menopausal problems have been established in various parts of the country. Contact the FPA for details.

Research into painful periods (also previously classed by some as totally psychosomatic in nature) has now identified one of the major causes, and drugs have been developed to counteract it (see page 147). To obtain help for these conditions, women need the confidence to realise they have a problem which *can* be treated, and to convince the medical world that this is so.

Menstrual facts and myths

The menstrual cycle is controlled by a balancing act between hormones (FIG 28). Their interaction ensures the synchronisation of the ripening and release of

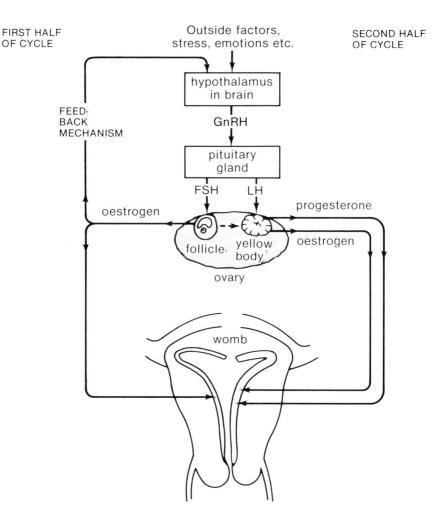

FIRST HALF
OF CYCLE

Outside factors,
stress, emotions etc.

SECOND HALF
OF CYCLE

hypothalamus
in brain

GnRH

FEED-
BACK
MECHANISM

pituitary
gland

FSH   LH

oestrogen

progesterone

oestrogen

follicle   yellow
body

ovary

womb

GnRH = Gonadotropic Releasing Hormone
FSH   = Follicle Stimulating Hormone
LH   = Luteinising Hormone

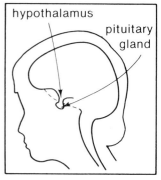

hypothalamus

pituitary
gland

Figure 28 The hormonal control of the
menstrual cycle, and the position of
hormonal control centres.

an ovum from one of the ovaries, (ovulation), with the growth and preparation of the lining of the womb to receive it, should fertilisation occur. The most significant event of the cycle is ovulation, but this is overshadowed in impact by the collapse of the unused lining and its visible passage out of the body as the monthly period.

During each cycle, changes occur:

i)   in the level of the controlling hormones
ii)   in the ovary
iii) in the lining of the womb (the endometrium)
iv)   in the mucus of the cervix
v)   possibly in the emotions and behaviour of the person.

Over the centuries many myths, taboos and fears have arisen about this menstrual flow. It has been attributed strange powers, mostly damaging, such as causing crops to fail, wine and milk to sour, cattle to abort, fruit to fall off trees, iron and bronze to rust and bees to die in their hives. Women have been made to feel unclean, untouchable, ungodly and unloved, while periods proceeded. It is interesting to speculate if such myths would have been generated if the flow had been white or colourless, and semen thick and red!

Variations on the cyclical theme
The start
The time of the first period (menarche) is linked with other pubertal changes (see page 124). The average age for menarche is 13. The timing may be influenced by excitement and stress, so teachers taking young teenage girls, on field courses, outings or trips abroad, can be fairly confident some will 'start' their periods on the top of the mountain or on the cross channel ferry. It is wise to be prepared for such contingencies.
The length of the whole cycle
This is influenced by both internal and external factors.

i)   Natural cycle lengths vary from about 16 to (rarely) 50 days, an average figure being 28 days. The menstrual 'clock' regulating this is in the hypothalamus.
ii)   Cycles are often very irregular at the beginning and end of the 30 years. Some girls have only 3 or 4 periods during their first year. 20% of 16 year olds have cycles lasting longer than 40 days [83]. Women approaching menopause may also have long gaps between periods.
iii) Once cycles have begun, they usually continue, unless the female loses weight, is very energetic, e.g. ballet dancers, athletes, marathon runners or joggers, or, on a very different level, she is suffering from starvation, or anorexia nervosa. In all these cases periods may stop.
iv)   Emotions, shock, pleasure, excitement, etc. can influence cycles, delaying or precipitating periods.
v)   Cycle length can be influenced by the presence of males. In all-female situations girls may have longer cycles, of 35 days or more. When in contact with the opposite sex, these may shorten, to nearer a 28 day length.

vi) Some females living closely together find their monthly periods become synchronised. Research in America [87] has shown this may be due to an ingredient in their sweat which acts as an external hormone, or pheromone.

vii) Night shift work, changing the 24 hour rhythm, can alter the pattern of cycles, as many female nurses have found.

viii) Air travel of any distance, also affects biological rhythms and may change the cycle, as does travel in space!

The length of the period

This can vary from 2 to 10 days or more, an average being 5 days. Over 90% of the blood loss occurs in the first 3 days however.

Heavy periods (menorrhagia)

The amount of blood lost varies very much between individuals and is possibly partly an inherited factor. It can be less than $20cm^3$, (about an egg-cup full) or as much as $500cm^3$ or more. The average amount is about 30–$40cm^3$. For any one woman the amount of blood lost does not vary much from one cycle to another, once these are established [88], so any change one way or the other, should be medically investigated.

Heavy periods are defined as a blood loss of $80cm^3$ or more each period. As women have no standards for comparison in assessing their loss, there is a wide variation in their perception of this amount. Heavy losses can be caused by:

i) a medical condition such as fibroids or polyps

ii) the use of an intra-uterine device

iii) a changing balance of hormones, as happens at adolescence or menopause.

However, in 50% of women no specific cause is obvious, and the losses cannot be related to specific hormone levels, ovulation, or the weight or cavity size of the womb [85]. It has been suggested a heavy flow is related to the amount of prostaglandin (see page 147) in the lining of the womb, the greater the amount, the heavier the flow.

Heavy blood losses are very inconvenient and may cause anaemia, so relief can be sought by:

i) diagnosis and treatment of any medical condition causing the loss

ii) the use of some types of contraceptive pill, or other drugs, which reduce menstrual flow substantially

iii) treatment with specific antiprostaglandin drugs, which have been shown to reduce excessive flow, [89] including that caused by intra-uterine devices.

Painful periods (dysmenorrhoea)

A National Opinion Poll survey [82] produced figures ('grossed up' to the nearest 0.1 million) showing that of 11.6 million females between the ages of 15–44 in the U.K:

i) 4.6 million never suffer from period pains

ii) 6.8 million (roughly 2 out of every 3) do

iii) 2.8 million of these are incapacitated to such an extent they cannot cope with a normal daily routine, and half a million women and girls are out of action for more than 2 days.

Painful periods are therefore a widespread problem.

Symptoms

Cramp-like pains due to contractions of the womb, exactly similar to those of labour, but up to 4 times stronger in some cases, headaches, faintness or dizziness, sickness and diarrhoea, backache, leg pains and overall clumsiness. The symptoms can vary from period to period, and may be worse in times of stress.

Causes

They may be caused or intensified by:

i) a medical condition such as fibroids, endometriosis or pelvic inflammatory disease. In such cases they will disappear when the specific condition is treated.

ii) the presence of an intra-uterine device

iii) neither of the above, in which case the condition is said to be 'primary', and was previously unexplained. New research, however, has shown there may be up to 8 times the quantity of prostaglandins in the menstrual blood of sufferers than non-sufferers.

In school

Menstrual pains can be crippling and should always be taken seriously. A rest room, hot water bottles, sympathy and advice on seeking medical help should be available, as well as an escort home if necessary. It is most distressing for girls to suffer in this way, and it is beholden on all of us to do whatever we can to alleviate the situation and ensure proper help is obtained.

Prostawhatsits?!

Prostaglandins are a family of chemicals made in many parts of the body, but particularly the womb. They were first discovered in semen, produced by the prostate gland, hence the name. They are made in minute amounts, and rapidly broken down, but are extremely powerful, and have many different functions. One action is to cause strong contractions of the 'smooth' muscle found in gut, blood vessels and the womb and they are important in promoting labour and childbirth. This may explain some of the symptoms of painful periods which were all produced as side effects when prostaglandins were used intravenously to promote labour in late pregnancies.

Help

Drugs are now available which inhibit the way the body makes prostaglandins. One such antiprostaglandin drug is the well known aspirin, others delight in the names fluf-enamic acid, flurbiprofen etc. These have been used successfully to treat women with painful periods, and with heavy blood loss [86]. The particular advantage being they only need to be taken during menstruation and when the symptoms are worst.

Combatting troublesome periods

i) General good health and sense, learning to relax to combat tension, the use of pain killers when necessary.

ii)   If these measures do not work satisfactorily seek help from a doctor.

Pre-menstrual tension: PMT
This can be experienced at regular times in any part of the menstrual cycle, but is most common in the second half, after ovulation, in the days just before a period, hence the name.

In addition to the effects listed on page 143 the symptoms may include a combination of a 'wound up' feeling, restlessness and lack of concentration, irritability, tiredness and apathy, depression, anxiety, forgetfulness, headaches, backaches, joint aches, bloatedness, water retention, breast tenderness, increased pressure in the eyeball, dizziness, weight gain, emotional outbursts and violence or moodiness. Women who suffer from PMT are therefore justified in feeling disadvantaged! Katharina Dalton has been the pioneer worker investigating this syndrome, and has suggested a lack of progesterone in the second part of the cycle may be one of the causes. Treatment is therefore possible [90] and numbers of women have gained relief in this way. For many women, relieving symptoms and being aware of the need to be extra careful during this time, may be sufficient to enable them to cope with the situation.

Special considerations in school
Half the female pupils may have some PMT symptoms at some time, 'mood swings' can occur even before menarche. Allowances can be made for these if necessary and a discreet record kept of lowered academic performance or disruptive behaviour if this seems cyclical.

Women teachers of course, are not immune to PMT, and may need sympathy or need to consider perhaps whether they tend to give more severe punishments or lower marks at certain times in their own monthly cycles.

Examinations can be spaced out for longer than a week, or have papers in two parts, at intervals, to lessen menstrual effect on performance. There may be more than the average number menstruating during exams of course, due to the stress effect [83]. Staff knowledge of the general level of the problem and interference with work for any particular individual, will be relevant here.

Climacteric and Menopause
Towards the end of the years of menstruation the hormone balance changes again, as the ovaries cease to produce their hormones. The feedback 'switch off' for the follicle stimulating hormone is therefore not present, and there can be larger amounts circulating. The average age for menopause (the last period) is 50, but the span is about 45 to 55. The changes, the climacteric, can take from a few years to nearly 7 to complete. Cycles without ovulation increase, and periods stop, either gradually, becoming lighter, and more spaced out, or both, or, less often, they end abruptly, sometimes in response to stress.

Symptoms which can be associated with menopause
i)   Hot flushes occur, which may be accompanied by sweating, and vary in incidence from very few a week to over 50 a day or night.
ii)   A lack of oestrogen may cause dryness and discomfort in the vagina which may be relieved by an oestrogen cream. Other effects may be loss of elasticity in the skin, narrowing of arteries, bones becoming more brittle and

stiffening or swelling of joints.

iii)   General symptoms may occur, similar to those of pre-menstrual tension: tiredness, irritability and depression being most common. Again understanding and tolerance are required, and if the symptoms are severe, hormone replacement treatment can be most successful. Psychologically a woman at this stage may need extra reassurance as she may be concerned about perceived loss of sexual attractiveness. Understanding is needed that sexual desire and magnetism does not stop at menopause. Many women at this stage find increased pleasure in sex, very much appreciate the lack of periods, and look forward to the future with confidence. Survey the number of successful women in their 50s and 60s who are attractive, active and interesting people.

Social effects of the menstrual cycle
Preparation for menstruation
The shock of menstruating with no pre-knowledge of this event is quite tremendous, and can affect feelings about each period, for a long time after. It is essential girls are told about the process in good time (see page 76) and they all know:

i)   who to go to in school, to get sanitary towels, this should be someone familiar to them, of a sympathetic and reliable nature,
ii)   that a period will start gradually, so they will not be 'caught out' in the middle of a class,
iii)   school management of the disposal of towels, tampons, etc.
iv)   arrangements for being excused from games or swimming if absolutely necessary. This will hopefully be a dignified process and neither mean sitting out in front of the whole class, nor 'telling a male teacher when you're on'.

Staff should be tactful if a normally prompt girl is late for a class, and not demand a public explanation. It does take time to adjust to the mechanics of sanitary protection, and school toilets are not always available in every block or floor.

Parental responsibilities
School arrangements for helping girls cope with their periods can be explained to parents and that it is most beneficial if they will comment on the event of menarche, and congratulate their daughter in a positive way on reaching womanhood. Her first period can then be a welcomed event, and not one to be ashamed or embarrassed about. The wider implications of sexual maturity should also be discussed with her at that time.

Some girls may not welcome menarche as it distinguishes them too much from former companions. Adjustments will therefore be more difficult and they may need some help in accepting the situation.

Cultural factors and menstruation
In nearly all cultures women have historically been made to feel impure and even dangerous, when menstruating. In some faiths such as Hindu, Muslim, Greek Orthodox the Jewish Orthodox, some women and girls may still be considered 'unclean' when they have their periods. They may be required to

observe certain practices e.g.

i)   They may have to go away from the rest of the family in a separate room.
ii) They may be barred from the prayer room, Mosque or Temple.
iii) They may not be allowed to perform any religious ceremony or ritual.
iv) They may not prepare food or touch anything from the kitchen.
v)   Married women may not be allowed intercourse during this time and may not sleep in the same bed as their husband nor 'make themselves attractive'.
vi) They may be required to perform ritualised bathing ceremonies at the end of the period.

The coil as a contraceptive method is sometimes resisted by women of these faiths, as it may prolong periods, and hence all the taboos which go with them [38].

Ironically, although menstruation may often not be discussed openly everyone in the family knows exactly who is having a period, and for how long.

Some e.g. West Indians and others, may believe:

i)   the woman's 'egg' is produced at menstruation, so avoiding intercourse at this time will prevent a pregnancy,
ii) a period gets rid of 'bad' blood so a heavy one is good (a contraceptive coil is often preferred [38]) otherwise the blood may go to the brain, causing headaches, or be damming up somewhere, with possible dire results.

Future prospects
The effect of the contraceptive pill on menstruation is significant. For women on some types of pill, blood loss is reduced. Research continues on the effects of taking particular kinds of 'the pill' continuously, so removing the need to menstruate for some part of the 30 years. As some pills mimic pregnancy, no periods or ovulation occurring, this would be returning to a primitive life style, only without the large family! The hormonal state of pregnancy may protect from problems associated with the breasts, ovaries and womb, as the incidence of these is higher in women who do not have children.

Menstrual hygiene
Scrupulous cleanliness during this time is advisable. Blood soaked tampons and towels, at body heat, are an ideal culture medium for bacteria! The vulva should be washed regularly and showers and baths taken even more frequently than usual. Sanitary towels and tampons should be changed regularly, several times a day. A wide range of sanitary towels and tampons is now available, so every girl should be able to find some, in combination, that suit her requirements at different stages of her period. How much more convenient they are than the folded linen napkins used by women in the early part of this century which had to be washed after use. We have a lot to be thankful for indeed.

Tampons
Some girls are able to use tampons from menarche and there are slim-line ones designed for young girls. They must be used according to instructions and the

girl must be reliable enough to change them regularly, and remember to remove the last one. Hands should be washed before and after insertion.

The benefit of using tampons apart from the convenience, lessening of odour and being able to go swimming, is familiarisation with the vulva and vagina, and being given 'permission' to touch this area.

The toxic shock syndrome: TSS

There have only been a handful of cases of this disease in the UK and no deaths have occurred. The problem was identified in North America in 1980, when several hundred young women, 90% menstruating, and using certain tampons, suddenly developed extreme symptoms of a high fever, vomiting, diarrhoea. etc. The cause seemed to be infection with one strain of a very common bacterium, *Staphylococcus aureus* (often found in boils), which can develop in menstrual blood. The toxic shock may be caused by the poison (toxin) produced by it. Research and discussion on contributing factors continues [91] but may include:

i) leaving a tampon or any other object, such as a barrier method of contraception, in the vagina for a long time (in the first UK case the tampon was in for 3 days);

ii) the use of very highly absorbent tampons, as because of their efficiency they may tend to be left in longer, or may slightly damage the vaginal wall by drying it;

iii) the use of some kinds of tampon applicators which might scratch the vagina.

None of these factors have been conclusively proved, but it does seem good sense to keep to the following guidelines for tampon use.

i) Use the correct absorbency of tampons for the heaviness of the flow, and change them about 3 times a day, but not so frequently the vagina becomes dry.

ii) Do not use super-absorbent tampons unless the flow warrants this.

iii) Vary the use of tampons and towels during a period, using a towel at night when the flow is lighter for example.

iv) Do not use tampons at other times in the cycle.

v) In the highly improbable event of any toxic shock symptoms occurring, remove the tampon and seek medical help immediately.

The risks of getting the disease are very small indeed.

Teaching about menstruation

A positive approach should be taken, with the naturalness of the event emphasised. Boys and girls should be taught together for the most part, unless there are particular reasons why this should not be so (see page 39).

The events of the menstrual cycle are complicated and involve new concepts:

i) of the ebb and flow of hormones in females;

ii) of the unique tissue, the endometrium, which can break down and 'bleed' and then renew itself to nourish the next potential fertilised ovum;

iii) that the most important event is the ripening and release of one of the

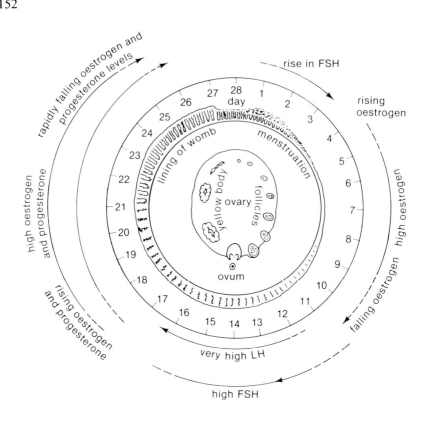

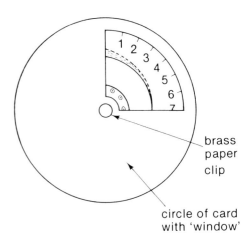

Figure 29   A visual
aid to understanding
the menstrual cycle.

thousands of ova (up to 500 000) present in the ovaries since before birth [61]. Only about 400 ova will be developed in this way, the others disintegrate.

The basic facts of ovulation and menstruation can first be illustrated with models and diagrams of the whole womb, Fallopian tubes and ovaries (page 130). Emphasise the 'lining' is only a very thin layer, from 3mm to about 6mm when at its thickest.

The next stage could be to abstract the events on to a circular or long diagram, see FIGS 29 and 31. The central circular disc in FIG 29, could be copied, mounted on card (yellow bodies coloured in!) and a larger circle of card with a quarter section 'window', mounted on top, so the cycle can be visualised in sequence.

Hormonal control

The hormonal changes in the menstrual cycle are complicated and full details are only needed for some examinations (see the figure on page 154). However, all children should know of oestrogen and progesterone, so they are more able to understand the working of hormonal contraception.

Male hormones

These are produced fairly continuously (FIG 32) rather a different pattern from the female variations (FIG 31). There is a slow feedback system between LHRH and testosterone. The male hormone hypothalamic/pituitary system is much less sensitive to being switched off than the female's, which is one reason why hormonal contraceptive research has not yet found an effective male hormonal contraceptive. So that's their excuse!

Male and female hormones are fascinatingly similar chemically, (see FIG 30) some synthetic progesterone hormones are actually derived from the male hormone.

Varied teaching activities

1. Groups could send off to one of the firms (addresses on page 158) for details of educational services, and examples of their leaflets, charts, etc. When all materials have come, each group reads their own pack and assesses content and presentation, for
 i)   understanding, how many long words are used?
 ii) diagrams and pictures, are these clear, accurate, attractive?
 iii) interest, etc.

Some of the diagrams in the leaflets are not very good, though all texts are sensible and reassuring.

A chart is filled in, showing what is provided by the various firms. Each group then reports to the rest of the class, and the material can be displayed.

At the end of all the activities the facts learnt could be summarised, and a quiz given:

i)   What are periods?
ii) When do they start?
iii) About how often do they happen?

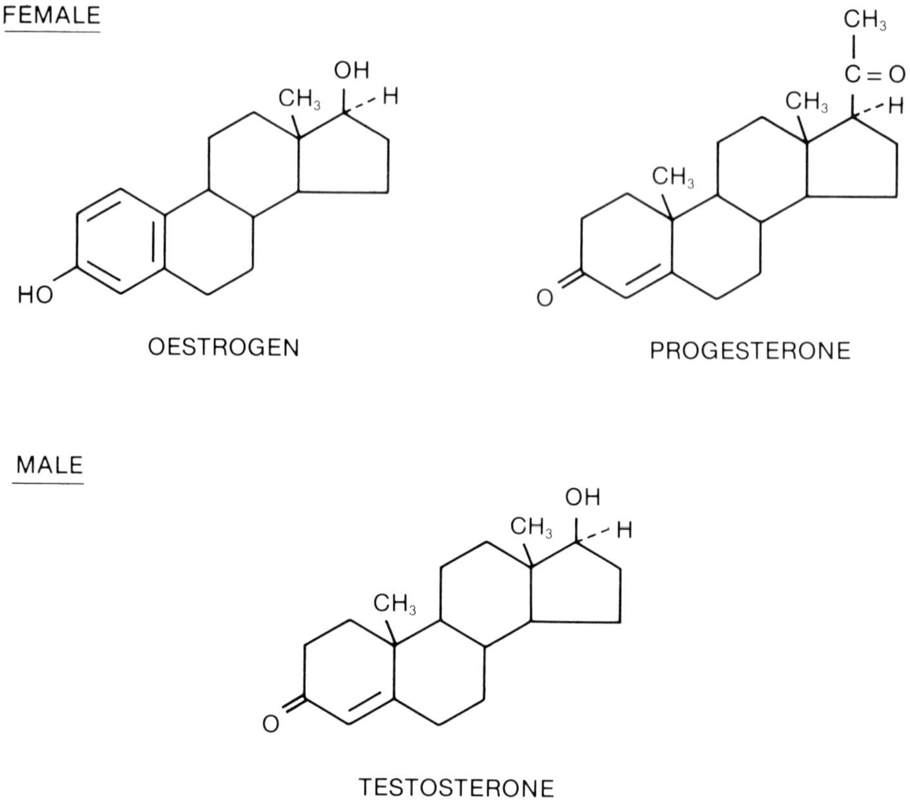

FEMALE

OESTROGEN

PROGESTERONE

MALE

TESTOSTERONE

Figure 30   Male and female hormones. They are chemically very similar.

iv)   Are they exactly the same for every girl?
v)   Do periods ever vary?
vi)   What things are available for use during a period?
vii)   Can anyone tell when a girl is having a period?
viii)   Can she bath and wash her hair at this time?
ix)   Can she exercise and do PE as usual?
x)   Can she go swimming?
xi)   Are periods uncomfortable?
xii)   When do they stop?

All boys and girls should be able to answer these questions.

2.   A particular leaflet can be obtained in quantity, so each pupil can have
one. They are then allowed x minutes to read it carefully. Two teams are
then chosen and have to answer questions based on the leaflet, set by the rest
of the class.
Points obviously not well understood, can be re-emphasised afterwards.

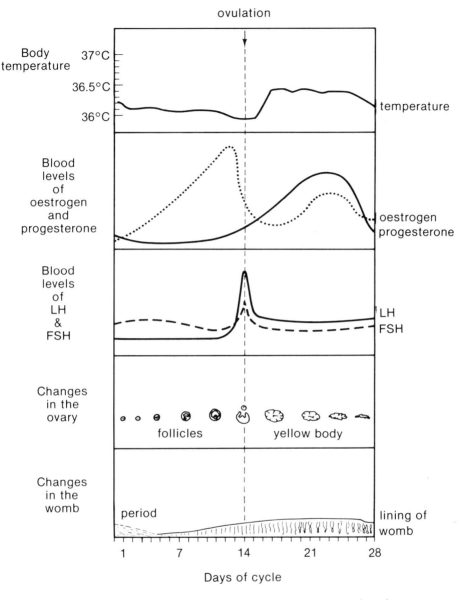

Figure 31 Summary of changes during the menstrual cycle.

3. Mood collages can be made, for both boys and girls, showing the variation normal in all adolescents, moody blues, lively yellows, peaceful pink, grumpy green? Some girls may find particular moods associated with certain times in their menstrual cycle, but not all will notice this feature.

4. Collect pictures of females of all ages, races and social class, and mount them in 5 big posters.

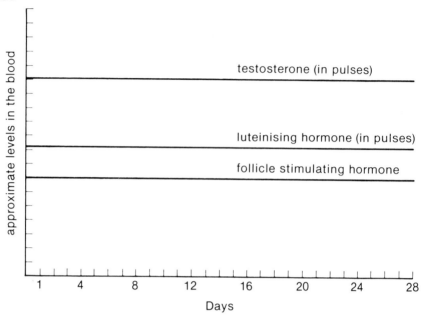

Figure 32   Male hormone levels after puberty, after K. Dalton.

i)   Age 0–9: These girls have not yet begun their periods.
ii)   Age 10–17: *some* of these girls have begun their periods,
iii) Age 18–45: all these women have periods (but see page 145).
iv)   Pregnant women: these women are not having periods at the moment. (They will again, 2 to 4 months after the birth, or longer if breast feeding.)
v)   Age 50 and over: these women have stopped having periods. (Choose happy, active types!)

This activity emphasises the universality of menstruation across all cultures, colours and classes, and has a 'join the group' approach which may be reassuring.

5.   Discuss the best way to record periods, and how important it is to do so. Ordinary calendars and diaries can be confusing to use unless children realise not all months have the same number of days! This means even if periods come at exact 4 week intervals (28 days) they will not arrive on the same date in the next month, though it may be on the same day of the week. Use old, unused calendars and diaries, or ones bought cheaply in July, to practise on. It is easiest to see the pattern of a cycle, if it is recorded on the type of chart shown in FIG 33. These are available from some firms (Libresse and Lilia White). Demonstrate what a 21, 28 and 35 day cycle looks like (FIG 33). Days of the period can be circled or crossed. N.B. The cycle is counted from the first day of bleeding, which will not usually be the first day of the month. Individuals can find out which type of calendar suits them best. The

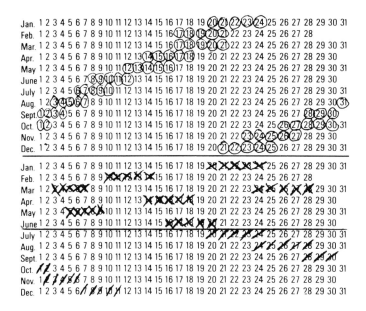

Figure 33   Recording a period: a calendar showing 21, 28 and 35 day cycles.

girls could mount and decorate a menstrual chart, boys could do one for relatives if they wished.

Set everyone a homework, to record a 7 day period every 30 days, or a 3 day one every 22 days, etc. on a menstrual chart, to see what the pattern looks like.

6.   Small groups prepare illustrated leaflets called for example:

i)   Myths and old-wives tales about periods. Collect these by interviewing older people (and see page 145).

ii)   How to help yourself or others during a period: exercise, sleep, hygiene, recording a period, etc.

iv)   What boys need to know about periods: the basic facts plus some possible difficulties, so they can understand females better.

7.   Older girls might be interested in the STOPP leaflet, *Steps Towards Painfree Periods*. See below. N.B. If you expect something to hurt, it probably will! 'Menstrual cramps' are often asked about quite early, as knowledge is passed on by older sisters and others. Periods are not likely to be painful for the first few years, perhaps because many cycles at this stage are anovulatory. However as some girls start periods aged 9 or 10, a few may be experiencing discomfort, by 12. It can be pointed out tactfully at some stage that exaggerating symptoms and feelings before and during menstruation, will not help anybody, and credibility and sympathy may well be lost for those that do.

8. Older children should be aware of the nature of pre-menstrual tension. The 'Mood Chart' from Kotex (page 159) has a summary of symptoms, which could be used for discussion of the help available for those with severe symptoms.

9. Individuals could write a letter to a 10 year old friend (either sex) explaining 'all about periods', These could be used later with classes of younger children as an introduction to the subject.

10. Those with a scientific bent might check the relative capacities of tampons of any one make. How much more does a 'super' or a 'super plus' absorb, than a 'regular'? Devise an experiment: equal volumes of water in measuring cylinders, lower in the tampons (for x minutes?), the final readings should prove illuminating. There is more to tampon design than just absorbency of course, and different makes suit different people's needs.

Resources for menstruation

Books, booklets and leaflets can be obtained from the firms mentioned below.

1. For teachers
   i) *Female Cycles* Paula Wedeger, 1978 Women's Press A survey of the wider implications of menstruation.
   ii) *Once a Month*, Katharina Dalton 1978 Fontana
   Fascinatingly anecdotal and informative.
   iii) *Telling them the facts*, Robinsons
   iv) *From fiction to fact*, Tampax
   Both these booklets provide guidelines for teachers.
   v) *Growing Up Young*, Kimberley-Clarke
   Specifically written to help parents and teachers of less able girls. It includes advice on the approach, vocabulary and methods of coping with periods, for slow learning girls.
   vi) On the Menopause:
   The Change of Life, HEC. leaflet
   The Menopause, HEC. leaflet
   The Menopause, Robinsons
   A Third of your Lifetime, 1978 Schering
2. For Children
   The book by Ruth Thomson *Have you started yet?* 1980 Piccolo, has a friendly, realistic, helpful approach.
   Some booklets and leaflets:
   i) *Growing up today* Libresse, Comic strip format of 'old wives tales' lead in to quiz and questions and answers.
   ii) *What's all this about growing up?* Lilia White
   iii) *Very Personally Yours* Kotex
   iv) *Your first period, Periods Without Problems, PMT* Robinsons
   v) *Steps towards pain free periods*, STOPP
   vi) *Tell me about periods*, Tampax
   vii) *Accent on You*, Tampax
3. Audio-visual aids
   On free loan from Random Film Library, made for Lilia White;
   i) *Girls of today* 10 mins. 16mm sound & colour For girls of 12 and 13, starting their periods.
   ii) *And Now you're a Woman*, For older girls, includes details of how to use tampons.

iii)   *Very Personally Yours*, 32 frames on menstruation and personal hygiene. Film strip, chart and teaching notes, made for Kotex Educational Productions Ltd.

iv)   *Growing up for Girls*, Robinsons. 38 colour slides with commentary on cassette.

v)   *It happens to us all* Kit for 9–13yr olds. Excellent coverage of physical and emotional changes in both boys and girls. Teacher's notes included. From Johnson & Johnson.

4.   Educational Services

The following firms and organisations provide educational services which may include: speakers; leaflets, booklets, fact sheets, wall charts; films on menstruation for younger and older girls; films strips; mother and daughter packs.

Most services are free, but there may be a small charge for large numbers of leaflets, or for visual aid material.

i)   Kotex Advisory Service (Kimberley Clark Corp.) Larkfield, Maidstone, Kent ME20 7PS

ii)   Libresse Advisory Service, P.O. Box 34, East Grinstead, West Sussex RH19 1UW

iii)   Lilia-White Ltd., Alum Rock Road, Birmingham B8 3DZ

iv)   Robinsons Hygiene Education Service, Wheat Bridge, Chesterfield, Derbyshire S40 2AD

v)   Schering Chemicals Ltd., Burgess Hill, West Sussex RH15 9NE

vi)   STOPP, 25, North Row, London WIR 2BY

vii)   Tampax Education Dept., Dunsbury Way, Havant, Hampshire PO9 5DG

viii)   Johnson and Johnson Schools Information Service, Slough, Buckinghamshire.

Resources on pubertal changes

1.   Film. *Then One Year.* (See page 109).
2.   Television. ITV *Living and Growing* series (see page 109).
3.   HEC Booklet *How we grow up. (*See page 110).
4.   Film strips or slides. *Adolescence Part 1. Puberty.* Camera Talks. 25 frames, tape, script. Useful charts, graphs and diagrams, of changes at puberty, emphasising the range of ages at which these occur. The script covers some emotional factors but teachers may find it more satisfactory to use their own commentary throughout.
5.   Slide set. *Understanding Sex.* Institute of Sex Education & Research. 48 frames, tape and script. This includes photographs of naked children and adults, with one family group where the 'father' is not an ad-man's dream of masculinity, but a nice 'average' chap. Teachers may again find it appropriate to select frames, and use their own commentary. It could be used in conjunction with 4. above, giving a blend of diagrams and realism.
6.   Chart. Research in Reproduction. Vol. 8. No. 6. Nov. 1976. IPPF *Puberty.* This summarises pubertal changes, with a scientific presentation of relevant statistics,

Books for teachers

1.   Tanner J. M. *Foetus into Man.* 1978 Open Books. Physical growth from conception to maturity. An invaluable source lucidly written, by a world expert on this subject.
2.   Tanner J. M., Rattray Taylor R. *Growth.* 1966 Time Life. This supplements the above book with many excellent photographs.
3.   Nuffield Secondary Science 3. *Biology of Man.* 1971 Longmans. Section 2. The Human Life Cycle, reproduction, growth and development, with many suggestions for work with pupils.
4.   Chandler E. M. 1980. *Educating Adolescent Girls.* George Allen & Unwin. Helpful analysis of emotional and physical factors affecting young girls.

Resources on hygiene

1. SCHEP. *Think Well*. Unit 7. *Get Clean* (page 106).
2. Schools Council. Home and family project (page 108).
3. Holt A., and Randell J. *Come Clean*. 1975 Cambridge University Press: Lively cartoon treatment of all aspects of personal hygiene which sets absolute standards.
4. Allen E. *Wash and brush up*. 1976 A & C Black. Well illustrated historical survey of personal hygiene.
5. *Leaflets.*
    i) HEC *Keep it clean*. A direct approach.
    ii) *Why a bidet?* The Council of British Ceramic Sanitaryware Manufacturers. Bidets are presented as 'sit on washbasins', and facilitate discussion of the need to wash one's under-carriage regularly.
6. *Some of your bits ain't nice*. An animated cartoon on personal hygiene for older teenagers, 15 +, available on 16mm film or video, on free loan from Concord Film Library.

Books for children

Health and Growth series. (See page 74.) Book 4. Section 2. How do you grow? A good approach to similarities and differences in growth rates, illustrated with photographs. Book 5. *How do you grow up?* The physiology and hormonal control of growth, emotional development and moods. Like all the books in this series, self help review tests are given at the end of each section.

Resources for female anatomy

Clear drawings of female anatomy are provided in:

1. *The facts of love* (see page 34) Excellent drawings sensitively presented, and always related to the rest of the body.
2. The minichart *A look at your body*, Brook Advisory Centre.
3. *Understanding* (see page 110) and flip chart *Understanding Family Planning* (see page 110) both of which are extremely good for relating female organs to their position in the pelvis.
5. Derek Llewellyn Jones. *Everywoman*. 1971 Faber & Faber. Background information on medical conditions which children might ask questions about during discussion.
6. *Male and Female* A set of 15 teaching cards 1983. FPA Education Unit. Very clear drawings and diagrams, well related to the whole body.

Male anatomy

Good drawings of male sexual anatomy can be found in the book *The facts of love* the Minichart *A look at your body,* BAC and in the series of cards *Male and female* on male and female anatomy, available from the Family Planning Association, Education Unit and in level three of *Fit for life.*

A model of a male or female torso with interchangeable sexual parts is now available. This is excellent, though expensive, and is available from Adam Rouilly, Sittingbourne, Hertfordshire, reference MT58(4S).

Chapter 7

RELATIONSHIPS

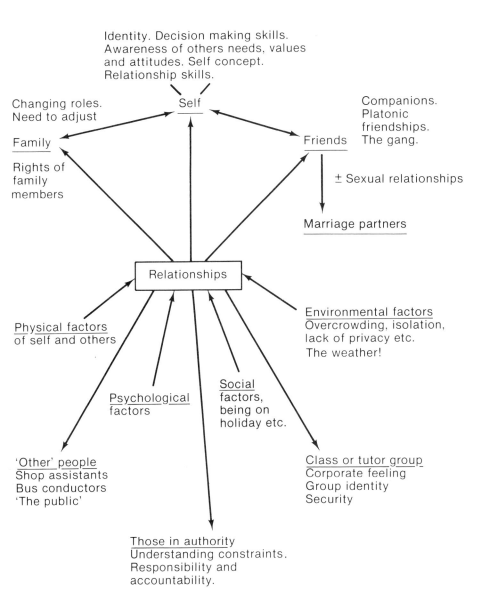

Identity. Decision making skills. Awareness of others needs, values and attitudes. Self concept. Relationship skills.

Self

Changing roles. Need to adjust

Family

Rights of family members

Companions. Platonic friendships. The gang.

Friends

± Sexual relationships

Marriage partners

Relationships

Physical factors of self and others

Environmental factors
Overcrowding, isolation, lack of privacy etc.
The weather!

Psychological factors

Social factors, being on holiday etc.

'Other' people
Shop assistants
Bus conductors
'The public'

Class or tutor group
Corporate feeling
Group identity
Security

Those in authority
Understanding constraints.
Responsibility and accountability.

Total dependence on family and other caring systems. ⟶ Independence ⟶ Interdependence. Cooperation, sharing.

Personal relationships

In a rapidly changing world, the art of being adaptable becomes increasingly important. Children will vary very much in their potential for developing relationship skills, but education should help each to blossom as much as possible. The very broad aims and objectives might be, to develop awareness and understanding of:

i)   what is meant by a relationship (without becoming too self-conscious about the process);

ii) the physical factors affecting relationships, such as
     personal looks, body image, clothes, age and sex
     being ill, tired, worried, under stress
     taking alcohol or other drugs;

iii) the need to develop relationship skills both verbal and non-verbal;

iv) the needs of other people, and yourself, in relationships, and the morality considerations in satisfying these;

v)   the different attitudes and values held by various people, and that growing up means you will have to decide what yours are, and may be asked to justify them;

vi) the fact that not everyone will react in the same way to any one situation, nor one person react in the same way every time;

vii) that relationships both short and long term can be successful! Good relationship images are important for credibility. Media coverage of unsuccessful ones is intensive, and can produce feelings of insecurity. Satisfying relationships may be less newsworthy, and perhaps grow best without constant scrutiny and analysis.

Relationship skills

These can start at the very basic level of social skills, 'what would you say?' in certain situations, as well as 'what would you do?'

Role play busy adults approached in various different ways for a simple request. 'I want ...' 'I've got to ...' 'I need ...' or 'Excuse me, but could I ...?' 'I can see you're very busy, but ...' Which is most effective in getting the desired response? List some 'magic phrases' that smooth the path.

Parents also need consideration. If you ask them about important things when they're preoccupied or just going out, they may well 'not listen'. Ask when you could talk about it perhaps. Does tone of voice count?

Other activities

Listening, responding (facially as well as verbally) agreeing, not agreeing, but diplomatically, (not shouting) praising, encouraging, sympathising at various levels, including about bereavements. Many people find it difficult to know what to say if something has gone wrong for someone, work out useful starting phrases again.

When writing, the 'tone' of communication in letters can vary, and have very different effects on the recipient. Try out some alternatives.

Children could write down anonymously, relationship situations they have found difficult to cope with. These could be used as a basis for selecting the most appropriate situation discussion material from the resources listed on page 174. Self-selection of the material by the children is another way of ensuring its relevance.

Evaluation
Short term
This can be done by the children themselves. Does this class/group, get on well together? If not, what can we do about it? Do we get on well with our teachers, dinner helpers, caretakers, secretaries etc. How can we help each other? This can also be assessed by teacher observation and recording of individual relationship skills, and the development of these over a given time.
Long term
Relationship skills can be assessed on termly or yearly reports. These could be in broad categories, and would indicate which children needed special help.

The clear identification of the need for such skills in this way, would help to confer on them some value and status.

Adolescent relationships
Adolescence is a time of sexual experimentation, and trying out different kinds of relationships. Tentative forays will be made, but rejection may be taken very seriously and can paralyse social development and lower self esteem for a while.

Public demonstrations of relationships may be exaggerated at this stage, partners being treated like an accessory to go with the latest outfit. There is much talk of 'who do you fancy?', and threats of actually *telling* them! Learning about relationships requires feedback, both verbal and non-verbal. How do people react to you, look at you, behave towards you? There is a need to find out ... 'Am I normal? Am I likeable?' and, after puberty, 'Am I sexually attractive?' (See FIG 34.)
Relationship with self
Self-image, identity and feelings of worth (or unworthiness), will colour every other relationship. It is advisable to try and become a person you feel you can live with for the rest of your life! Feeling good about yourself matters!

Appearance
As we are animals dominated by the sense of vision, and appearance is the most easily identifiable characteristic, it is not surprising this tends to be the focus for teenage rating systems. Look, feel, good. But who decides if you do look good? Briefly revise work done in earlier classes on advertising (page 79) and gender role (page 84) and develop a similar survey on the more sophisticated concept of body images. At the moment it seems 'men' are supposed to be muscular, tall, craggy-jawed, broad-shouldered, slim-hipped, keen-eyed, virile (leaders, innovators and decision makers) whilst 'women' must be slim, young, with flawless skin, long legged and with a certain size and shape of breasts, (also acquiescent, home-loving, pleased by small gifts and cleanliness).

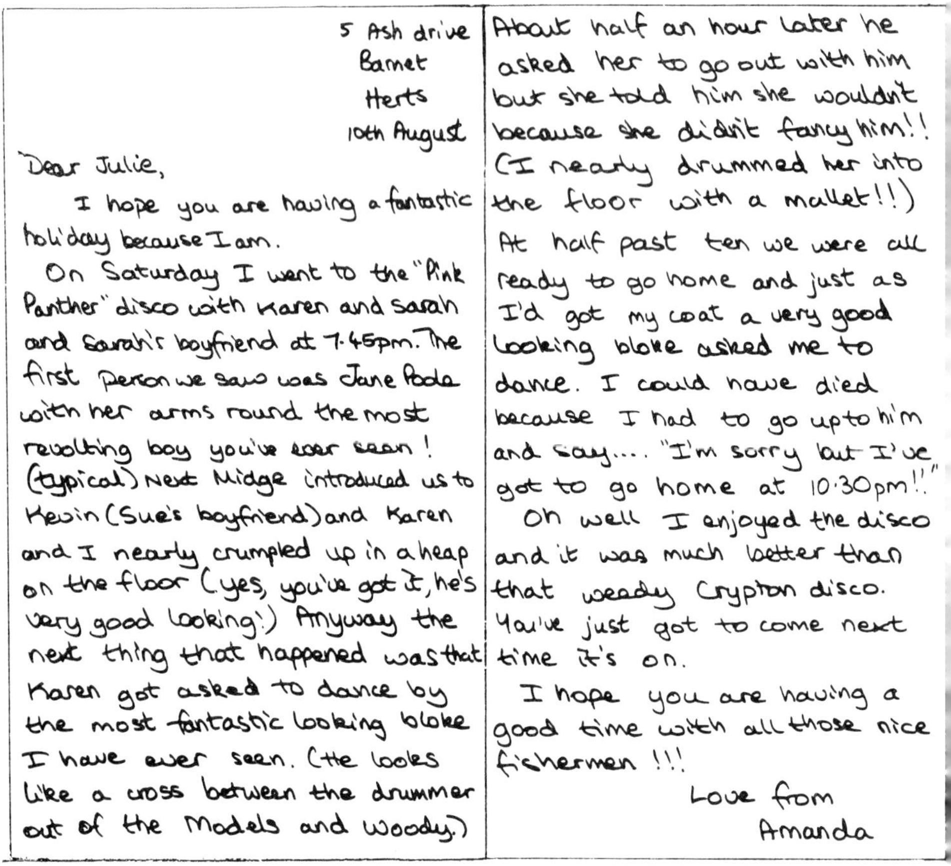

5 Ash drive
Barnet
Herts
10th August

Dear Julie,

    I hope you are having a fantastic holiday because I am.

On Saturday I went to the "Pink Panther" disco with Karen and Sarah and Sarah's boyfriend at 7.45pm. The first person we saw was Jane Poole with her arms round the most revolting boy you've ever seen! (typical) Next Midge introduced us to Kevin (Sue's boyfriend) and Karen and I nearly crumpled up in a heap on the floor (yes, you've got it, he's very good looking!) Anyway the next thing that happened was that Karen got asked to dance by the most fantastic looking bloke I have ever seen. (He looks like a cross between the drummer out of the Models and Woody.)

About half an hour later he asked her to go out with him but she told him she wouldn't because she didn't fancy him!! (I nearly drummed her into the floor with a mallet!!) At half past ten we were all ready to go home and just as I'd got my coat a very good looking bloke asked me to dance. I could have died because I had to go up to him and say.... "I'm sorry but I've got to go home at 10.30pm!!"

Oh well I enjoyed the disco and it was much better than that weedy Crypton disco. You've just got to come next time it's on.

I hope you are having a good time with all those nice fishermen !!!

        Love from
          Amanda

Figure 34   Letter from one fourteen-year-old to another.

How do we know this? From teenage dolls of extraordinary proportions, and because the media carefully select their real models from the tiny minority of the population who have these characteristics. The super-normal sign-stimuli of their 'perfect' parts are guaranteed to rivet our attention. Some models even specialise in portraying one body part only. They devote much time to preserving and enhancing these natural assets. Of course, it's their livelihood. No harm in that? Only if we ordinary mortals are daft enough to believe this is real life (make up and hair adjusted between takes?) and is one we should all aspire to. Only if it makes us discontented and feel ashamed or inadequate when presenting ourselves. How many of us *are* intimidated by 'beautiful people', even by those so perfectly groomed creatures at cosmetic counters? How many of us spend much time emulating them?

Personal beauty is highly valued in all cultures, but so are other characteristics less easily or speedily identified. Collect information on fashions in body images, and historical and cultural differences. What shapes were selected by artists etc. for permanent record on pots, paintings or photographs? Who selects the 'perfect' image of the time?

One particular danger is that various pressures may lead to adolescents developing a false perception of their own body image, leading to *anorexia nervosa*, which 1 in 200 teenage girls (mostly from social classes I and II) were found to be suffering from in one study of nine schools in England.

Faces

The face is usually the most important communicating part. Liaise with a drama group for a session about make up. Collect pictures from magazines showing a make-up sequence which starts with the model with all features obliterated. What is the effect of having no eyebrows, lashes, or lips? Expressions are difficult to read. Why?

Eyebrows

These are used in greeting (quick flash up and down), quizzically, ferociously, in surprise etc. All these expressions are enhanced by emphasised eyebrows. Collect pictures of famous eyebrows ... Cleopatra, Greta Garbo, Angela Rippon, Denis Healey, Boy George...

Eyes

Probably *the* most expressive part of the face. We search for meaning in the eyes (and mouth). 'Look at me when I'm talking to you!' Eye make-up, our white eyeball (other primates do not have this) and the use of hands, fans, etc. all emphasise eye movements, which give vital clues in conversations. No wonder we feel uneasy if someone's eyes are hidden by dark or mirrored sunglasses, goggles or masks.

Staring

Eye gaze length is partly culturally determined. Young children stare, disconcertingly, until taught not to do so. Some races hold eye contact longer than others. West Indians may do this fractionally longer than some Europeans, which can be misinterpreted as being rude or defiant. In other races, women particularly, are taught to lower their eyes 'modestly', but this does not mean they have no feelings or spirit.

Pupil size

It seems we respond instinctively to the size of the pupil in the eye. If someone is very interested in a conversation, their pupils dilate. In one study, students given a choice of otherwise identical pictures of faces, selected those with the largest pupils as being the 'nicest'. We are also attracted to large eyes (a feature of baby faces).

Spectacles

In the past these have collected derogatory remarks such as bookish, fussy, old four-eyes, men never make passes ... at girls wearing glasses. Even

Superman puts them on when disguising his attractions. In one survey [58] 1 in 5 children were supposed to be wearing glasses. Few were. We do need to educate for acceptance of spectacles. Many children will need them for the first time at puberty, (page 121). Explain we shall probably *all* need to wear them before the end of our lives. Some people just get more practice than others!

Modern frames can be most attractive, and are far preferable to screwed up, peering faces, or offending your friends by not recognising them across the street! Other people do not notice glasses nearly as much as the wearer feels they do. Many cannot remember if someone usually wears them or not. They become totally part of a person's face, and are accepted as such.

Collect and mount pictures of glamorous and famous people wearing glasses, and encourage and praise children who need to wear them, to do so.

Mouths

The other most communicative part of the face? Test this statement. Volunteers cover the top part of their faces, and try to convey non-verbal messages to the class (anger, fear, pleasure, dismay, questioning, considering). Then lower the cover so mouths are hidden, and eyes alone are used. Which is least ambiguous? What happens when eyes and mouth give different messages at the same time?

Noses

Not usually terribly mobile but they can convey some messages, and give an overall facial image which can be misleading e.g. haughty, distinguished, pert, sharp etc. Sniffing is another culturally controlled behaviour pattern, in some cultures it is perfectly polite to sniff frequently!

Facial expressions

These are made with our uniquely primate face muscles. No non-primate animals can move their faces in such a way. They rely totally on body language. It is important in relationship education to learn how to read expressions, as some children have found to their cost. It *is* beneficial to develop and practise this art.

Body language

Posture and dress are other vital components in our personal communication system. Desmond Morris has made a detailed study of this area, and in his book *Manwatching* [93] gives endless fascinating examples.

Clothes are used to emphasise mood, occasion, personality, rank or sexual attractiveness. Parents worry about the last function, fearing teenagers 'dressed to kill', may unleash behaviour patterns they cannot cope with. Girls probably worry most about the size, shape and position of their breasts. After all, many comedy programmes exist on one main theme ... 'The girl with the big ...?!' Large-breasted girls often get lots of attention, which may be very unwelcome, though some have made their fortunes this way. The danger here is that size erroneously becomes equated with femininity, so those less 'well-endowed' (a derogatory phrase in itself) unjustifiably feel they cannot be sexually attractive. The range of form should be emphasised, from Twiggy to Dolly Parton, the actual size and shape of breasts being determined mainly by genetics, like other parts of the body.

Other characteristics
Continue to develop an understanding of the value of other qualities than looks. It may be an uphill struggle, most teenagers would rather just be beautiful, but personality does count!

Continue the personal identity search (SCHEP 5–13 page 108) and arrange activities where individuals can present their likes, dislikes, fears, joys and interests, and list ways in which they have succeeded. Define and discuss more abstract qualities such as being thoughtful, considerate, appreciative, calm, courteous, loyal, humorous, committed, inventive, imaginative, patient etc. Which of these would be useful in communicating, and which characteristics would be desirable in a long term partner? How many of these then, have you got yourself, or are developing?! When it comes to choosing a partner remember some spectacularly beautiful people have had spectacularly unsuccessful relationships.

Voices
Sign stimuli are not just visual. How do people react to very aristocratic voices, cockney voices, 'country' accents etc. What assumptions do we make about the owners? Try reading the same statement in many different accents. Does this change its effect?

How good are you at listening? Try and develop this communication skill. Silence is not the same as listening, it may just mean someone is waiting for the chance to say what they feel, or is thinking of something else together!

Role play various types of conversations, some where people are just talking at each other, some where a good response is made; pick up points about what the person really wants to talk about.

Be a conversation watcher (not eavesdropper!) and analyse how people are reacting to each other. Can you tell what kind of relationship they have with each other? These might be of close friend, acquaintance, working, business, dominant etc.

How important is 'small talk'? Can you chat easily with a wide range of people? Read, Berne E. *The games people play*, 1970 Penguin, for more sophisticated concepts on communication, and the psychology of human relationships.

Relationships with the family
These are constantly changing during adolescence, young people often racing to join the adult world, while parents may be anxious about increased freedoms.

To get the balance right during the gradual transition of adolescent to adult can be difficult. Some families cling to their 'children' too long, others may precipitate them into the grown-up world too soon, withdrawing support and interest after puberty, 'now you're old enough to look after yourself.' A lead in to discussions on changing roles could be the Health Education 13–18 Unit *Coming of Age*, for children of 13–14. This has sections on *How I have coped with change, Seeing Myself Now*, and *Rights and Responsibilities*. It lists the ages at which young people are legally entitled to various activities and follow up work develops understanding of the responsibilities which go with each new possibility.

You and your family: This survey of 16 year olds [58], confirmed in general, found 4 out of 5 got on well with their families, particularly with mothers (86%). Fathers achieved an 80% rating but brothers and sisters did less well. Ask individuals to write down the points below on separate sheets of paper anonymously, and as a voluntary activity in case current family problems are causing distress.

i) Things they like about their family such as a welcome home, a feeling of being loved, home comforts, being listened to, security, being able to be 'yourself', relaxing, having fun, holidays, visiting relatives, sharing, belonging, love of family members, having an 'identity' etc. These are the needs which are satisfied by the family.

ii) Things the family disagrees about such as clothes, hair styles, time to be in and go to bed, which TV programmes to watch, boy or girl friends, keeping bedrooms tidy, being nagged at, a feeling of being the least liked member of the family (NB. About one third of children share a bedroom, and up to 8% may share a bed [58] so many lack privacy, and a place to do homework or hobbies, or just be alone.)

See which are the most common likes and dislikes about families. These could be portrayed in pictorial chart form. Discuss reasons why parents' values may differ from the adolescents, why they need to know where their children are, and when they are coming home etc. Are there disagreements about the amount of independence teenagers feel they would like? Use the Schools Council Moral Education Project *Lifeline* (see page 174) for discussion on all aspects of relationships.

Parental involvement

The family likes and dislikes charts could be used at PTA meetings to show how the children generally feel and that they *do* like their parents, even if they don't always show it. Parents might be asked informally and anonymously to write down family situations they find pleasant or, trying e.g.:

i) Pleasant feelings about adolescents:
    enjoying their increased awareness of adult activities
    liking them as companions, as well as loving them as offspring
    shared activities, and shared pleasures
    watching them grow in confidence
    the increased possibility of genuine help from them
    increasingly shared sense of humour
    pride in their achievements etc.
These are feelings of being successful as a parent.

ii) Points of friction:
    using the home as a hotel
    never clear up or help

are self centred and selfish to extremes (moody, bad tempered?)
have no consideration for others (use of bathroom)
show no interest in other members of the family
stay in own room, only emerging to be fed and watered

These are feelings of failing as a parent or family or of losing a family member.

iii) Other points of friction:
interest exclusively centred on 'gang' activities of a dubious nature
choose amazingly unsuitable companions
play unbelievable 'music' far too loud etc. etc.

These are value judgements of the older generation.

Discuss the universality of such feelings and how these characteristics may be partly due to young people's need to begin to detach themselves from their families. They may unconsciously do this by generating antipathy in order to feel they want to go, and they don't need their families any more. Their behaviour may also reflect the discovery we all make during adolescence, that our parents have clay feet, and can no longer be viewed as the omnipotent beings of our early childhood.

If parents are able to understand these feelings, and discuss them with their children, compromises may be possible, and a less drastic transition period ensue. Parents do need to set standards and guidelines and give help and support while their children learn to cope with anger, disappointment, sorrow, frustration and loneliness, as well as joy, delight and happiness. All such emotions, experienced in quick succession during adolescence are very much a part of growing up. A firm but negotiable line on important issues is necessary, and is appreciated by teenagers retrospectively. The compromises might be on dress, pierced ears, tidy rooms etc. these are really only of temporary importance and not usually permanently damaging!

It seems it may be necessary to suggest to parents, of all classes, that satisfying children's material needs, though hard enough to do in some circumstances, is not really quite enough. There are great benefits in continuing to take an interest in their children after puberty and in spending time with them learning of their emotional needs, showing affection, listening to them, and discussing their beliefs and values. Boredom has been cited as the root cause of many anti-social activities, so teenagers need to be helped to develop legitimate interests. This becomes increasingly relevant in times of reduced employment prospects, when they may stay with their families much longer than 'expected', causing new family tensions, and need to work out a different kind of relationship.

Relationships with friends

In European cultures these may come under the following categories, with a progression of involvements either way, or all going on at the same time.

Group or gang

Belonging to an identifiable teenage group can ease the transition from family member to adulthood. The groups are often specifically designed to exclude younger children and grown ups. The need to conform with the group may be absolute, and involve dressing in very specific ways, meeting at certain places etc. Such minutiae of belonging are vital and should not be ridiculed or questioned. Identity and acceptance by the group may depend on such niceties.

What does need to be discussed, are the pressures on individuals within the group, to conform in certain behavioural ways, and how to develop the skills necessary to extricate yourself if these begin to conflict with your own values and beliefs. It is so easy to be unthinkingly swept along in the comfort of a 'concensus' opinion, and a protective group identity. Suggest it may be wise to pause occasionally and consider if you still want to be identified with that particular group. What could you do if you did want to break away? Would you need any help?

There is often a progression from single to mixed sex groups, where boys and girls can learn about each other from a secure base, with the support of the same sex friends available if necessary. As girls mature earlier than boys, their interest may however be orientated towards older specimens of maleness, and not to their contemporaries. A 1983 survey [178] found 38% of 14 to 19 year olds had a special boy or girl friend, 54% went out sometimes with the opposite sex, and 19% never did.

Intimate groupings

These are smaller groups of two or three close friends. Girls' groups tend to spend much time talking about personal relationships of all kinds, boys are perhaps more often more possession and activity orientated. Perhaps both groups would benefit from a wider topic base, and discussion on the types of things they discuss! What values and attitudes do these show?

When discussions include qualities needed in a friend, consider the value of friendships with the same sex, throughout life. For some, these will be the only sort of relationship wished for, but heterosexuality need not be the exclusive occupation some youngsters make it. Many children feel more at ease with members of their own sex, because maturity differences mean it is less likely they can form heterosexual relationships with members of their own age group. The meaning of 'platonic', can be explained, and that it really is possible to be 'just good friends' (this term has been used in derision on many occasions). For children who believe this is not so, it adds yet another pressure to be sexual, when they may really not wish to be.

Sexual relationships

In many countries children are becoming sexually active earlier than previously. The search for sex may be for a variety of reasons:

i) developing from a real 'love' relationship, (this is the image teenagers prefer and they may see all the following categories in this light);
ii) to satisfy a need for love and affection not gained from the family as a sexual affair may mimic this for a while;
iii) as a search for identity;

iv)   to demonstrate to parents and others that you are grown up;
v)   to conform with perceived group behaviour;
vi)   to get attention;
vii)   for curiosity, to find out what all the fuss is about;
viii)   because it is 'expected' (see below);

Pressures to be sexual
These may come from many different sources.

1.   Parents, particularly of boys, may even boast about their offspring's activities, the parents living vicariously through their children.
2.   The media: sensational headlines and plays, about teenage orgies and permissive parties give the impression all adolescents are sexually active. Consider media stereotypes of a sexually active person. Images of aggressive looking females, fully able to cope with all approaches, manly types drinking alcohol, attempting to 'relax' a female by its use? The messages are not very deeply hidden. At what age do children perceive these stereotypes?
   On the positive side, an increasing number of magazines for females have responsible articles on relationships and sex, which partly help to redress the images given by the advertisements they carry.
3.   The peer group. Pressure from this source can be intense. There is a need for more research into how teenagers view their sexually active peers. Studies on young people's images of young smokers and alcohol drinkers [98, 99] suggest they may associate smokers and drinkers with being:

i)   more popular, extrovert and fun
ii)   good to be in the same group with
iii)   tougher
iv)   more grown up and sophisticated
v)   of a higher status
vi)   more likely to succeed
vii)   more able to get on with adults.

They may also associate such attributes with those perceived to be sexually active. If this is so, it is not surprising that some wish to identify with this image, in the sadly mistaken belief that by being sexually active, they will miraculously acquire all the other 'desirable' characteristics.

Of significance here is whether this image is the same for boys and girls. How are sexually active girls spoken of? The words used on these occasions are often highly disparaging: tarts, sluts, will give it to anyone, spread-legs, fallen woman ... what are the masculine equivalents?

Dual standards
The new sexual 'freedom' seems very much weighted in favour of males. They apparently gain increased opportunities for sexual activity, with little or no loss of face or status. For girls the messages are very mixed. 'Be your own person, be sexual if you wish', but if you are you may well be looked down on, called

names, and described in ways making you feel guilty, disturbed and anxious. Girls perhaps on the whole do take sexual relationships more seriously than boys, and early on read into them signs of abiding love and commitment. They are often in love with the idea of being 'in love', so if sex is apparently required of this state ... they may conform for that reason.

What are adolescent expectations of a sexual relationship? A survey of the most popular reading matter for teenagers shows that magazines and books read by girls tend to be romantic, love and relationship orientated, promising deep emotions after very few encounters and on minimal information about the hero. Heroines are allowed to be sensual and ever so feminine, but not actually sexual ... Boys' materials are more varied, oscillating between hobby orientated journals on motor bike maintenance, rock music, etc. and, a variety of 'girlie' magazines. These last portray females solely as bodies, and infer there is an unlimited supply of such nubile creatures, just waiting to be sexually helpful, after the briefest of introductions.

When boys and girls do start to go out together then, their images of what might ensue can be very different! (And yes, there can be romantic males and sexually orientated females.) It is illuminating to explore male and female images presented in this way, and try and judge how far they are divorced from reality.

Loving and caring teaching approach HEC/FPA
Use the 5 part Trigger film *Loving and Caring* [16]. Each part, to be used separately, is less than 10 minutes. There are excellent teachers' notes accompanying the series.

1. *Boy and Girl*
Simon is trying to persuade Sandra to have sex with him. She does not feel ready for this stage, and is confused and anxious about the situation.

Discussion after this film might include the effect of a boy and girl spending a long time together, alone, in a comfortable room. Causing someone to be sexually attracted to you can be a test of your power over them perhaps.

Who could Sandra and Simon go to for advice, other than the friends and parents shown in subsequent reels?

2. *Boys talking*
Discussion between Simon and three friends, reveals their very different outlooks on girls and sex. One has no interest in either which the apparently sexually active Brian finds suspicious. The spectrum of attitudes portrayed, may help children identify similar characteristics in their contemporaries, and analyse them more carefully in the future.

3. *Girls talking*
Sandra asks for help from her friend, who reinforces her right not to be sexual, and raises the question of moral values. They are joined by Claire, who puts the opposite view.

There are many follow up discussion points from this sequence.
i) What exactly is meant by 'moral values'? The term 'moral' is not well

understood by many teenagers as it requires powers of abstract thinking some are only just beginning to develop.

ii)   The value of sex in a relationship, and the idea it will vary from couple to couple, and does not come in standard measures. Is it important partners put more or less the same value on sex? Why?

iii)   Does a sexual involvement mean more for girls than for boys? Are girls ready for a long term relationship earlier than boys? What are the possible positive and negative influences of sex on a relationship?

4.   *Mother and daughter*

Sandra's mother attempts to find out what is worrying her daughter, but her unfortunate approach does not prove very productive.

This sequence is extremely valuable for showing the need for good communication skills, and in highlighting the very different assumptions made about relationships by the two generations. What skills are needed for good communication? What is meant by 'open-ended questions'? Would these have helped? List other examples of poor communication about feelings. How could these have been avoided?

5.   *Parents talk*

Sandra's parents meet those of boastful Brian. The two women discuss ways of helping teenagers, but Sandra's father becomes alarmed at the uncaring, sexist attitude to girls shown by Brian's father.

Discuss how far parents' attitudes to sex are likely to influence their children. Does this include reactions to them telling and laughing at 'dirty' jokes? What other attitudes to sex might have a negative effect on relationships? In what ways do parents try to protect their children, 'Lock up your daughters?' Indeed so in some cultures. This acknowledges the potential power of sexual urges, and assumes that adolescents will not be able to control them.

'What *are* my parents afraid of? Don't they want me to have a boyfriend?' asked one 14 year old girl.

Discuss what these factors might be.

i)   The belief that a sexual relationship would be more of an involvement, could distract them from school work and might lead to deeper hurt and anguish if broken off. Jealousy and anger are powerful emotions. A switch back of ecstasy and despair may not lend itself to a very comfortable life style.

ii)   They feel that 'people' will talk about their daughter in a derogatory way, which may well 'spoil her chances later'? This assumes she has no choice, and the values of the modern generation are the same as the last. Do all young men today expect to stay virginal and marry virgins themselves? Some young people will indeed still want to keep to these standards, and their right to do so should be emphasised.

Adolescents who can communicate well with their parents are less likely to try an early sexual experience [22]. So it is most important parents try and voice their concerns, and rather than issue dire warnings about 'don't do anything I wouldn't do' or insist on a certain magic hour to return by, as if a sexual experience only took place 'after 8'

Resources

Discussion material and schemes of work
1. *Understanding Others* TACADE (See page 83)
2. *Living Well* Health Education Council Project, 1977 Cambridge University Press. Specifically designed to develop decision making skills and 'coping strategies' in small group and discussion situations.
    i) *And how are we feeling today?* Peter MacPhail. Teacher's notes and 35 cartoon cards plus discussion questions illustrate situations particularly relevant to adolescents.
    ii) *Who Cares?* Martin Rogers. 43 natural dialogues of adults in supportive situations with young people.
    iii) *Support Group* Claire Rainbow. 35 cards, illustrated by photographs and drawings, situations in which adolescents might need help.
3. *Lifeline* Schools Council Moral Education Curriculum Project 13–16. 1972 Longman.
    i) *In other people's shoes* Peter McPhail. The teacher's guide is invaluable for the rationale of relationship teaching, and detailed advice on using all the material, and how to adapt it for different ability groups. There are three sets of cards:
    Sensitivity. 46 cartoon cards of situations covering many aspects of relationships, particularly between parents and children;
    Consequences. 58 small cards each with a statement describing a negative situation, either from a moral or safety point of view
    Points of view. 36 illustrated, coded, work cards, depict potential conflict situations, including varying attitudes to sex.
    ii) *Proving the rule* Hilary Chapman Illustrated booklets help pupils explore relationships. 1. Rules and individuals. 2. What would you expect? 3. Who do you think I am? (on personal identity.) 4. In whose interests? (includes groups and gangs.) 5. Why should I?
    iii) *What would you have done?* Booklets on events of international major unrest.
    iv) *Our School* A handbook on the practice of democracy by secondary school pupils.
4. *Good for you.* Series II. Health Education Curriculum Units. ILEA. *Personal relationships.* A useful analysis of a sequence of teaching for personal relationships. Each section gives objectives, teaching points, suggested activities and resources.
5. *Lifeskills teaching programmes* 1 and 2 and background book, lifeskills teaching. Lifeskills Associates. Barrie Hopson and Mike Scally. A personal skills development programme to help children adjust to new situations. Nearly 200 exercises and classroom activities are presented in loose leaf binder form, and include, how to make, keep and end relationships.

Television
1. *ITV*
    i) *Good Health Series* (page 72). Useful as discussion starters for 12 and 13 year olds.
    ii) *Starting out.* Age 14–16 This new five part series focuses on one particular family coping with unemployment, leisure, choice of career, vandalism, loneliness, friendship, being in love, marriage and family life in general. Teacher's notes are available.
2. *BBC*
    i) *Scene* Age 14–16 A series of plays and documentary films, over all terms, and with a two year sequence. The situations shown, such as alcohol at teenage parties, or of how to present sex education, stimulate discussion on a wide range of social and relationship issues. Teacher's notes are provided.
    ii) *16 Up. Series 2* This series in the Young Adult Project, includes health education, sex and personal relationships, and self help.

Radio
i) *Lifetime* Age 13+ Autumn term. Spring 14+ Summer 15+. A series of plays and documentaries, over 3 terms on a wide range of relationships e.g. bullying, staying out late, sexual opportunities, getting married, roles in a family etc. Two books, Lifetime 1 and 2, give the text of the plays. Available from Cambridge University Press.
ii) *Teenage magazine. Wavelength.* Age 15+ A weekly magazine programme with interviews, letters and opinions on many topics relevant to adolescents.

Books
i) *Adolescence. Generation under pressure.* Conger J. 1979 Harper & Row. A very readable and well researched survey of the situations faced by adolescents today.
ii) *Counselling Adolescents in School.* Jones A. 1977. Kogan Page. Expert advice on the role of counselling primarily for girls, and on ways of organising this in a school situation, with case histories and children's comments.
iii) *It's a great life* Baldwin Dorothy. 1979. BBC Publications Helps Children understand some of the situations they may be involved in from the years 15 to 25.
iv) *1976. The two of us* Holt A. and Randell J. Cambridge University Press. Aimed at less academically able children, this investigates many different kinds of relationships, by photographs, drawings and charts.

Chapter 8

HUMAN SEXUALITY

Human sexuality is complex, varied and influenced by many factors, one of which is a learning process. If all the educational inputs have been negative, 'don't touch', 'don't look', 'don't do it' it is not surprising that confusion arises when adolescents do become sexually aware.

A standard view of human sexuality has been as IT. This refers to sexual intercourse between a husband and a wife, for the purpose of having children. It was developed, very understandably, in a pro-population ethos, where contraceptives were not available, 'adolescence' did not occur, women were regarded as property, and illegitimate children had no rights, nor a caring system available for them. Any form of non-reproductive sex, or sex outside the married state, was therefore considered unnatural. The 'curve' of human sexuality according to this model would seem to be as shown in FIG 35a. For all other human activities and pleasures the distribution might be considered likely to be as shown in FIG 35b.

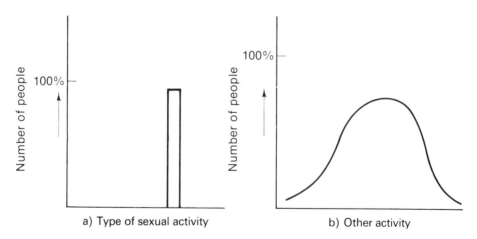

a) Type of sexual activity   b) Other activity

Figure 35   The range of human sexuality.

There are several disadvantages of the first model.

i)   Any sexual activity other than IT, may be viewed as wrong and cause intense guilt and anxiety.

ii)   Certain performance specifications are required, such as an erect penis, without which you cannot do IT, and have therefore failed.

iii)   If anyone does not enjoy this activity, even within a marriage, they may well become disillusioned and frustrated. As research [77] [102] suggests only about 30% of women gain their greatest sexual pleasure from unaided intercourse, many relationships must have been adversely affected by such restrictions. (A high proportion of women prefer additional stimulation of the clitoris area to complete their satisfaction.)

iv)   No consideration is made for the sexual needs of unmarried people, who now form a larger proportion of society.

Questions about IT

The most usual questions that children ask about intercourse are:
Will it hurt?
How long does it take?
How do you know when to stop?
How many times do you do it each night?
What does it feel like?
Can you do it during a period?
Can you do it when you're pregnant?
How do you actually do it?

Will it hurt?

There are several considerations here.

i)   Worries about the hymen being broken, causing pain. The varied nature of the hymen can be explained (page 135) and that in most cases it is stretchy enough to allow a penis to enter the vagina with no difficulty. In a very few cases it may tear slightly, and bleed a little, which may be sore for a short while, until it heals again. It is obviously sensible to be gentle and considerate on the first intercourse and not to rush the procedure. The female should feel she is in control of the situation.

ii)   If a female is not sexually aroused enough, her body may not be ready for intercourse, so this might be uncomfortable for her.

iii)   Some medically treatable conditions such as a very retroverted womb or an infection can cause pain for a woman during intercourse. For males intercourse is not likely to be painful unless, as very occasionally happens, the foreskin is too tight to allow a full erection. This can be remedied by a simple operation. The vagina is soft and does not contain any hard ridges (or teeth!) which could possibly hurt.

iv)   The sexual arousal process depends on reflexes more likely to occur when the body is in a relaxed state (controlled partly by the parasympathetic nervous system, which also primes the body for sleep). In this condition blood moves to the pelvic and genital regions, to prepare them for sex. The opposite system (influenced by sympathetic nerves, and the hormone adrenaline) prepares the body for 'fight or flight'. In this case blood is directed away from the pelvis, to the limbs, and this may block the sexual arousal process at any stage, tending to switch on the escape reaction of the body instead. So fear and worry ...

... of not being ready for this stage, of being hurt, losing virginity, of someone coming, of being overheard, of pregnancy, of being ridiculed or found inadequate in body or performance, of catching a disease ...
and guilt

... due to early learning that sex is dirty or an animal instinct, or of not being married, or that nice females are not sexual, or of being under-age, or with someone else's partner, or that parents wouldn't like it ...

... can all have a turn-off effect which may make the experience a negative one and might suggest it was an unwise decision to become involved in such circumstances. (Some people find guilt sexually exciting, so this would obviously have an opposite effect for them.)

Other questions about 'IT'

How long does it take?

James Bond usually looks at his watch and murmurs something about there being half an hour before the plane leaves ...! The answer is, it depends. Intercourse *can* take only a few minutes, or much longer, due to the 'plateau' stage, explained later. Variability again, due to differences between partners, the occasion, particular circumstances for any one person, or partners, and so on.

How do you know when to stop?

When either partner feels like stopping, which may be after the climax stage, or before. For males the ejaculation stage will probably mean they do not want to become aroused again, but they may still want to continue to give their partner pleasure if so wished.

How many times do you do it each night?

The frequency of sex varies for any one couple, and may be once or twice or more a night (or day of course, darkness is not a necessary component of sex) or once a week, or once a month or less, depending entirely on their desires. Sexual drive (libido) varies between individuals and for any one individual in their lifetime. There are no 'set' patterns or requirements.

What does it feel like?

It feels different for everyone, but descriptions of the climax, for both sexes have included arrows soaring into the sky, waves of pleasure from the toes up, and a feeling of melted butter in the veins. Many people agree a climax is a release of mounting tension and sensitivity, but not everyone has specific climaxes.

Can you do it during a period?

Yes, this would be possible but this is not a form of contraception and some religions do not allow this. See page 150.

Can you do it when you're pregnant?

This is indeed possible and some women feel a high level of sexual desire during pregnancy. Others do not, so again it varies with individuals. Some conditions

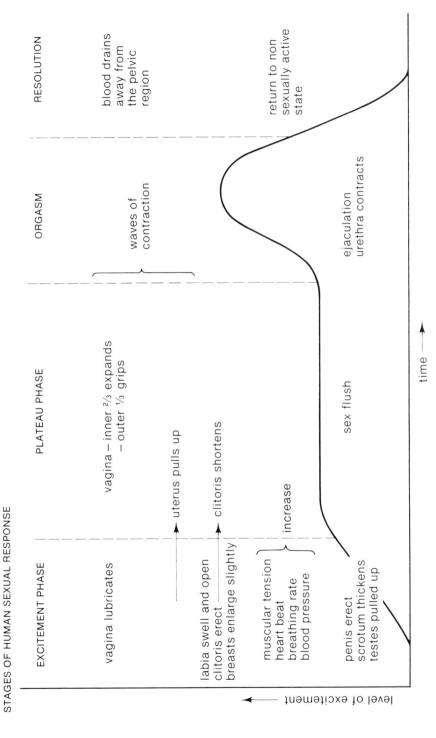

Figure 36 Human sexual response, after Masters and Johnson, 1966, *Human sexual response.*

in pregnancy may make intercourse unwise (the threat of a miscarriage or any bleeding for example) a doctor would give advice on this. (An ever increasing bulge may suggest experimentation with positions, see *Woman's body; An Owners Manual* [100]).

How do you actually do it?

Carefully, and with regard for the partner's wishes. It is important to communicate about these, and not make assumptions about which way 'is best'.

How *not* to do it, thoughtlessly, selfishly, hurriedly, furtively, mechanically, and with no regard to the emotional and physical consequences to oneself or one's partner.

Human sexual arousal

The pioneer work of Masters and Johnson [101], in the mid 1960s, elucidated the physiology involved. Their work suggested four main stages in the process. These can be described in a matter of fact way with reference to FIG 36 on the previous page. The film *Sexuality and Communication* (page 21) provides a very good description along these lines, for teachers to pre-view.

Both sexes may feel relaxed and sleepy after intercourse. This does not mean they have been drained of energy (semen only contains about 9 calories (K cals) per cm^3, so the $5cm^3$ or so produced will not represent any great loss).

The sexual process may be slightly different for males and females. Evidence suggests there may be a continuum:

More quickly aroused	Slower arousal
Visual stimuli dominate	More influenced by skin sensations
More focussed on the genital region	from various parts of the body
Pleasure gained at all stages, but	Pleasure gained at all stages, with or
particularly from the climax	without a climax
Less influenced by the environment	More influenced by the environment
Possibly less linked to affection and love	More linked to affection and love,
Learning process relatively quick.	learning process slower.

There will be many intermediate conditions between these, but *in general* terms males tend to be on the left, and females on the right of the spectrum.

Factors affecting sexual arousal

The partner

Sexual attraction is a very individual matter, of the 'chemistry' between two people. For women particularly, it seems sexual arousal is more likely with someone they feel emotionally involved with.

Sexual arousal can also occur through masturbation, individuals having their own preferences for stimulation techniques.

Individual differences

There is a great variation between individuals both physiologically, and from early learning about sex. If partners have any difficulty in their sexual relationships both the FPA and the NMGC can offer help.

Age

Sexual performance may slow down with age, but octogenarians of both sexes are still able to find it pleasurable. Females tend to require a longer learning process than males, so their pleasure in sex may in fact increase over the years.

Hormone level

The level of male hormones in both sexes, may affect sexual desire. So far, ease of sexual arousal has not been linked to any particular part of the menstrual cycle [103]. Being on 'the pill' can cause a lack of interest in sex in a few women, and has been a side effect of some of the trial contraceptive pills for males. In all these cases, however, it may be difficult to distinguish between hormonal and psychological effects on libido.

Fear, anger, guilt

See page 178.

Alcohol

Alcohol is a depressant. In small amounts its first effect is to relax the body, depress the 'common sense' learning centre of the brain, where decisions are made about suitable behaviour. This actually promotes confidence but sensible inhibitions may already have been supressed. Moderate to heavy drinking can prevent sexual arousal altogether, for males, causing 'brewers droop'. There is an HEC poster ... *there's one part every beer can reach.* It is important to be aware of these effects, and for females particularly not to become 'drunk in charge of a body', and perhaps wake up ... pregnant. Anaesthetising one's vital parts may not perhaps be the best preliminary to successful love-making anyway.

For suggestions on education about the use of drugs in general see *Free to Choose* TACADE [32].

Particular considerations

Although many stages in the sexual arousal process are involuntary and 'cannot be helped', others are very much under the control of the will. There are myths about being 'carried away with passion' or 'we couldn't help ourselves', which are absolute nonsense. An erect penis and a lubricated vagina do not perform on their own, they are attached to thinking bodies, and their owners do have responsibility for them. Most people can tell when they are beginning to be sexually aroused, and should take the decision then about the path to follow. It will not hurt bodies not to continue with the process, it can be stopped at any stage, so another myth, 'I've started so I'll finish'! is also false, though it should be clearly understood the further along the sequence goes, the greater probably will be the urge to continue. Constant arousal and subsidence without a climax may leave blood congestion causing aching, so is not so advisable physiologically. The other consideration is feelings. These may be very hurt if there has been an assumption of sex, which is then rejected 'at the last minute'. A sexual tease, male or female is not appreciated. Communication about intent, verbally, as well as non-verbally is vital.

As the sexual arousal process is a complicated one, it is unrealistic to suppose every part of it will necessarily be highly satisfactory for both partners on the first occasion. It is important to communicate about the stages reached, so the needs of both can be considered. As this involves learning, might it be wise to choose the person you were going to learn with rather carefully? What sort of relationship would provide some degree of security and trust?

Some boys can be alarmed at the intensity of sexual arousal at adolescence, which may be triggered by 'innocent' people, objects or thoughts. Understanding is needed that this is normal, and is the way the body practises the system. Nothing need be done about it. There are classic ways of distracting oneself.

Masturbation may provide relief for some. Fright can have side effects, 'Is impotence common at puberty?! asked young apprentices.

Girls tend not to have such sudden specifically sexual urges, though some may, but can feel overwhelmed with longing for a romantic partner. They too though should be aware of the physical effect of 'maleness' or 'femaleness', which can be a powerful force, and 'make you want to go on'.

Questions of Morality

It is likely adolescents will ask direct questions about the morality of sex outside marriage, and it is wise to have worked out a response.

The exact way in which such questions as those in FIG 37 are answered, depends partly on the context in which they are asked. In a class discussion it is important to avoid global assumptions e.g. that all teenagers want to be sexual, or not, and to be sensitive to the pupil's varied backgrounds. It may be that parents are not married, or have 'boy- or girlfriends' etc. so tact is required.

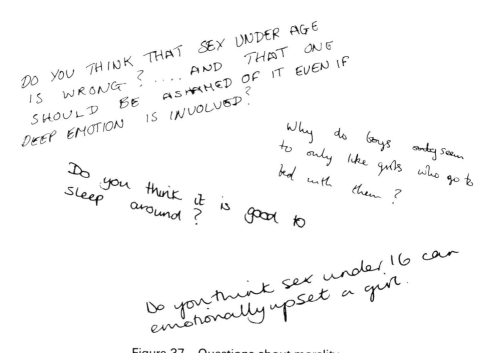

Figure 37   Questions about morality.

The reasons for the 'age of consent' being 16, can be discussed again (see page 96) and that it was introduced as a protective measure, with emotional upsets included in the consideration.

The phrase 'sleeping around' does suggest a very limited value being put on sexual activity. What is that person trying to prove? It may be agreed the benefits of such a life style do not outweigh the considerable disadvantages.

Individual children in private may reveal much more about their situation and, possibly, that they are looking for help, either not to start, or to stop, sexual activity. A clinic nurse who followed up one girl's apparent dissatisfaction with all contraceptive methods, ascertained she really did not want to be sexual, and did not even particularly like her boyfriend. It was explained she had rights in the matter too, and she returned to say 'I told him the nurse said I didn't *have* to have sex,' and he said '... OK'!

There are undoubtedly young people who are having sex as part of a relationship, and have no associated problems. Those that do seek help are often very uncertain of their attitudes and seek some guidelines. The teacher is then acting in a short term 'counselling' role, and providing the opportunity for value clarification and decision making, which should not extend beyond a few short sessions. Alternatives can be outlined in a non-judgemental way and possible consequences identified and discussed. In many cases the pupil will be seeking reassurance on factual matters. The child should feel able to come back again for more help if necessary, but unless a teacher has had very specific training in counselling, a long term support system will not be a viable prospect.

Sexual alternatives

The questions that children most often ask in this area are:

Is masturbation harmful?
How do girls masturbate?
What is oral sex?
What is a homosexual?
What do homosexuals do?

Masturbation

This subject has already been mentioned, pages 52 and 81 but at this stage, the spectrum of opinion can be discussed.

i) Masturbation is entirely unacceptable at any time. Advice to adolescent boys might then be 'It would be a serious sin if a person deliberately and with full realization of what he was doing, used the sexual parts of his body to produce the flow of seed, or made this likely to happen' [108].

ii) It is acceptable as part of development but if continued after marriage is detracting from 'true' sex, i.e. 'cheating your wife.' (Not usually expressed as 'cheating your husband' as until recently women's masturbation was not well documented.)

iii)   It is a normal part of sexual development for both sexes, and can be continued in addition to sex with a partner, if so desired.

iv)   It should be actively encouraged in children, as part of the learning process. A women's group (Sheba feminist publications) have produced a booklet advocating this approach.

If you became a parent what might you say to your children about masturbation? Most people believe that like other sexual activities masturbation should be a private event. This may have to be explained to small children and some less able or mentally handicapped people. It does help to acknowledge that masturbation is pleasurable, but being socially acceptable is also important.

How do girls masturbate?

As girls do not need to touch their genitals in order to urinate, the idea of them handling themselves at all seems surprising to some. There has been a strong social prohibition on girls touching their genitals. An analogy between the clitoris and the penis, can be made, and that both are liberally supplied with nerve endings, which can evoke sensations in the pleasure centre of the brain (in the hypothalamus). The clitoris can in fact be too sensitive to be directly touched in early arousal stages, so of the 60% to 80% of females who do masturbate [105] the majority of these (about 84%) rub the whole area of the clitoris and labia, or the soft mound of tissue over the pubic bone (the *mons veneris*) with fingers, or some other object. This then leads on to a more direct stimulation of the clitoris. Less than 2% of women masturbate solely by

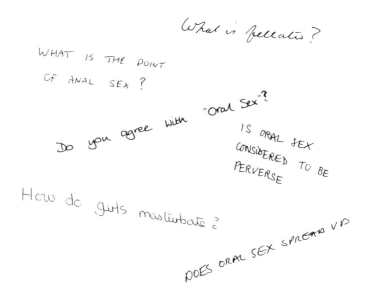

Figure 38   Questions about sexual alternatives.

putting something in the vagina [77]. Hite has suggested masturbation may be the basic expression of sexuality, and sex with a partner is secondary. The vast majority of boys masturbate and learn about their body sensations in this way so why should this not also apply to females?

Masturbating a partner to climax, as may happen in heavy petting, can be an alternative to sexual intercourse. Some girls have found masturbating helps to relieve menstrual cramps.

Oral sex

Questions about oral sex rate high on the list of those most dreaded by teachers. To some people such activity is beyond belief and very shocking. It may, however, be the only form of sexual expression for someone who is paralysed, and many others also find it pleasurable. The partners kiss, caress and stimulate all parts of the body including the most sensitive clitoris (as in cunnilingus) or the penis (as in fellatio) using their mouths and tongues. If a male reaches orgasm in this way, semen will be released into the partner's mouth, where it can either be swallowed or spat out. If swallowed by a female it will not cause pregnancy, as the sperm will be killed by the acid in the stomach, and anyway have no method of reaching an ovum, from this part of the body. Hygiene obviously needs consideration, but fresh semen or vaginal secretions are clean, like saliva. It *is* possible to pass on a sexually transmitted disease in this way and STD clinics will take specimen swabs for culture from the mouths and throats of people who prefer this method of sex.

Nobody should ever be forced to take part in oral sex against their will (it can be a feature of rape) as human variation again means wide spectrum of acceptance and non-acceptance of this particular activity.

Homosexuality

If children's early questions about homosexuality have been answered in context (page 81) they will already have had some help in dispelling the myths surrounding it. Homosexuality, as in heterosexuality, can involve not only a physical relationship, but emotional commitment, love and respect between partners. The sexual side is frequently overemphasised which is why the term 'Gay' may be preferred. In a class situation it must always be remembered that among the pupils will be not only children who are already aware of a permanent homosexual orientation, or who will realise this in the near future but also:

i) Children who are temporarily homosexually orientated, having an emotional or physical relationship with a member of the same sex (by the age of 15, 60% of boys [52] and 33% of girls [105] have experienced at least one act of homosexual play);

ii) children from families where one of the members is homosexual (the majority of gay people have heterosexual brothers and sisters);

iii) children who will in the future become parents of homosexuals;

iv) children who are, or will be bisexual (attracted to both male and female, sometimes termed ambisexual);

Table 11   Changes in thinking on homosexuality.

Homosexuality	
1957 **The Wolfenden Report (110) Recommendation of legality for homosexuality**	Compiled over three years, by a committee appointed by the House of Lords and headed by Sir John Wolfenden, this report suggested homosexuality should not be an offence under criminal law for consenting adults in private.
1957 **Homosexual men are identical in psychology to heterosexual men**	Hooker (111) established there was no difference in psychological adjustment between homosexual and heterosexual men. This finding has been further substantiated by recent research.
1967 **Homosexuality is legal in the UK (now including Northern Ireland) for females from the age of 16, and males from the age of 21**	The Sexual Offences Act (1956) was reformed, so sexual activity in private between consenting males over 21 became legal. Homosexual women have never been subject to legislation in this country (except in the armed forces where, like male homosexuals, their sexual orientation constitutes grounds for discharge from the services)
1973 **Homosexuality is not a psychiatric disorder.**	The American Psychiatric Association removed homosexuality from the list of mental afflictions.
1975 **Recommendation for non discrimination on the grounds of sexual orientation.**	The NCCL Report on Homosexuality and the Teaching Profession (12). Analysis of replies from LEAs in England and Wales, on the employment of homosexual teachers, showed a general improvement in attitudes, suggested a positive image of homosexuality would be beneficial to all, and proposed legislation outlawing discrimination on the grounds of sexual orientation.
1976 **There are no physical differences between homosexuals and heterosexuals.**	West (112) affirmed there is no consistent research showing any systematic physical difference between heterosexual and homosexual males, or heterosexual and homosexual females.
1976 **The 'seduction' theory of homosexuality is unsubstantiated**	No research has been able to explain why some people become heterosexual, some homosexual, and some bisexual. The orientation seems to occur very early, probably by the age of 5 or even by 2 (115). Adolescents have therefore been pre-programmed many years before, and do not choose their orientation at this stage, but may confirm it. It is therefore extremely unlikely that homosexuals can be "recruited". Christopher (38) details four examples of findings (in 1957 and 1976) that homosexual experiences of boys or men do *not* change heterosexuals into homosexuals. These experiences may be gained in 'facultative homosexuality' in all male communities such as of prisoners, sailors, or boys boarding schools, where there is no choice in the sex of the partner. Homosexuality is, therefore, not catching.
1976 **Suggestion that information on homosexuality should be included in all programmes of sex education.**	The NCVYS discussion report (114) suggests there should be more concern about the quality of any relationship rather than the physical sexual component, and that the aim should be to combat myths and false stereotypes and educate for knowledge about, and acceptance of, homosexuality.
1979 **Acceptance of homosexuality by some members of the Christian Church**	Working Party Report from the Board of Social Responsibility. This board received evidence and discussion findings from the Methodist and Anglican Churches. The final report advocated, and indeed pleaded, for acceptance of homosexuality as a variation of human sexuality, as those who are so orientated "have no choice but to be homosexual".

v)   children who will become parents of bisexuals;

vi)   children who will marry partners who subsequently show a homosexual or bisexual orientation;

vii)   children who know homosexuals and bisexuals (we *all* do).

All these groups are going through our education system. What are they going to learn which will help them understand the nature of different sexual orientations, combat the rigidly stereotyped portrayals of homosexuality so frequently seen on television, and allay fear and anxiety caused by misunderstanding and ignorance?

The reports on the opposite page show a progression of thinking away from ideas of homosexuality as deviant, punishable, a mental condition to be pitied, a downright sin, or something to be 'cured' of, towards the view that this sizeable minority of the population show a natural variation of human sexuality, and should be able to take their place in society with dignity, a good self image and a positive outlook for the future.

This evidence can be used to discuss the discrimination and prejudice still shown towards homosexuals. Why is media coverage so intensive and suggestive, if homosexuality is an accepted variation, is legal, and the person concerned has not committed any offence? What *value* does society seem to put on sexual orientation if this is put above all other considerations of character, personality, loyalty, efficiency and talent? In the light of the above reports such attitudes can only be seen as taking 'sex' right out of context as *one* aspect only, of human relationships. Legal discrimination is shown in the age of consent for homosexual men remaining at 21. A male soliciting a male commits an offence punishable by imprisonment, whereas there is no such 'offence' for female solicitation of males.

Further discussion material is provided in the tape/slide set *Homosexuality. A fact of life*, available from the Campaign for Homosexual Equality. This contains a 50 slide sequence, tape commentary and script, student's booklet and teacher's guide, all most sensitively and professionally presented.

The sequence begins with a discussion of human variety, and Kinsey's analysis of sexuality as a spectrum of at least seven categories, covering all combinations of heterosexuality or bisexuality and homosexuality. The frequency of homosexuality is approximately 1 in 20 or 5%, which in the UK is equivalent to 3 million people or the population of Wales, (though not all Welsh people are gay!).

The next sequence, of colour drawings, portrays the story of Dave, who realises he does not feel attracted to girls, and Sue, who has a gay companion, Jane. Dave is very confused, and subsequent slides explore his dilemma of wanting to be honest and conforming, but knowing he does not feel the same way as his friends or brother. All the images he sees are of heterosexuality. Sue is under pressure at home to find herself a boyfriend rather than 'spend so much time with Jane.' Dave wonders who he could go to for help, but is hesitant, as all his previous learning about homosexuality, from stereotyped images, indicates very negative future prospects. The next sequence explores sexism, and fixed ideas of gender and friendships.

Sue and Jane are happy in each other's company though forced to be secretive about it, but Dave is very lonely and has no way of identifying a possible partner. There follows an explanation of the need for specific meeting places for homosexuals. Following slides depict 'aversion therapy' used to try and change sexual orientation, but the explanation is given that in the majority of cases this does not work, as feelings are set so early. Dave is shown contacting a national organisation, Friend, offering help and support for homosexuals, and later meets a local CHE group; and at last begins to relax and feel accepted.

Ignorance, fear, hate and violence are shown as chain reactions putting intensive pressures on homosexuals, but the final slide shows Dave with friends, and the hope that he too will be able to establish a happy relationship in the future.

Most of the questions and discussion raised by this presentation are answered in the accompanying teachers' booklet, which gives full research references, and an extensive bibliography. Particular points which might be discussed.

i) The generally greater acceptance of friendships and more freedom of expression for affection between females. Lesbians have not had such vindictive feelings directed towards them, although they too can be assaulted. Physical and verbal abuse can be very real hazards and of course militate against honesty and openness.

ii) Parents may not have had any education about homosexuality, and may need help in adapting to the situation, if one of their children is homosexual.

iii) The sexual part of a homosexual relationship can be overemphasised, and will be valued differently by different couples. Individuals do not always take either a 'masculine' or 'feminine' role but vary lovemaking, using techniques of mutal masturbation or oral sex, or sometimes of anal intercourse. This last behaviour is still illegal for heterosexuals, even if man and wife, (they could face a maximum penalty of life imprisonment) but is legal between consenting males over 21, in private.

Anal intercourse is another expression of sex some people have difficulty in understanding. The pleasure giving parts of the body do however extend round to the anus. Watching small children fill nappies or potties will testify that the act of defacation can be a pleasurable event. It is not socially acceptable however, to talk about this very natural function, nor the satisfaction it sometimes provides. Questions about piles (haemorrhoids) may arise at this stage. Of course they would make anal intercourse uncomfortable, but they are not caused by the activity. Just as for other methods of sex, sexually transmitted diseases can be conveyed by anal intercourse, and doctors warn the sphincter muscle may be damaged [113].

iv) Because a person is homosexual it does not mean they do not wish for a family, nor are incapable of a caring relationship with children. There is no evidence that being brought up in a lesbian or male homosexual household has any effect on the subsequent sexual orientation of the child. The majority of homosexuals have presumably been brought up in heterosexual families.

Homosexual couples, like others, would keep sexual activities private, and ordinary expressions of affection and caring between two people are surely good images. Maddox [116] discusses in detail the desire felt by many homosexuals to become parents, and other reasons why some entered marriage.

Because of present prejudices it would be advisable for a senior, heterosexual member of staff to present the programme outlined above. There are still people who would interpret a discussion about homosexuality led by a homosexual, as being a 'recruitment drive', and of a threatening nature.

It is beneficial for staff from the sex education team to meet homosexuals, and discuss the attitudes they encountered at home and at school. As with so many minority groups, apprehension is lost once individuals are known as people, and not just because of a label on one aspect of their lives.

It is helpful for the team to be aware of certain points.

i) Homophobia, an intense expression of dislike of homosexuals, can sometimes be the result of an unacknowledged homosexual orientation in the person concerned.

ii) Many homosexuals go through an 'identity crisis', when they realise their orientation. Some may try to combat this by very obvious heterosexual relationships, or by getting married. Such strategies may lead to broken relationships. If images of homosexuality could be presented in more positive ways, acceptance might be so much less of a trauma for all concerned, but until the many respectable and respected homosexuals in the community feel able to declare their orientation and join those who have 'come out', such images will be difficult to find.

iii) Adolescents who do not have any interest in the opposite sex are not necessarily homosexual. It is not obligatory to 'have' a boy- or girlfriend just to be like the others. Many people wish to be independent, or in a group, for part or all of their lives.

Further information on homosexuality and support groups for homosexuals and their families can be obtained from:

The Campaign for Homosexual Equality (CHE) 274 Upper Street, London N1 2UA Tel. 01.359.3973.

Friend, c/o CHE, 22 Great Windmill Street, London WI.

Gay Christian Movement, 3M Box 6914, LONDON WC1N 3XX

Parents' Enquiry c/o Rose Robertson, 16 Honley Rd, Catford, London SE6 2HJ.

Albany Trust, 24, Chester Square, London SW1.

Resources

i) *Understanding Human Sexual Inadequacy* Belliveau F. and Richter L. 1971 Hodder. Two journalists translate the scientific language of the work of Masters and Johnson and with the author's consent give an explanatory version for the non-medical world.

ii) *Our bodies ourselves.* Phillips A. and Rakusen J. 1980 Penguin. Revised version of the American Boston women's health collective, handbook on all aspects of women's health.

iii) *Women's body. An Owner's Manual.* Diagram Group. 1977 Paddington.

iv) *Man's body. An Owner's Manual.* Diagram Group 1977 Paddington.

v) *Sex for beginners.* Trimmer E. 1983 Answers to questions from teenagers.

vi) *Learning to live with sex.* Burkitt A. 1980 revised. FPA A glossary of many of the words teenagers wish to know about.

Chapter 9

POPULATION GROWTH AND FAMILY PLANNING

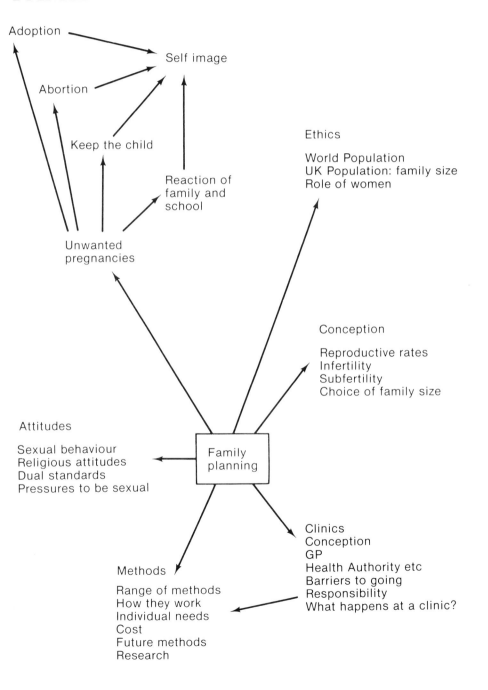

Adoption

Self image

Abortion

Keep the child

Reaction of family and school

Ethics

World Population
UK Population: family size
Role of women

Unwanted pregnancies

Conception

Reproductive rates
Infertility
Subfertility
Choice of family size

Attitudes

Sexual behaviour
Religious attitudes
Dual standards
Pressures to be sexual

Family planning

Clinics
Conception
GP
Health Authority etc
Barriers to going
Responsibility
What happens at a clinic?

Methods

Range of methods
How they work
Individual needs
Cost
Future methods
Research

Population growth

For any individual the growth of population seems gradual and is not perceived as the dramatic 'explosion' of headline news. Even in the UK, however, where the growth rate over the last century has been relatively slow, older people recall fields, and woods pre-dating roads and buildings covering them today. Any local history, geography and land use studies give substance to these anecdotes, and are a very effective way of teaching about population changes, and multiplied over the country as a whole they do constitute dramatic and accelerating change within the lifetime of any one person. People pressure is impinging on everyone. Population growth is probably the single most important factor which will affect the quality of life of every individual in the future. The evidence is overwhelming [179].

Revise visually the meaning of one million; use rice grains, sand, 1m² of mm squared paper etc. Then consider one billion, = 1,000 million.

From the evolution of humankind to the year 1820 the world population slowly rose to 1 billion people.

Today the population of China alone is now over 1 billion!

Within the next 100 years the world population rose to 2 billion people
Within the next 30 years the world population rose to 3 billion people.
Within the next 15 years the world population rose to 4 billion people. (this was recorded in March 1976.)

The world population figure for mid 1982 was over $4\frac{1}{2}$ billion people. This recent rapid rise can be displayed graphically as in FIG 39. The 1980 United Nations estimate for the year 2000 was a world popualtion of 6119 million people. These figures are astronomical and difficult to grasp. One very effective visual aid is *Population Dots*, available from Concord Films Council. This very short film shows a world map, with dots representing millions of people, and a heart beat sound track. Dots are added at the correct rate with a base line showing the year. The extremely rapid recent growth rate is clearly demonstrated.

Growth rate

To understand why a population grows, consider the difference between the birth rate, and the death rate, usually expressed as births or deaths per 1000 of the total population in any given year.

The birth rate of the UK in 1982 was 14.

The death rate of the UK in 1982 was 12.

As there were more births than deaths, there was a slight increase in the population, amounting in this case to 0.2%, one of the lowest in the world. Other factors affecting the population of any country will be the numbers of people leaving through emigration, (e = exit) and the numbers entering through immigration (i = in!) Percentage increase is again difficult to visualise, so population increase is often expressed in terms of how long it would take for the population to double. Population doubling time, in the UK would be 462 years, which sounds a long time, but the UK is already one of the most densely

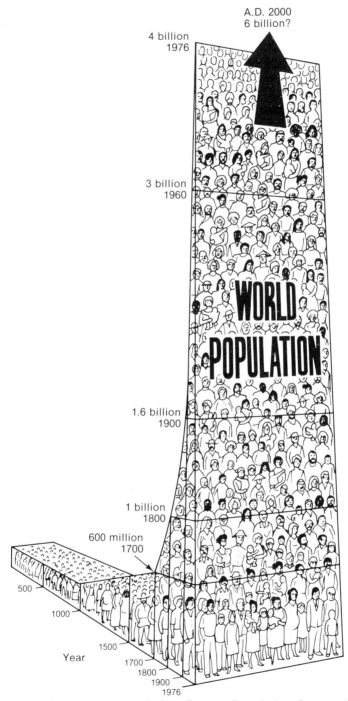

Figure 39   Growth and population. From a *Population Concern* leaflet.

Table 12   Population density.

Country	Population Density (People/KM^2) 1980 except where specified
EUROPE United Kingdom Netherlands Belgium Germany (Fed Rep) Italy France Spain	228 (1979) 345 325 245.8 – 98 –
ASIA Bangladesh Japan Sri Lanka India Pakistan	588 309 219 194 95
AFRICA Egypt Nigeria Kenya	40.0 (1978) 83.5 27.3
LATIN AMERICA Colombia Brasil	23.4 14.3
USA	23
CHINA	102
USSR	11.9

populated countries in the world (4 times that of China) so any increase will have a noticeable effect (see above table).

Some other developed countries also have very slow growth rates, though very few, Denmark, Luxembourg, East Germany and Hungary have a 'Zero' growth rate [118].

A useful aid for appreciating the difference in rates, is a metronome. Set it to 90 ticks per minute (Larghetto). This is the world death rate. For each tick, somewhere in the world, someone dies. A sobering thought. Now set the metronome at the fastest beat (Presto-prestissimo), probably the maximum is 208, but it should be at 230, to represent the world birth rate. Pause for thought about the significance of the different rates. 140 extra people are added every minute, or (roughly) two extra people for each heart beat. 700 million extra people each year. The difference between the two rates is the world population

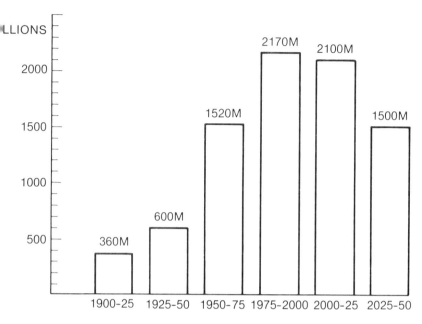

Net additions to world population at 25-year intervals 1900-2050 (Salas, 1981).

	Population in millions	Natural Increase annual %	Population 'Doubling Time' in years	Life Expectancy at birth in years	GNP in US$
World	4,585	1.7	40	60	2,620
More developed countries	1,152	0.6	116	72	8,130
Less developed countries	3,434	2.1	33	57	680
Africa	498	2.9	24	49	770
Asia	2,671	1.9	37	58	920
North America	256	0.7	95	74	11,240
Latin America	378	2.3	30	63	1,910
Europe	488	0.4	187	72	7,990
USSR	270	0.8	88	69	4,550
Oceania	24	1.3	55	69	7,600

Figure 40   Additions to world population.

growth rate, in 1982 this was shown to be down a little at 1.7%, with a world population doubling time of 40 years. Between 1980 and 2000 annual world growth rates of between 1.8 and 2.0% are predicted, with the greatest increase ever being added from 1975 – 2000 of 2170 million people.

Only when the two tick rates are equal will the population eventually show zero growth.

There are two ways of achieving this

i) To increase the death rate, (wars, starvation, epidemics, accidents caused by overcrowding etc.)
ii) To decrease the birth rate.

Remember:
A population growing at 1% will double every 70 years
A population growing at 2% will double every 35 years
A population growing at 3% will double every 23 years
A population growing at 3.5% will double every 20 years

This is exponential growth, the percentage increase being added each year to the total, so the next increase is on that already augmented figure. Work out the difference between compound interest (exponential growth) and single interest, over 5 years, for any particular sum of money!

Now consider figures given on the *World Population Data Sheet* [118] available from the IPPF. Every country is listed, and figures include:

Population estimate for mid-1982 in millions

Crude birth rate and death rate.

Natural increase (annual)

Population doubling time in years (at the current rate)

Population projected to the year 2000 in millions

Infant mortality rate (annual deaths of infants under 1 year per 1000 live births in a given year)

Total fertility rate

Population, percentage below the age of 15, and above the age of 65

Life expectancy at birth in years

Urban population percentage of total population

Labour force engaged in agriculture, in percentage of total population

Per capita gross national product in 1980 in US dollars.

The division between the 'rich' North and poorer South countries can be clearly seen. Which continent has the highest increase rate? From FIG 40 this is Africa, and from the detailed chart [118] the country is Kenya, with a 3.9% annual increase, a doubling of the population in 18 years. The *average* number of births to women in Kenya at the moment is eight.

What other factors are important?

The actual size of the population determines how many are involved in the percentage increase. The proportion of the world's population in different continents will change when the rates of growth are different.

The density of population in any one country, the proportion living in cities, urbanisation, the movement of people into cities, all put increasing strain on their country's services. This trend has been continuing, particularly in the South.

The facilities available nationally for food, water, housing, clothes, education, and medical care are vital factors.

The age structure is important, particularly how many of the population are under 15, or over 65, and therefore have to be 'supported' by the 15–65 year old age group. These proportions can be shown by drawing pie diagrams from the given data ($1° = 3.6\%$ see FIG 41). The larger the 'dependent' proportion of the population, the more difficult it is for a country to support them.

The age dependency ratio i.e.

$$\frac{\text{Population under 15, plus population 65 and over} \times 100}{\text{Population aged 15–64}}$$

is high in less developed continents such as Africa, where 45% of the population is under 15, and 3% over 65, whereas in more developed countries only 23% is under 15, though the proportion over 65 is high (and increasing) at 11%. The age structure is expected to change by the year 2000.

		1980	2,000
Percentage of the population over 65	Developed Countries (North)	11%	13%
Percentage of the population over 65	Less developed countries (South)	4%	5%

Population momentum

This is an important concept because it explains why many populations will not suddenly stop growing, even if the fertility rate (the number of live births per 1000 women aged 15–44) is at replacement level. Previously higher fertility rates may mean an increased number of women in the childbearing age groups each year, and hence total births will continue to exceed total deaths for two or three generations, or 50–70 years.

The population handbook [117] gives clear explanations of the many other factors affecting population growth and change. The age and sex structure of populations can be shown in population pyramids, and the long term effect of an expansive profile, as increasing numbers reach maturity, can be envisaged.

The many serious implications of population growth are being considered by responsible governments. Population limitation has been found to be linked to general socio-economic development, education, the role and status of women, and cultural and religious beliefs and the effectiveness of government family planning campaigns.

What can be done?

After discussion (as above) of the factors involved, the class could work in groups, as delegates to an international conference on population growth, and draw up a list of recommendations. Compare these with The Colombo Declaration (Sept. 1979) from the International Conference of Parliamen-

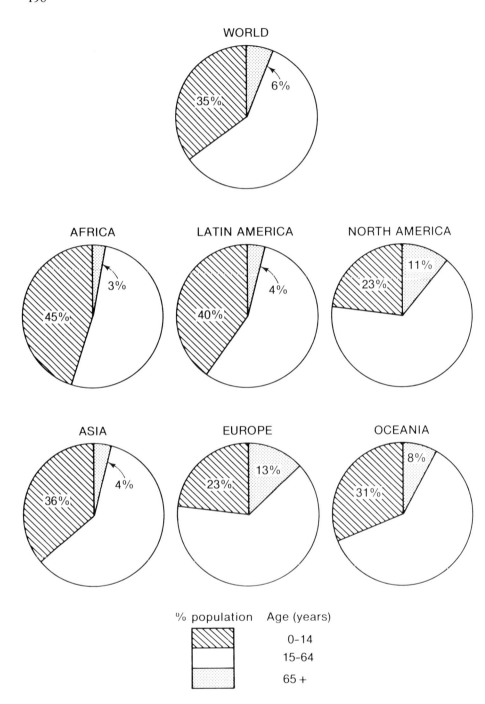

Figure 41   The percentage distribution of age.

tarians on Population and Development, which among other things called on all governments to:

i)   strive to close the wide economic gap between rich and poor countries,

ii)   formulate and strengthen population policies as an integral part of socio-economic development plans,

iii)   ensure the basic right of people to decide the number and spacing of their children, and ensure they have the information and means to do so,

iv)   promote the role and status of women in the family and society, to enhance their access to education, employment, health services and financial credit,

v)   support increased research into safer, more efficient and more widely acceptable techniques of fertility regulation.

The full text of the Colombo Declaration and useful leaflet *A Growing Concern*, is available from Population Concern, the fund raising and educational organisation associated with the Family Planning Association. Another international conference at Santo Domingo (December 1983) on Voluntary Contraception, made similar pleas in their declaration reported in the IPPF Medical Bulletin Vol. 18 Feb. 1984.

Do people actually want to limit their families? *The World Fertility Survey* (WFS 1972) started collecting information from many countries, and since 1974, has found:

i)   in developing countries half or more of all married women of childbearing age wanted no more children, but only half were using effective family planning,

ii)   a high percentage of women questioned did not wish for their last child or current pregnancy,

iii)   one third of women questioned said their ideal family size was less than their actual one,

iv)   the wish for no more children is high in all socio-economic groups, whether urban or rural.

This evidence suggests attitudes towards having large families have changed (more children now survive infancy and life expectancy is rising) and many families would be willing to change their behaviour and use effective contraception if it was available. The motivation for an immediate lowering of population growth rates appears to be present. The survey found there has been a sharp fall in the birth rate in many countries in the 1970s, by as much as 15–50% in some. In a few – such as Bangladesh and Pakistan with only a small drop, however, only 10% of women were using contraception. The main factors helping people to have smaller families were found to be:

i)   some basic education and work outside the home for women,

ii)   women using contraception effectively,

iii)   increased age for marriage (which lengthens the intervals between generations),

iv)   increased wealth and better living conditions,

v)   effective government sponsored family planning policies.

Reports stress the need for education for women, but it is equally necessary to involve the men, so they can share the responsibility for family limitation. The situation in the developed countries appears to be more stable, with low growth rates. However, as many are quite densely populated, and are not self sufficient, they may still need an integrated population policy. Some people suggest countries with contracting populations may face social difficulties, but it is certain, those with ever increasing ones will. It must also be remembered that at the moment, every child born in the 'rich North', consumes about 30 times as much as one born in the 'poor South'.

Strasbourg Conference

At the European Conference in Strasbourg (Sept. 1982) all countries agreed the basic right of individuals and couples to decide freely and responsibly on the number and spacing of their children should be fully respected. This implies free access to family planning services. In the UK, surveys have shown that in spite of free contraceptive services, as many as one third of all conceptions are unwanted, and there are at least 160 000 abortions every year. There is surely no room for complacency.

The International Planned Parenthood Federation

The IPPF, is a voluntary organisation linking the work of independent Family Planning Associations in 108 countries. It offers specialist advice to governments wishing to increase their family planning services, having experts on standards of care and the efficiency and quality of contraceptives. Part of the IPPF role is to liaise with WHO, UNESCO and UNICEF. The educational aspect of their work is fundamental and they supply up to date information on family planning services in nearly all countries.

The 30th Anniversary issue of *IPPF in Action*, gives details of their very varied work. A catalogue of all their publications, periodicals, research papers, books, leaflets, posters and wall charts, is available.

Family planning

The general idea of family planning will already have been established (pages 87–95). The majority of teenagers at school will not wish to be sexually involved with a partner for some years, but others will already be starting sexual activity.

Both boys and girls of this age, will benefit from an understanding of:

i)   The need for contraception, within and outside marriage,
ii)   the motivation and attitudes required for people to 'accept' the idea of the risk of becoming parents, if they are being sexually active,
iii)   the provision of contraceptives from family doctors, clinics, and chemists etc.
iv)   the different types of contraceptives, their relative effectiveness, advantages and disadvantages, and correct use.

It has been suggested [124] that teaching about contraceptives should be only in the context of marriage and not given to children under the age of consent.

This opinion could be discussed with parents, and also:

i)   the number of extra-marital pregnancies, 70,000 in one year, (40% of those aborted) [47]
ii) the pressures on the young to be sexual
iii) that many adolescents have myths about conception and contraception
iv) the educational premise that information is best assimilated before it is needed
v)   that only 20% of teenage mothers in a recent survey [177] had used any form of contraception, and one quarter became pregnant again within a year of having their first baby
vi) the survey [59] which found that information on sexuality was viewed by teenagers as neither dissuading nor encouraging them to have sex before marriage
vii) that only one third of babies born to girls under 20 are conceived within marriage [177]

It might then seem a responsible approach for parents and teachers to co-operate to ensure all young people are aware of the four areas of understanding previously suggested.

Teacher sensitivity is needed during this teaching to the background of pupils and parents, and the views of different religious and cultural groups on contraception.

Possible teaching approach
The need
Remind pupils of the right not to be sexual, and that many people will wish to wait until marriage before being so. This choice does not usually promote media coverage. Revise the facts of conception, and that this is what sexual organs and behaviour are biologically designed for.

Use this quick quiz for self assessment perhaps.

i)   When does a girl's body begin to make ova? (*At menarche*)
ii)   How often is an ovum produced after this? (*About once a month*)
iii) It is possible to tell exactly when this happens? (*See page 92*)
iv)   When does a boy begin to make sperm? (*At puberty, when ejaculations begin*)
v)   How many sperm can be released at one time? (*300–500 million*)
vi)   How long can sperm stay alive in a female's body? (*Up to 5 days*)
vii) Can the ovum be fertilised without full intercourse? (*Yes, if any of the sperm are put near the entrance to the vagina, they may find their way up to the ovum.*)
viii) When should contraception be used, if conception and a baby are not wanted? (*On every conceivable occasion!* Do all young people understand what a 'conceivable occasion' is? Possibly not, as there were 34 000 abortions to girls under 19 living in England and Wales in 1981.)

Motivation and attitudes

Why are the abortion numbers so high, when contraceptives are available free, to anyone who needs them? Use the FPIS poster *There are 8 methods of birth control . . . and this isn't one of them.* Showing the back view of a couple, their arms round each other, but with fingers crossed. They could be envisaged as newly married or steady partners, or they could have just met at a party.

Why have they got their fingers crossed? Ask for some suggestions.

Don't they know they're going to have sex?

Are they 'not sure' how far things will go?

Are they both drunk?

Haven't they talked about sex to each other?

Why not?

Do they take each other for granted?

Are they too embarrassed?

Didn't they understand about sexual attraction and arousal?

Haven't they considered the value of sex in their relationship?

Why haven't they got contraception before this?

What might the boy (man) be thinking?

It's chicken to use contraceptives?

It would spoil his fun?

Contraceptives are too expensive?

It's up to girls to get themselves fitted up?

Show the *Pregnant Man Poster* (FPIS) with the caption 'Would you be more careful if it was you that got pregnant?' Discuss the joint responsibility for family planning. N.B. Some boys and men do not believe it is their job to 'take precautions', so it's as well this view is aired. Revert to the original 'couple' poster.

What might the girl (woman) be thinking?

I'm not really being sexual, because I'm a 'nice girl'?

I'm too young to get pregnant?

It can't happen the first time?

I'll have a really hot bath straight afterwards?

I hope he'll be careful?

I don't really want to, but I suppose everyone else is, and I might lose him?

I'll sneeze and jump up and down after. . .?

I'll be all right if I don't 'enjoy' it?

It can't happen to me?

Isn't this romantic, it's lovely being in love?

We don't really want a family yet, but I guess it doesn't matter as we're married?

I didn't get pregnant last time so I must be sterile?

Perhaps some of the other 34 000 young couples also thought these things? What advice could be given to them? Groups could then write down suitable guidelines which might include the idea that if you don't use contraceptives you may be choosing a parent for your child. Discuss the HEC advertisement campaign to help young people accept responsibility for being sexual, (reviewed in the Health Education Journal Volume 41 No. 1 1982).

Note to teachers

A high proportion of adolescents do not use contraceptives until six months or a year after their first intercourse [126]. In Farrel's [2] sample, two thirds of the sexually active teenagers said they had not used a contraceptive method on every occasion, a small number (8%) had never used any method, and of these, the majority were young, working class boys.

The more stable the relationship, the more likely it is that a reliable contraceptive will be used [2] [123] possibly as the sexual part of the relationship then becomes more 'acceptable'. The time of highest risk of an unwanted pregnancy in a relationship appears therefore to be at the very beginning of sexual activity. It has been estimated that 20% of teenage pregnancies in the USA for example occur in the first month of sexual activity [126]. See page 96, for identification of other 'high risk' groups. It is appropriate therefore to emphasise that the first occasion of sexual intercourse is a high risk one. To make this point the comic *Too Great a Risk*, available from the FPIS can be used. It tells the story of a girl in a stable relationship, who fears she may be pregnant. Most teenagers become involved in the storyline and it is helpful for less able children who find other presentations too academic. Many discussion points are raised by the story. For children with a good reading ability the FPIS leaflet *Straight facts about sex and birth control* is a useful follow up to the comic.

Another comic *Don't Rush Me* (available from Wandsworth Council for Community Relations) is enjoyed by adolescents of all races, but is particularly appropriate for use in areas with a high West Indian population. A background booklet on the evaluation of the use of the comic, and with suggestions for discussion topics, is available from the Community Relations Commission.

Both comics are very professionally produced, with a romantic imagery clothing very fundamental facts. Teenagers find the format most acceptable, and identify well with the characters.

Other potential high-risk scenarios can be discussed, such as being away from home, on holiday, with a gang, at an all-night disco or party with alcohol etc. With older children, or youth groups a selection of the posters from ICARUS might be used. Some are very hard hitting so discretion is needed for choice of poster for use with any particular group. Some of the titles are:

Yours because you never asked.

A warm night, a borrowed car, and three pints of light ale.

Heard the one about self control?

What advice might the group offer to a committee planning a campaign to make teenagers more aware of the long term consequences of sexual behaviour?

The sound tape *Hello Gorgeous* from the Brook Advisory Centre Education department, starts with a ten minute interview with an unmarried teenage mother from Birmingham. Her rich accent and obvious sincerity are extremely effective for promoting audience sympathy, and many of the issues of teenage sexuality can be raised in discussion afterwards.

Provision of contraceptives

Discussion of the couple on the poster or any other hypothetical couple. Suppose this couple were married, or had talked about their relationship and felt they might want to have intercourse, thus being honest with themselves and taking responsibility for their future. Where could they have got contraceptives?

i)   From their own family doctor.
ii) From a family planning clinic.
iii) From a clinic specialising in advice for young people, such as a Brook Advisory Centre.
iv) From a Youth Advisory Service Centre, some clinics run these.
v)   From a chemist shop.
vi) From machines dispensing sheaths.
vii) From mail order firms.

Why might they not have done this? Perhaps they were afraid of what people would think of them? Discuss the ambivalent attitude shown by a society promoting sex from hoardings, films, television and teenage magazines, but not 'allowing' young people, particularly girls, to feel able to plan, responsibly, to be sexual. Guilt feelings can prevent acknowledgement of real facts.

Perhaps they were not sure how to make an appointment? Explain it is exactly the same procedure as for all the other clinics already discussed. Perhaps they don't want their parents to know?

Parents' attitudes to contraception

Sadly some of the most usual questions asked by teenagers are 'How can I get contraceptives (or an abortion) without my parents knowing?' To promote understanding of the changing attitudes to sexual behaviour from one generation to the next, arrange a debate, forum, or interview with volunteer grandparents, parents and teenagers (or these could all be taped). This may enable adolescents to realise the tremendous changes that have taken place in talking about sex, the roles of men and women, attitudes to and availability of contraceptives, and so on, in the past 20 years.

Many parents are more 'liberal' than their children perceive, and some would much prefer their adolescents to be protected rather than vulnerable if they insist on being sexually active, and would welcome the chance of discussing the situation with them.

Will the Doctor tell my parents?

Stress the complete confidentiality of all services, even for those under 16, but explain the Doctor will suggest it would be a good idea if the patients themselves could tell their parents, and would discuss this possibility with them.

Will it be a man or woman doctor?

In many clinics and GP groups there is a choice of doctor. Many doctors at Family Planning Clinics are women.

Can I take a friend?

Almost certainly, friends and partners are welcomed at most clinics, and this

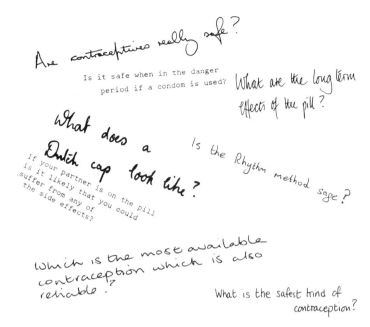

Figure 42   Questions about contraception.

can be asked about when the appointment is made.

What happens at a clinic?

Explain the routine followed, including form filling (done by the clinic personnel) the questions that will be asked, e.g. about the date of last period and possible blood pressure and weight checks etc.

Apprehension about pelvic (vaginal or internal) examination can be allayed, they are often not now done on the first visit. Reassurance about this procedure also comes from previous teaching (page 135).

Types of contraceptive

The actual choice of any particular type of contraceptive, and motivation to use, and continue using it, involves a complex interaction of medical, psychological, religious and social factors.

Teaching about contraceptives

(See page 95) Teachers will realise it is not their role to influence specific choices, by discussing the merits of one particular pill over another for example. The following approaches can be helpful:

i)   Talk about the various contraceptives in a neutral way, saying something positive about each one, as well as discussing possible disadvantages.

ii)   Explain specialist advice on contraception can be obtained freely from FP clinics and GP surgeries.

iii) Dispel myths and fears about contraceptives so 'consumer' perception of the method is as accurate as possible.

iv) Suggest different methods may suit different individuals or couples at various times, some methods can be used together, and it may help if both partners are happy with the one chosen.

v) Explain the correct use of each method is vital to its efficiency rating.

vi) Suggest any method is better than no method. There is a danger that if 'the pill' for example, is perceived as the only safe method, a couple without immediate access to it may take a fatalistic view, and not take any contraceptive precautions at all.

vii) In the absence of any method, or if sexual activity is not desired, even if contraceptives are available, the oral contraceptive '*NO*', should be used. This undoubtedly has side effects, which if not anticipated might involve anger, frustration or possible 'loss' of a partner. However these will only be temporary, and do not involve the most important factor, parenthood. Other side effects are the chance to think things over, and get help and advice if necessary.

Explore ways of saying 'no', verbal and non-verbal, in a way which does not threaten a relationship, nor infer rejection of the sexuality of the partner.

The contraceptive methods most often used by teenagers, according to Farrel [2] are withdrawal, the sheath, and the pill, so these might be considered first, particularly as the first two can be used without a medical consultation and hence discussion and instruction about the method may not take place.

Withdrawal (Being careful)
This is a widely used method for all age groups, so it is helpful to discuss it seriously, and put it in perspective. It involves the man taking his penis out of the vagina very near the time of climax, so the actual ejaculation takes place outside the woman's body.

Advantages

i) It does not involve any planning, except at the very last moment, and does show some degree of a caring attitude to pregnancy avoidance.

ii) It is free, but so are all the other methods.

Disadvantages
It requires considerable control on the part of the man, whose high level of sexual arousal will mean the biological reproductive system will be at maximum revs, and he has to judge the moment before 'ejaculatory inevitability'. A few drops of fluid are usually released from the penis well before the main ejaculation, and the man has absolutely no control over this. These can contain many millions of sperm. The woman may feel anxious, if not confident the man will be able to 'withdraw' in time. This may mean she will not enjoy love-making as much as she could.

Efficiency
Not very great, because of the factors mentioned. It has been suggested it may be about 50% efficient [128]. That is, of 100 women using the method for one

year, half would not be pregnant at the end of the year.

Myths

That it is a reliable method. The effectiveness will partly depend on the relative fertility of the couple, which is likely to be high in late teens and early twenties, and partly on practice of the method. Unfortunately during the 'practising' conception may occur.

The sheath

(This is also known as the condom, skin, protective, French letter, rubber, Johnny). This is a thin rubber sheath worn over the penis during love-making, so all the sperm are collected in the end and not released into the vagina. Sheaths are obtained rolled up, in small plastic or metal foil packets. They can have added lubricants or spermicides, and specially tested ones have the British Standard Kite mark on the pack (and yes, they can be coloured and have sculpted surfaces 'to increase pleasure' but check the quality of these).

Correct use is essential

How many packets have full instructions, and how many people are good at following written instructions?!

i)   Sheaths are very strong but have been made thin to allow maximum sensation for the male, so care must be taken not to tear or snag them, with nails or rings.

ii)   A few centimetres are unrolled, and the tip of the sheath pinched, to get rid of the air (which might form a bubble, stretching the rubber) and to make a space for the sperm to collect in.

iii)   The rest of the sheath is then unrolled onto the erect penis, well before actual intercourse, so the few drops of fluid and millions of sperm released early, can be caught. After the climax the sheath must be held on at the base of the penis, which should be withdrawn while still erect, so the hundreds of millions of sperm are kept in the far end, and cannot swim out round the rim.

iv)   Each sheath must only be used once.

v)   For extra safety a spermicide should be used as well, in case of leakage or the small possibility of the sheath tearing.

Advantages

i)   They are easy to obtain and are a male responsibility method.

ii)   They are free from Family Planning Clinics.

iii)   They can be bought from chemists and barbers, from vending machines in pubs and garages and from mail order firms, all with anonymity.

iv)   They help protect both partners from sexually transmitted infections.

v)   They help protect women from cervical cancer.

vi)   They can be seen to be used, and hence are a visual reassurance care is being taken.

vii)   The process of putting them on can become part of love-making.

viii)   They have no side effects (unless someone is allergic to rubber) and do not change body chemistry.

ix)   They are a suitable choice of contraceptive when sexual intercourse is relatively infrequent.

Disadvantages

i)   They may slip off, particularly after the climax, when the penis has lost some erection.

ii)   They may tear or split,

iii)   They may lessen sensation for the male slightly, though this can be helpful if the man is very sensitive.

Efficiency

If used correctly, with added spermicide, they can be 97% effective.

Myths

i)   That they seriously lessen sensation. Unlike the original sheaths made of leather or linen, modern ones are very thin. Prolonging intercourse may in fact give more pleasure, not less, to both partners.

ii)   People, such as the government, stick pins in them to keep up the birth rate, or make sure a girl is 'punished' for having sex, by becoming pregnant. Show an unopened pack, and how it is possible to see any pin hole made in it! Anyone can examine a pack before use, to confirm it has not been tampered with.

Chemicals

These can be obtained from FP clinics free, or from chemists. They are specifically designed to kill sperm, hence the term spermicide (cf homicide, fratricide, suicide ...). They are 'delivered' into the vagina in many forms, foaming tablets, soft jellies, creams, or aerosol foams. These last are first squeezed from their container into a smooth plastic 'applicator', which is then slid into the vagina so the spermicide can be placed high up, near or over, the neck of the womb.

Also C-film which is placed over the penis or put into the vagina, is one form of spermicide. This is not to be confused with 'cling film', excellent for other things, but which has no such chemicals and does not form an effective sheath either!

Chemicals alone are not a very safe method but must be used with a sheath, (where they may also aid lubrication and lessen the likelihood of tearing), and with the cap and can be useful as an additional method for couples using IUDs. There is evidence that spermicides have a protective effect against some sexually transmitted diseases.

The following methods can only be used after consultation with a doctor, so there will be some discussion and explanations of the method then.

'The Pill', Oral contraception

Between 50 and 80 million women in the world are using hormonal contraception (more than 3 million in this country) and this is the chosen method for more than 75% of older teenagers attending Family Planning

Clinics. There are many different types of contraceptive pill, which must be used according to the instructions, which will vary slightly for the various kinds, as explained by the doctor or nurse. (Mother's comment to teacher 'I can't think why Angela 'got caught', I gave her a pill every time she went out with her boyfriend'!)

There has been much publicity given to possible side effects of hormonal contraception, most relating to earlier much higher levels of the chemicals used in such pills over 20 years ago. Doses are now a tiny fraction of the earlier ones, and a wider range of synthetic hormones is available for use N.B. 'Natural' molecules of the hormones cannot be used because they are rapidly broken down by the liver, and are said to be not 'orally active', so the chemistry has to be changed very slightly to make them effective when taken in this way. A high level of monitoring is still maintained, so women on 'the pill' are asked to go for regular weight and blood pressure checks, and for questioning about headaches, which should always be taken seriously, or other pains. Many side effects, such as slight nausea, get better as the body gets used to 'the pill', in a similar way that it 'gets used to' a pregnancy, which has a similar contraceptive effect! (No extra conceptions occur when intercourse takes place during pregnancy, as no ova are released.)

Intensive long term studies on the side effects of hormonal contraceptives suggest that not only are they very safe, but that they confer extra benefits, over and above that of not becoming pregnant. So far these have not been given the same publicity as the early disadvantages.

Types of contraceptive pill
The combined pills
There are many low dose varieties of combined pill now available, each containing an oestrogen and a progesterone, usually taken for 21 days at a time. In one type of combined pill, the amount of the two hormones is the same balance in every pill. The contraceptive effect is threefold: by preventing ovulation, by keeping cervical mucus thick and impenetrable to sperm, and by minimising the thickening of the lining of the womb.

In another type of combined pill, the biphasic or triphasic pill, the balance of the two hormones is varied in two or three stages during the 21 day course, in a way which mimics the body's natural cycle, and enables a lower dose of oestrogen to be used.

In all types the 'sudden' loss of the pill hormones during the pill-free week, causes the lining of the womb to break down, in 'withdrawal bleeding', with often not so great a blood loss as during a real 'period'.

The mini pill, or progesterone only pill
This type of pill contains only one hormone, a progesterone, which is taken every day without a break. It is only slightly less efficient than the combined pill, and its main action seems to be in keeping the cervical mucus thick, so sperm cannot reach the womb. Ovulation may be supressed in some cycles and the womb lining may also be affected, so it would not be supportive to a fertilised ovum, should one occur.

The advantages of oral contraception

These include the ease of taking the pills, which does not have to be related to the time of intercourse, and their very high efficiency in preventing pregnancy. Combined pills are virtually 100% efficient when taken correctly, and the progesterone only pill only slightly less so, at 98% efficient.

Extra benefits of using oral hormonal contraceptives

i)   Less problems with periods, risk of iron deficiency anaemia down 50%, incidence of painful, heavy and irregular periods, and pre-menstrual tension, significantly reduced.

ii)   Reduction in cancer of the womb.

iii)   Reduction in breast diseases, (benign tumours show a 50–75% reduction) For the possible effect on breast cancer see below.

iv)   Ovarian cysts are virtually eliminated.

v)   Ovarian cancer may be reduced.

vi)   There is less risk of rheumatoid arthritis, (down 50% in some studies.)

vii)   Less inflammation of the Fallopian tubes.

viii)   Less pelvic inflammatory disease (PID) (which can be 10–70% less after one year on oral contraception).

ix)   Reduction in the number of ectopic pregnancies where the embryo implants in the Fallopian tube or elsewhere, instead of the womb.

Evidence from many sources about these benefits has been summarised by Ory [129] who estimates the use of oral contraception in the USA has prevented at least, 50 000 hospitalisations annually.

The disadvantages of oral contraception

The pill and cancer

Much publicity was given to two studies published in the Lancet (October 1983) one from America [180], the other from Oxford [181], suggesting a possible link between some types of oral contraception and the incidence of breast and cervical cancer. At a London conference of doctors [185] held to discuss those findings, both studies were thought to be equivocal, and 'cause and effect' not entirely proved. The American study on breast cancer was criticised for the telephone interview technique used, and for the questionable reliability of the test used to determine the progesterone potency of the pills implicated. In discussing the paper on the claimed relationship between oral contraception and cervical cancer it was regretted that the research did not take account of the age of first sexual activity, level of sexual activity and number of partners of the woman studied, as these factors are known to be a consideration in cervical cancer development.

The Committee on Safety of Medicines was also not convinced by the causal links suggested in the Lancet papers, and saw no reason for women to stop taking their pills immediately, but did recommend the use of lower dose pills where possible, and regular screening for cervical cancer.

The International Medical Advisory Panel of the IPPF (November, 1983) also evaluated the Lancet papers, and the known beneficial effects of oral

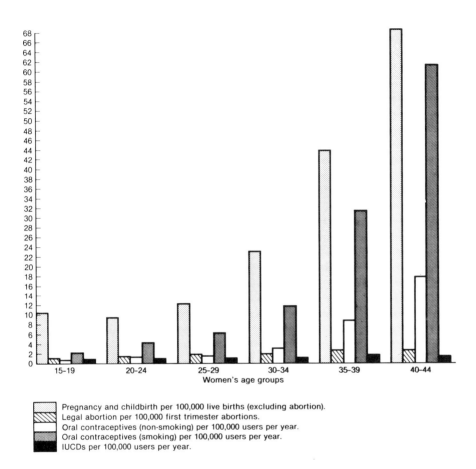

Figure 43   A comparison of mortality rates associated with different methods of birth control and childbirth. Source: U.S.A. data Tietze, C. et al (1979) Int. J. Gynae. Obstet. 16, 456.

contraception, and decided there was insufficient information to recommend modification of existing practice. (IPPF Medical Bulletin, 6 December 1983).

It is helpful to explain to the children that as it is very difficult even for experienced members of the medical profession to interpret the results of epidemiological studies, as so many variables have to be taken into account before real 'cause and effect' links can be made, it is very important not to be panicked by sensational headlines in the popular press, which often exaggerate possible effects and present them as proven facts. It is always wise for anyone concerned with any aspect of any drug to seek the advice of a doctor. The FPA has produced guide sheets and fact sheets on oral contraception, which include the recommendation for all women using it to check their breasts regularly and have cervical smear tests every 3–5 years.

The pill and side effects

The main side effect of the combined pill is to slightly increase the rate of blood clot formation, which could cause heart attacks, strokes or other thrombosis problems. These risks are increased for older women, and for those that smoke. Other concerns are that there may be a delay in the start of fertility after stopping oral contraception, and there is a very small risk that if a woman becomes pregnant while taking the combined pill, the developing foetus might be affected.

The progesterone only 'mini-pill', seems very free from side effects except for those causing irregularities of the menstrual cycle, and these may decrease with time in some women.

Certain types of drug may interact with some types of oral contraception, so it is important a doctor knows of all the medications taken by a patient. For relative actual mortality rates per 100 000 users per year, see bar chart FIG 43, where in no case are the methods shown to be more dangerous than the condition they are used to prevent, i.e. the risks of pregnancy and childbirth, which are, naturally, not given publicity. A comprehensive summary study of hormonal contraception factors is given in Population Reports, from the John Hopkins University [135].

All patients on oral contraception should discuss the relative risks of the different types, in detail, with their doctor. There are some contra-indications to taking 'the pill', so it is important for teachers not to talk as if they were suitable for all women. Another factor is the reliability of the user. Missed pills do matter, particularly with low dose pills, and instructions then usually include using an extra form of protection till the end of the cycle (or for 14 days of taking the progesterone only pill).

Discuss with children the social and psychological factors also involved, such as the importance of effective family limitation on a world scale, or of possible personal feelings such as that a girl on the pill is 'free to anyone', or that some women may resent being put 'at risk' perhaps not fully appreciating how relative these are.

Finally, perhaps explain that research continues, to find the lowest possible dose of hormones which will give effective contraceptive protection, while altering body chemistry by the least amount.

The Cap

There are several different types of cap, each acts as a barrier to sperm reaching the womb. The diaphragm can be demonstrated using the ortho-pelvic model (page 133). A cap must be initially 'fitted' by a doctor, who will select the right size. The woman is shown how to use it, and given training until she is both competent and confident. It must be used with a spermicide for maximum efficiency.

Advantages

i)   There are no side effects (unless there is an allergy to rubber).

ii)   It can be placed in the vagina, with the spermicide, up to three hours before intercourse. It cannot be felt by either partner.

iii)   A major advantage is that like the sheath it may help to protect from cancer of the cervix.

iv)   It is 97% efficient when used carefully and with a spermicide.

Disadvantages

The woman must feel happy about touching her vulva and inserting the cap correctly. She must also have a suitable environment in which to do this, and to remove it not less than eight hours after intercourse for correct checking, washing and storage. It should not be left in the vagina for much longer than this.

Myths

That it is difficult to use. With experience it only takes a few seconds to insert a cap correctly.

The coil (IUD, Loop, IUCD)

This is the *intra-uterine* contraceptive *d*evice or something placed inside the uterus (womb) to prevent conception. A range of shapes of plastic and plastic plus copper wire are available. They are inserted into the womb, by a doctor, through a narrow tube about the width of a drinking straw. This can be demonstrated using an overhead projector, and a transparency with an outline of a womb, actual size (FPA teaching card no 12 see page 160.) It is fascinating to see the 'coil' first disappear into the applicator tube, so this can be slid up the neck of the womb, and then reappear and regain its shape. The threads attached can be shown protruding from the cervix, where they can be regularly checked by the woman.

Advantages

i)   High efficiency, from 96–100% [131] depending on the type of coil and age of the patient. Once inserted the coil is effective immediately (hence its action as a 'morning after' device) and for years after, and no more action need be taken.

ii)   It is very suitable for women who have had a child (as it is easier to insert) but some types can be used for those who have not.

iii)   It is easily removed, by a doctor, if a pregnancy is desired.

Disadvantages

i) A coil may cause heavier periods, more vaginal discharge or cramp like pains. It may be rejected by the womb, and passed out (expulsion).

ii) It may aid the spread of pelvic infections if already present or caught later.

iii) Devices with copper wire have to be renewed every few years.

iv) Should a pregnancy occur there is a greater chance of a miscarriage or an ectopic pregnancy.

v) Very rarely the device may go into the wall of the womb, causing a 'perforation'.

Myths

Some people have the idea that coils are huge, made all of metal or can 'get lost'. Seeing and handling the very small, light devices will help here. Research continues into new shapes, and some coils have an added hormone, which is slowly released.

Sterilisation

This is nearly 100% efficient. Why not 100%? Because very rarely (1 in 1000) the tubes may join together again. Also, in a female, an ovum might have been in the lower part of the Fallopian tube, which is why other contraceptive precautions are needed right up to the time of the operation, and perhaps for one month after.

Advantages

i) It is very effective, for the female almost immediately, and for the male after two successive semen samples have shown no sperm are still present.

ii) No more action is needed. At least 100 million couples in the world have used sterilisation as a method of contraception, and it is increasingly in demand (Fifth International Conference on Voluntary Surgical Contraception, December 1983).

Disadvantages

i) It must be considered irreversible, so is only suitable when both partners are sure they will not want more children. Research continues on ways of making the operation more reversible.

Myths

Sterilisation lessens masculinity, femininity or sex drive, or causes ova and sperm to accumulate (in fact they dissolve and disappear).

The rhythm method

This is explained in some detail, on page 92. There are a variety of methods used to try and find the probable time of ovulation, and the efficiency of the method varies accordingly.

Advantages

i) It may be the only acceptable method for some couples with very strict religious or personal beliefs. Training is available for those wishing to use this method.

ii) It may help to space the children in a family. New thermometer design, or 'temperature probe' may assist accurate temperature recording, and new methods of detecting mucus changes, hormone levels and changes in the cervix are being researched so women can be trained in 'fertility awareness'.

Disadvantages

Very few women have absolutely regular cycles, and even they can be influenced by illness, excitements and changes in routine, making it very difficult to accurately predict ovulation.

The 'unsafe' days, when intercourse may not take place, require careful calculation, and can mean abstinence for 15–19 days or more of the cycle. One survey gave an average figure of 17, for 'unsafe' days [132].

Myths

That the method can be used 'instantly' by avoiding intercourse at 'about the middle of the cycle', with no calculations, records kept, or mucus change determination etc.

The shot, the injectable, the jab

This has been in use for mullions of women in the world for 15 years or more. There are two types of progesterone hormone being used in this way.

Advantages

This method has high efficiency and no other method need be used. It does not affect breast feeding, and like the 'mini' pill may be useful if a woman is sensitive to oestrogens.

Disadvantages

i) It may cause disturbances to the menstrual cycle, and irregular bleeding.

ii) There may be a delay in returning to fertility of up to one year after use.

iii) Depression and weight gain are other possible side effects.

'Morning after' contraception

(See page 92.) This may increasingly be used as it has been cleared by the Committee on Safety of Medicines to back up a known contraceptive failure (torn sheath or slipped cap), or unprotected intercourse, though not routinely. Contact the FPA BPAS or BAC for more details.

Breast feeding

Breast-feeding does have some effect on fertility, but is only effective as a contraceptive if suckling occurs at relatively frequent intervals, such as at least five feeds a day, each lasting for at least 10 minutes. This keeps the level of the milk-producing hormone prolactin, high enough to stop ovulation. In mothers who do not breast-feed their babies, ovulation returns within three to six weeks of the birth. The capacity to breast-feed does not depend on the size of the breasts, by the way, which is a question children sometimes ask. Human breast milk has recently been found to have an antiseptic effect on certain gut parasites, and so helps to prevent diarrhoea in babies.

Future methods
Hormonal methods
Research is proceeding into new ways of delivering hormones into the body, such as:

i)   once a month, or once a week pills
ii) microcapsules, thousands of minute biodegradable capsules injected into the blood stream providing a steady release of hormones for 6 months to a year, or longer,
iii) pellets, implanted under the skin, to release hormones such as the natural oestrogen,
iv) sniffing from a nasal spray may enable hormones such as GnRH analogues (page 144) to be taken directly into the cerebro-spinal fluid and hence quickly to the brain and hypothalamus,
v)   IUDs and vaginal rings and intra-cervical devices, which contain slowly released hormones acting locally, rather than systemically.

Spermicides
Research continues into chemicals which either kill sperm, or inhibit the enzyme normally released by them which enables them to fertilise the ovum, and also for new ways (creams, jells, foams) of delivering these into the vagina.

Prostaglandins (see page 147)
Synthetic versions could be used in a vaginal pessary, or tampon, either after unprotected intercourse but before the next period, or, if a period was late, to cause 'menstrual induction'.

Vaccination methods
These are being developed to counteract

i)   the human chorionic gonadotrophin (hCG) produced on implantation,
ii) the zona pellucida region around the ovum, making it impenetrable to sperm.
iii) the sperm themselves (some women naturally develop an immune response against their partner's sperm).

Barrier methods
New types of cap, or sponges, for insertion into the vagina, are being developed.

Male methods
Hormones have been used to try and 'switch' off the production of male LH and FSH, and hence testosterone and sperm development. So far these have not proved consistently successful, and have also sometimes produced side effects, such as nausea and loss of libido. A nasal hormone spray might also be possible for men using GnRH analogues, as for women.

Maturation of sperm in the epididymis, has been interfered with by using chemicals, either directly injected into the testes, or to form a plug in the sperm duct, or by taking a chemical orally. Gossypol, a phenolic compound from cotton plants has been tried in China for this last purpose, but there have been many side effects and a high toxicity shown in experimental animals.

Research goes on into methods of preventing the so called 'capacitation' changes which sperm need to undergo in the female tract to act effectively.

Note to Teachers

Two particular factors have affected research into male reproduction control.

i)   It has proved very difficult to reverse male hormone production, as there is no natural 'switch off' mechanism, as in the female cycle. Immediate prospects of a universal 'male pill' therefore seem unlikely.

ii) When sperm production or maturation is supressed, this process must be reliably completely successful. Because of the 110 million of sperm usually formed per day, if sub-lethal damage occurred by using a contraceptive chemical, enough mutant or abnormal sperm might survive to be capable of fertilising an ovum, leading to an abnormal foetus.

Methodology

Because the details of the contraceptive methods change, it may be advisable to use contemporary posters, actual contraceptives (sheaths and transparent caps show up well on an overhead projector) current leaflets and slides, rather than relying solely on a film, (though three are listed later). It may be helpful to have a speaker from the FPA or BAC initially, who could perhaps help in a team teaching situation, where the teacher does some of the explanations.

Remember there will, sadly, probably always be a few young people who cannot initially be helped by contraceptive education as they have a need to become pregnant to prove they are grown up, or feminine, or have a 'role' to identify with, or for gaining attention, or that they are not in control of their lives ... and other most complex reasons. Those who are motivated to take responsibility for their behaviour in the future, will benefit from accurate knowledge and a chance to discuss alternatives openly.

N.B. It is obviously highly desirable to keep any contraceptive kits and materials in immaculate condition, and attractively presented. Any item showing signs of educational fatigue should be renewed at once.

Resources
Population studies

1.   FPA fact sheets Available from the Family Planning Association
     B1 (0) World Population Statistics
     B5 (6) Population Statistics – Sources
     B3 (7) Population and Medical Statistics
     B4 (17) The age structure of the population of Great Britain
     I1 (4) Birth rate trends
     I3 (9) Births by Age of Mother and Legitimacy
     B2 (14) Population Background
2.   1982 *World Population Data Sheet*. Population Reference Bureau Inc., USA, and from IPPF.
3.   1979 *Family Planning in Five Continents*. IPPF. Details of government policies, public and private family planning programmes, sex education provision, and government legislation.

4. 1980 *Women in Society.* A wall chart on the health, education, employment, political and legal status of women in 128 countries. IPPF.
5. *Population Handbook.* Haupt A. & Kane T. T. 1978 Population Reference Bureau Inc. USA, and from IPPF.
6. *Population Today.* McGraw E. 1979. Kaye & Ward Ltd. Very visual presentation of the major factors affecting population growth.
7. *Proposals for a National Policy on Population.* McGraw E. 1981. Population Concern. Discussion on a national policy on population in the UK.
8. *The Shape of Things to Come?* Population Concern. The future needs of five countries with expanding populations, India, China, Mexico, Kenya and Egypt, projected to the year 2000.
9. *Changing fertility in the Developing World, and its Impact on Global Population growth.* Hall, Ray 1984. Geography. Vol 69 Part 1 Jan. 1984

Contraception

1. *Resource list on Family Planning.* HEC.
2. FPIS LEAFLETS, Background information for teachers. See their order form for recent titles including fact sheets and information sheets.
3. *Brook Advisory Centres* The education department provide many leaflets, with clear line drawings, fact sheets, and discussion sheets, such as on relationships with parents, teenage marriage, unplanned pregnancy etc.
4. *BPAS material* The British Pregnancy Advisory Service can supply leaflets on topics such as 'Morning-after' birth control, vasectomy, female sterilisation, vasectomy reversal operations, and a booklet on post-coital contraception
5. *Wyeth.* Fold out card leaflet on oral contraceptives, their mode of action and effect on the normal menstrual cycle. Attractively presented coloured diagrams explain the working of the combined and triphasic combined pill, the progesterone only pill, and show the relative risks of some birth control methods.
6. *Multicultural materials* The FPIS produce leaflets on family planning, in several Asian languages and a booklet on family planning in 5 languages and English is available from Wyeth, and LRC.
7. *Books and reports*
   i) *Contraception, A teacher's guide.* Andrew S, Jenks J, Long Z. 1975. ILEA. A most helpful summary of resources for teaching about contraception, children's questions, a description of methods and notes on sex and the law.
   ii) Guilleband J. 1980. 2nd Ed 1983 *The Pill.* Oxford University Press
   iii) *'Woman's Own' Birth Control.* Smith M. 1980. Hamlyn.
   iv) *Natural Family Planning: A teacher's handbook.* Marshall J. 1978. Catholic Marriage Advisory Council.
   v) *Contraception* Kane, P. A *Which?* consumer association publication.
   vi) *Family Planning, guide to methods.* IPPF.
   vii) *The case for the condom.* Cossey D. BAC.
   viii) *Men, Sex and Contraception.* FPA.
8. *Pharmaceutical companies providing educational material.*
   i) *London Rubber Industries,* North Circular Road, Chingford, London E4. A wide range of information on barrier methods.
   ii) *Ortho Pharmaceuticals,* Saunderton, High Wycombe, Bucks.
   iii) *Searle Laboratories,* P.O. Box 58, Lane End Rd., High Wycombe Bucks, HP12 4HL.
   iv) *Schering Chemicals,* Education Service, Pharmaceutical Division, Burgess Hill, West Sussex RH15 9NE.
   v) *Syntex Pharmaceuticals* Ltd. Syntex House, St. Ives Rd., Maidenhead, Berks SL6 1RD.
   vi) *Wyeth Laboratories,* Taplow, Maidenhead, Berks.
9. *For use with children*
   i) Comics such as *Too great a risk.* (see page 203) FPIS. and *Don't rush me.* (see

page 203). Wandsworth Council for Community Relations.

ii) Booklets e.g. *Family Planning.* Wyeth. Clear line diagrams and simple explanations of all the main methods, *Introducing Contraception. IPPF* and *Starting the Pill,* Schering, which clearly explains the benefits and the risks.

iii) *Flip chart* Family Planning. Wyeth. Enlarged version of the booklet diagrams. Very clear simplified drawings (but relate womb to actual size and position, see page 130).

10. *Leaflets for older children.*

i) FPIS leaflets, see item 2

ii) *Safe Sex: Contraception.* Brook Advisory Centre. A leaflet summarising all the main methods.

iii) *What you need to know about the sheath.*

iv) *What you need to know about spermicides.* BAC

11. *Films*

i) *Responsibility.* 16mm Colour. 20 mins. Eothen for LRC Productions. 1976. Specifically made for teenagers, this film puts contraception into the context of personal relationships, and behaviour choices, by using cartoon and real life scenes. Teacher's notes available. From Guild Sound and Vision.

ii) *To Plan your Family.* 16mm Colour. 10 mins. British version 1970, Boulton Hawker. All the methods are discussed, and the reproductive organs shown by means of coloured drawings. Could be used as a lead into, or summary of, family planning. Teacher's notes. Obtainable from Concord Film Council.

iii) *Conception and Contraception.* 16mm Colour 25 mins. 1980. Schering. Colourful drawings and animations show conception, menstruation, fertilisation and pregnancy, there is discussion on the reasons for contraceptives, and a description of all the main methods. A presenter's guide, with the film text and background information is available, and associated booklets reinforce the information given in the film. Available from Vision Associates.

Chapter 10

PARENTHOOD

Gestation and birth

Leading on from work emphasising the importance of choosing whether or not to become a parent, the pressures to 'achieve' parenthood could be discussed, and that there may be couples who will not wish to have children, ever. Leaflets are available from the British Organisation of Non-Parents, BON [137] with questions on 'am I parent material?', and case histories of couples who have chosen not to have a family.

An advisable plan for people who *do* wish to become parents could then be formulated and that it should start with preconception care, so both parents can be as fit as possible, to prepare for the pregnancy (see page 97).

Conception

Revise the facts of conception, the most likely time to conceive, and that although only one sperm actually penetrates the ovum when fertilisation occurs, many hundreds of sperm are needed to ensure this can happen, by removing the layer of cells round the ovum. It does not really pay to get to the ovum first! Better to be about, perhaps, 256th?! (and that one was *you!*)

Subfertility

About 10–15% of couples will have some difficulty in conceiving, and might seek help if this has not happened within about a year, for a couple where the woman is under 30, and about 6 months if over 30. They can then have a series of tests where possible reasons for the problem may be identified, which in about half the cases will be found to be in the man and half in the woman.

There are many causes of infertility, some related to overall health. The Wynns [138], have suggested that between 23 and 54% of women attending fertility clinics in hospitals may be very underweight, which can cause a lack of periods, and disrupted cycles. Also the quality of diet, amount of smoking and drinking alcohol, in both men and women, can affect fertility. Other causes may be of a more complicated physiological or psychological nature, so expert help may be needed. This can involve, for a few, fertilisation of the ovum outside the mother's body, and implantation into her womb. For others, artificial insemination, either by husband or donor, may be possible.

Further information is available:

i) 'Which'? publication 1972. 'Infertility', Consumers Association.

ii) British Pregnancy Advisory Service leaflets. Infertility Investigation, Sperm Counts and Semen Analysis, Artificial Insemination AIH, and Artificial Insemination AID, which includes discussion of the legal position of children conceived by this method.

Unplanned pregnancies

It is clear that great emotional and physical difficulties can occur if a pregnancy is not a planned event, and the girl or woman does not seek pre-conception or ante-natal care. This is perfectly illustrated by the real life interview with 'Susan', on the *Hello Gorgeous* tape (page 203). The feelings of another girl who finds she is unwillingly or unwittingly pregnant are explored in the film sequence from the 3 part series *If Only We'd Known,* on free loan from Concord Films council, or Central Film Library, Part 1 *Debbie and Linda:*

i) 8 minute discussion trigger (and see page 225). Prime the class that 16 year-old Debbie is not necessarily going to get good advice from her older friend Linda. Extensive teaching notes and a work card set are available from the HEC or the Spastics Society, who jointly produced the films. The various options open to Debbie and her boyfriend Terry can be detailed, and the advantages and disadvantages of each discussed.

ii) A five minute documentary follows, showing another girl, Fiona with her sympathetic, family doctor. He confirms she is pregnant, giving her a pelvic examination (always done with a nurse present if the doctor is male). This is an extremely useful sequence, as fear of such an examination may prevent some women seeking advice early, particularly in a first pregnancy, as they may not have had one before. A similar examination is not usually necessary again until late in pregnancy.

Previous teaching, about the soft, stretchy, vagina, the idea of touching the vulva area (for tampon/cap insertion etc.) will all help generate confidence in this simple, quick procedure. If occasionally in P.E. lessons, relaxing exercises can be done, in the lying on back, knees bent and apart, position, this again would help make the occasion more acceptable. Every woman is advised to have cervical smear tests done regularly, whether or not she has a baby.

See page 225 for details of part II and III of *If only we'd known.*

Perinatal and Infant Mortality

The film series, *If only we'd known,* was made in response to general concern in the health care services, and voluntary organisations for handicapped children, about the factors affecting the perinatal and infant mortality rates in the UK. These terms are defined as deaths occurring as shown in FIG 44.

222

Actual rates and numbers

The perinatal mortality rate in England and Wales is now dropping, with a 10% fall between 1979 and 1980. However at 13.3 [139] it still does not compare very favourably with other North European Countries such as

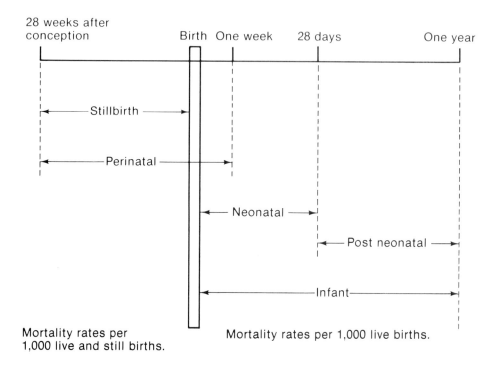

Figure 44   Perinatal and infant mortality rates at different stages.

Sweden, (with 9.4 in 1978). The infant mortality rate has also dropped, from 12.8 in 1979 to 12 in 1980, but this is higher than for any other country in North Europe except for Ireland [118]. Infant mortality rates for every country are given on the World Data Sheet [118]. It has been estimated that 9000 to 10 000 babies in England and Wales die, in the perinatal and neonatal period each year, and that from one third to one half of these deaths are preventable [140].

Why is this number so high?

Table 13   Comparison of perinatal and infant mortality rates in different groups.

Perinatal & infant mortality rates, per 1,000 total births England & Wales. 1979. OPCS Monitor DH3 81/1		Perinatal Mortality	Infant Mortality
Age of mother	Under 16	33	34
	16–19	19	20
	20–24	15	14
	25–29	13	11
	30–34	14	11
	Over 35	21	14
Social Class Legitimate births.	I	10	10
	II	12	10
	III	14	11
	IV	17	14
	V	19	19
Number of Children.	First born	16	11
	Second children	11	11
	4th or more.	23	17

Contributing factors

The following factors affect perinatal and infant mortality rates in England and Wales.

A birth weight of 2500g (5lb 9oz) is considered low and such babies are at a greater risk of death or handicap. It can be due to babies being born too soon, i.e. prematurely, or full term babies which have not grown enough. Various factors have been implicated, e.g. smoking, drinking alcohol, some infections, poor nutrition, stress, an unwanted pregnancy, a previous pregnancy loss, and low socio-economic status of the mother.

i)   Low weight babies 2500g (5lbs 9oz) or less are at a greater risk of death or handicap [141].

ii) The British births survey in 1970, showed about 17% of perinatal deaths, were due to the mother becoming pregnant again too soon, before her body had fully recovered from the previous birth.

iii) Higher mortality rates are found among illegitimate babies, and those of single, unsupported mothers are nearly twice the rate of those of married mothers [139].

iv) The perinatal death rate is nearly five times higher in children of mothers receiving only late ante-natal care, than in children of mothers attending early [142].

v) Congenital defects. Certain types of defects occur at a steady rate, only increasing in incidence if the mother is over 35. Other conditions can be caused during the pregnancy by infections such as Rubella (see page 199) drugs such as alcohol, or a poor diet lacking in vitamins.

Action needed

The need for effective pre-conception, ante-natal and post-natal care is clear, and education could help a great deal to promote an understanding, acceptance and effective use of the services available. This can be done in a positive way, with reassurance about the benefits to be gained rather than a close examination by pupils of the previous statistics, which might cause them anxiety and fear.

Health Authorities have been trying to improve the take up of ante-natal care for some time, and many have been able to do so in spite of financial and other difficulties.

The Government has set up a Maternity Services Advisory Committee, which in its first report stressed the desirability of a more flexible approach to ante-natal care and suggested the setting up of local Maternity Services Liaison Committees. A teacher from the sex education team could perhaps keep in touch with such a committee, and be able to act on identified educational priorities for schools. Its second report emphasises that a woman having a baby is not ill, and recommends she be allowed to discuss a 'birth plan' giving her preferences.

Classwork

Revise the benefits for both parents-to-be of going to a doctor or clinic before, or early on in a pregnancy.

i) They get emotional support, and adapt to the idea of parenthood,

ii) They make friends who will be having their young families at the same time,

iii) They can be reassured on physical matters, both about the baby and the mother,

iv) They get the chance to learn about forthcoming changes, and correct self help,

v) They prepare for the birth process, so confidence can be increased,

vi) They get information on maternity benefits, free dental treatment, etc.

vii) They know any possible problems can be identified early, and preventive measures can be taken.

Read from the report *Towards Healthy Babies* [141], which suggests that probably over one quarter of mothers in the UK are not receiving their first ante-natal check until well after the third month of their pregnancy. Why might this be? Show the HEC poster ... *don't wait for your baby to prod you into going to the doctor* again, and ask the class to work in groups, to list reasons which might prevent expectant mothers, or fathers, from seeking help.

i)   They may not be aware of the pregnancy (revise the signs and see page 253).
ii) They may not want to accept the pregnancy (as in *Hello Gorgeous*, page 203).
iii) They may not know that checks are needed early, or who to go to for these.
iv) She may be afraid of the examination involved, or the medical profession in general.
v)   They may not be bothered, no motivation? Where do responsibilities for parenthood start?

Now list ways in which such people could be helped, and see how many are similar to those suggested in the reports [141, 146].

i)   Practical help with transport to and from the ante-natal clinic, or GP, who may have ante-natal sessions.
ii) Avoiding long waits at the clinic, by having a realistic appointments system.
iii) The provision of evening and week-end clinics.
iv) Being looked after by the same doctor, nurse or midwife each time, so a relationship can be built up. Community midwives can be involved in this way. Sometimes in a 'Domino' (Domiciliary in and Out) system, including only a 6 hour stay in hospital after the birth.
v)   Involving the expectant fathers, as they also need support.
vi) Creche facilities at the clinic for pre-school children brought to the ante-natal clinic.
vii) Refreshments being available, and a friendly social atmosphere.

Won't all this cost a lot? Possibly, but far less than the cost of looking after handicapped children, put at £373 000 for care for life [141] or premature babies which could have been prevented (some can not), or the cost in human unhappiness this can cause.

Could the school help in any way? Perhaps in the last two areas mentioned, by collecting and repairing toys and books, or volunteers, boys and girls, helping with toddlers or pouring teas?

Expectant fathers

Involving expectant fathers can be followed up too. Might fathers feel 'left out' with all this attention being focussed on the mother? What do they feel about and expect of the pregnancy, birth and fatherhood? Do they realise special care and help may be needed? Use *If Only We'd Known* Part II *Clinic Talk*. This 6 minute film shows Debbie at the ante-natal clinic and the concern shown by her boyfriend Terry, who wants to be involved.

After discussion (see teacher's notes and work card) show Part III, *Sarah and Eric* (4 minutes). Eric is not very sympathetic when his wife tells him the clinic has suggested she must rest for a week. He tries to persuade her to go on working right up until the birth of their (second) child.

From this can come discussion on the rights of pregnant women at work, such as for paid time off to go to the ante-natal clinic, the extent of maternity pay and leave, the right to return to the job up to 29 weeks after the week of the birth, the maternity grant, now not contributory, and so on. Show how to use the HEC *Pregnant at Work*, and *Pregnancy. What you need to know*, leaflets to extract this information. One report showed employers were not always aware of provisions needed for maternity care, though some were supportive and helpful.

Preparation for pregnancy and birth

There are a large number of teaching approaches possible here, but it is not suitable to try and give the whole ante-natal course in school! A selection of important stages is needed to further understanding of the facilities available locally, and nationally.

Real Experiences

Enlist the help of mothers and fathers to be, the National Childbirth Trust has local members willing to help. They might be able to visit the school at various stages of the pregnancy or when breast feeding, to explain their feelings, what ante-natal care they had had, the parentcraft classes provided locally, and so on. They may agree to be interviewed at home, by a small group of children who could record answers to questions previously decided by the class and teacher. Sensitivity and tact are required here. If several different couples could be recorded, a range of experiences and feelings could be collected over the years.

Ante-natal clinics

i)   Doctors, midwives or nurses might spare the time to come and explain the running of the local clinic.

ii)   Photographs could be taken showing the facilities, the staff, and, with their permission, a group of expectant parents at a 'relaxation' class.

iii)   Small groups of children might be able to visit for a short time, or help in the way already suggested, (page 225).

Preparation for Parenthood

This course for schools produced by the National Childbirth Trust, Newcastle-upon-Tyne in 1980, has excellent material giving detailed guidelines for selected class work. Foetal development, normal pregnancy, ante-natal preparation, labour and birth and the new family, the responsibilities, commitment and problems of parenthood are all explained. Visual aids are suggested, and work sheets included for evaluation.

Background notes for teachers

The expected date of birth

It is never possible to say exactly how old the embryo or foetus is, because the precise days of fertilisation and implantation will not be known. The length of the pregnancy is dated from the first day of the last menstrual period (LMP), and is taken as being about 40 weeks or 280 days (a little longer than the well known '9 months'). A range of between 37 and 42 weeks, 259–293 days is however considered normal [51].

Conception may have taken place at any time during or after that menstrual period, if intercourse occurred, but as the most likely time for this to have happened is the middle of the cycle, the foetal age is usually taken from this mid-point, and so is two weeks younger than the weeks of pregnancy (see FIG 45). There can be some confusion when labelling drawings and diagrams, so it is advisable to give both the weeks of the pregnancy (sometimes called the post menstrual weeks) and the weeks of foetal development. There will be some variation in the size of a foetus at any one stage in a pregnancy due to several factors:

i) the time of conception, which as explained above may vary by up to 3 weeks

ii) the growth rate of the foetus, which will vary a little within a normal range,

iii) the genetic size of the baby at 'full term', which can vary, and is also influenced by the size of the womb, which restricts foetal growth in the final stages of pregnancy [51]

iv) whether or not it is a multiple birth.

Doctors can check the size of the womb at about the 10th week of pregnancy when it may have enlarged sufficiently to be 'felt' over the top of the pubic bone. The size of the foetus can be estimated when it has grown large enough to be detected by feeling through the abdominal wall, and if necessary earlier by an ultrasonic scan.

Hormonal changes during pregnancy

When an ovum has been fertilised in the Fallopian tube, it divides to form a minute blackberry-shaped hollow ball of cells, which is slowly moved down to the womb, and embeds in the lining. Part of this ball of cells forms the actual embryo, and part the chorion. This last structure immediately produces a hormone, human Chorionic Gonadotropin, hCG, (very similar in effect to LH). Its action is to maintain the corpus luteum (yellow body) and to increase its size, and hence its production of hormones, particularly progesterone. The lining of the womb therefore remains thick, and does not collapse, as it would at menstruation. The presence of hCG hormone in the blood, and subsequently in the urine is one of the first signs of pregnancy, and its detection forms the basis of the 'pregnancy test'.

The chorion develops into the placenta, which gradually takes over the role of producing hormones from the corpus luteum, which then slowly withers. The placenta manufactures large amounts of progesterone (which has a calming effect on the body) and other hormones, which maintain and develop the pregnancy.

Growth in the mother

The changes in the mother's body are gradual at first, but foetal growth accelerates in the middle 'trimester' (i.e. the middle 3 month period) and then slows down again at the end of the pregnancy.

Table 14   A breakdown of growth during pregnancy, accounting for the mother's gain in weight.

Growth During Pregnancy	
The womb	From pear-sized and about 60g (2 oz.) to more than netball sized and weighing 1,000 g (approx. 2 lbs. 3 oz.)
The baby	From less than a full stop, and a minute fraction of a gram, to about 45 – 50cm (18 – 20 inches) and 3,300 g (approx. 7 lbs. 5 oz.)
The placenta	From nothing, to a flat cake like organ about 20 cms (8 inches) diameter of 676 g (approx. 1 lb. 8 oz.)
Blood volume	This increases in the mother by about 40% weighing about 1,568 g (approx. 3 lbs. 8oz.)
Fluid	Up to 1 litre of this is amniotic fluid round the baby, and extra fluid is retained in other parts of the mother's body, ie. 2,240 g (approx. 5 lbs. 0 oz.) in all.
Breasts	Increase in size in preparation for breast feeding, of a least 448 g (approx. 1 lb. 0 oz.)
Fat stores	These can accumulate in the mother 2,016 g (4 lbs. 8 oz.)
Total	11,248 g about 25 lbs.

The overall weight gain is substantial and consists of increases as in the table above.

These figures are only typical, and will vary from person to person. For more realism bring in an $11\frac{1}{4}$Kg (25lbs) equivalent in potatoes or packs of sugar. Get each child to lift this weight and assess the effect of carrying it around each day. No wonder expectant mothers need extra rest, and may tire quickly towards the end of their pregnancies!

Nutrition

Because the mother must supply the 'raw materials' for all the growth listed previously, how much, and what she eats is obviously of great importance. It must be adequate in both quantity and quality. What might be particularly necessary?

A class might be able to suggest the need for iron, to make all the extra blood; protein for muscles and other tissues; calcium for the baby's bones and teeth; vitamins, needed by both mother and child . . . etc.

When a woman is pregnant her body switches to a 'priority selection' system in favour of the baby. This means all the necessary items will be extracted from the blood by the placenta, and the mother will get what's left!

Contrary to popular belief however, her teeth are not affected, though dental treatment is free during this time, If a mother enters pregnancy underweight, or tries to 'slim', during it, the baby may not be able to grow properly, (even though given top priority by the body) and the mother's health will also be affected. Such people are obviously 'at risk'! The opposite, putting on too much weight, should also be avoided, and 'eating for two – adults' is not required. Advice on suitable foods and quantities will be given by the doctor, nurse or midwife, and weight checks are done at ante-natal clinics to make sure all is well. Expectant mothers do sometimes get cravings for certain foods and conversely some may 'go off' favourite foods or drinks. It is not known why this happens though the physiological changes in pregnancy do alter perceptions of smell and taste, as many women will testify.

Smoking in pregnancy
Why might this not be such a brilliant idea? Not because it 'stains the baby yellow' as one exam answer suggested!
Some facts
Discuss these too when smoking and drugs are considered in health education in general.

i) Smoking in pregnancy lowers the birth weight of the baby on average by about 200g (7oz). The heavier the smoking, the lighter the baby. Twice as many babies of smokers as non-smokers come into the high risk, low birth-weight category, probably due to lack of foetal growth, rather than being born too soon, though there is an increased risk of this as well.
ii) Recent research, documented in a report by the Spastics Society, has shown that mothers who have smoked for more than 6 years, are very much more likely to have pregnancy problems due to difficulties with the placenta.
iii) Children of mothers who smoke heavily during pregnancy may have an increased risk of being mentally or physically retarded, well into childhood.

The effects of smoking are many, but include that of the inhaled carbon monoxide, which joins with the red blood cells better than oxygen does but is no use in respiration for either the mother or the baby. Smoking three cigarettes, quickly, can lower the oxygen carrying capacity of the blood by one tenth. Nicotine is known to cause small blood vessels to narrow, so those in the placenta may also be constricted in this way; not good conditions for a healthy baby.

For anyone wishing to become a parent it would seem sensible to try and give up, or lower smoking well before conception, and certainly to give this top priority during the pregnancy.

Discuss the HEC poster *'Do you want a cigarette more than you want your baby?* How else could expectant mothers be helped to stop smoking?

Other research (JAMA 1983. 250, 499) suggests a strong link between smoking and cervical cancer, another good reason for giving it up.

Alcohol in pregnancy
Alcohol is a depressant, which affects the nervous system: it easily crosses the placenta, and circulates round the baby's blood in the same concentration as that of the mother. Even small amounts may have some effect on the developing nervous system. Doctors at a London hospital [163] have recently

found that women in social classes I–III who have more than 10 alcoholic drinks per week (one drink defined as a unit of 10g of alcohol, i.e. approximately 1 glass of wine or 1 measure of spirits, or half a pint of beer) are more than twice as likely as light drinkers (5 drinks per week) to have a low birth-weight baby. This effect may start before, or in the very early weeks of pregnancy. Women in all social classes were found to be over three times more likely to have low birth-weight babies if they both drank heavily, and smoked. The National Council of Women have documented evidence [164] suggesting that heavy drinking during pregnancy, either daily (possibly at the 6 drink level) or less frequent but heavy, or only occasional but very heavy 'binges', can all lead to damage to the developing child (the foetal alcohol syndrome). Such babies tend to be physically abnormal, and mentally retarded [141]. The NCW report stresses the need for LEAs to recommend that schools and colleges include in their curricula teaching about the effects of alcohol and other drugs on the unborn child.

In all work on foetal development, teachers should emphasise it is during the first three months of pregnancy that the organs, limbs etc., of the child are differentiating, i.e. becoming distinguished from each other, and the foetus is particularly vulnerable to drugs and infections reaching it through the placenta. It is therefore extremely important that a woman knows when she is pregnant, and has planned for this event.

Birth

Children have a great deal of knowledge about birth, of abnormal, difficult or unusual births that is, such as multiple births, Siamese twins, births in cars and planes, delivered by policemen, or, with no help available etc! They seem to gather these impressions from an early age, and have recently added equally amazing ones (to them) of naked women standing up, and the baby being born 'on the hard floor' as one girl put it. There have been many birth sequences shown on television, and not all parents have either known their children have been watching, or felt able to discuss the process with them afterwards. It would therefore seem very appropriate to emphasise that the vast majority (75%) of babies are born normally, and parents can get help in training for this event.

Normal birth

Explain the mother's body has been getting ready for the birth for 40 weeks, (from as long as Easter to Christmas). The preparation inside the body is helped by the hormone relaxin, which softens the ligaments of the pelvis, to make it more flexible, and also softens the neck of the womb so it may open more easily.

The mother knows when the birth process has started, and 'labour' has begun, when one or all of the following happen:

i)   She can feel the womb contracting, at regular, but long intervals, about 20 minutes or so. (It may in fact have been 'practising' these contractions during the previous months.)

ii)   She has a 'show' of pinkish mucus, which has come from the cervix.

iii)   Less often, she feels a leak or gush of fluid from the vagina which means the membranes round the baby have broken, and its private swimming pool is beginning to drain out.

The birth process: The first stage

Because the cervix has remained closed during pregnancy to 'keep the baby in' as it were, the first thing that must happen is for it to enlarge and open. This can be demonstrated using a baby doll inside a child's polo necked sweater. (Turn the sleeves inside, as they are the wrong end to be Fallopian tubes!) Show how the cervix, the 'polo' neck, has been closed, by bunching it together, and then how it will be gradually pulled open, and up, by the muscles of the womb. Give small pulls on the jersey at regular intervals to simulate this action.

Explain this process can take some time, hours and hours, especially for a first birth, as the cervix will not have been open before (as with a brand new jersey!). The mother cannot actively help at this stage, except by relaxing, walking around if she wishes, keeping occupied, reading perhaps. When the contractions are closer together, at about 5–10 minute intervals, it is wise to be where medical help can be given if necessary, as the transition to the next stage may be near.

The second stage

The muscles of the womb now begin to contract in a different way, so they are squeezing down on the baby, which is therefore pushed strongly, through the wide open cervix, down the stretching vagina, and out!

The mother can help during this process by reinforcing the action of the womb by pushing hard herself with her abdominal muscles, while keeping the vagina and pelvic floor muscles relaxed, as she may have been taught to do. This is tiring work, real 'hard labour', but it does not usually last nearly as long as the first stage, perhaps from a few minutes to half an hour or so. The muscles of the womb are not under voluntary control, the mother cannot 'decide' when they are going to contract next, but they are the most powerful of all human muscles, (better even than those of Mr. Universe!) and are designed specifically for pushing out babies! Mothers can often now choose which position is most comfortable for them during this stage.

The third stage

The womb contracts again after a few minutes, to push out the placenta and membranes, the 'afterbirth', which will be checked to see none remains inside. It is much larger than many people expect, and has had the vital role of absorbing nutrients from the mother's blood, and passing waste products back, through the millions of tiny villi, which have total surface area of about 11 square metres.

The womb continues to contract over the next few days and weeks, and reduces in size rapidly back to its original pear shape.

The father's role

The father can help a great deal during the birth, if both he and the mother wish, by sharing in her experience emotionally and physically, by keeping her company, perhaps rubbing her back if it aches, and in the final stages helping her concentrate on the breathing control system they may have learnt together, so she feels in control of the situation.

The new baby

More people are now accepting the ideas of Leboyer [151] that it helps the baby if it can be born into a peaceful atmosphere with dimmed lights, and quiet sounds, and the reassurance of being placed at once in contact with its mother's body, to be gently supported and held. The 'bonding' between mother, father and child can begin.

The umbilical cord is cut when it has finished pulsating, and all the blood from the placental villi has returned to the baby's body. In some cases it may be medically necessary to give the baby help with its breathing before it is held. For about 10% of deliveries the parents will be advised the safest method would be by Caesarian operation.

Teaching about birth

A sequence of slides showing all stages of birth has been selected by the National Childbirth Trust, from the Camera Talks sets *Birth a shared experience*, and *Tranquil Delivery*. It is explained, with a commentary, in their *Preparation for Parenthood* course book for teachers (page 250).

It is helpful to talk about the birth process first, and then use the slides, so questions can be answered as they arise. Beware of children feeling faint, even at this stage. Without precipitating mass hysteria explain how usual this is (often for the boys) how to recognise the feeling and put the head down! Stress there is no disgrace in feeling faint, it is a normal human reaction for some, when any medical matters, or blood are discussed.

Questions may arise on:

i) where it is 'best' to have a baby, at home or in hospital
ii) the tests done during pregnancy
iii) induced births (1 in 3 of all births at the moment)
iv) whether the father should be present or not
v) forceps delivery, breech births, Caesarian births, episiotomy
vi) pain relief techniques, these are very important for promoting confidence so explain research continues for new methods, such as the 'obstetric pulsar', which makes use of low voltage electrical current on the mother's back, to counteract any pain
vii) monitoring the state of the baby during the birth
viii) the position of the mother for the birth
ix) if it will be possible to hold the baby immediately after birth
x) whether breast feeding or bottle feeding 'is best'.

Most are discussed in detail in the valuable publication for BBC TV. *That's Life*: called *Having a baby, advice and information sheet*, prepared by the Spastics Society, March 1982, and available from them. Each situation is discussed in context, and the pros and cons for a decision either way are given.

It is advisable for teachers to take a fairly 'neutral' line in answering such questions. It would be lovely to think every woman could have a 'natural' birth, if she wished, in whatever position suited her best, but there are many reasons why this may not always be possible.

Suggest perhaps that every birth is different, the best will be done under the circumstances, and we can all help to make sure that this is so, and that the wishes of parents are given value.

Some societies working towards such a goal are:

i) The National Childbirth Trust, 9 Queensborough Terrace, London W2 3TB.

ii) AIMS, Association for Improvements in the Maternity Services, C/o E. Cockerell, 21 Franklin Gardens, Hitchin, Herts.

iii) Active Birth Movement, 32 Cholmeley Crescent, Highgate, London N6.

Resources
Preparation for pregnancy
Your baby, week by week, Spastics Society or HEO. This cheerful chart, gives an illustrated check list for all the pregnancy stages, and a timetable of the 40 weeks of development, and six weeks after birth.

Material from the local health authority, such as the flip chart *Pregnancy Care*, published by the West Midlands Regional Health Authority, The cover shows ultrasound scanner being used to monitor foetal growth. Children are very interested in this process which is also demonstrated in the film *Birth, an everyday miracle,* BBC, though use this with care as there are some negative attitudes shown as well.

The 1984 *HEC* major publication on pregnancy and the first few weeks of parenthood, providing reassurance for expectant parents is called *Pregnancy*. This is beautifully produced, and was a response to parents' questions.

Foetal Development
In addition to the material above, slides or films showing foetal development are *The First Days of Life* slide set, by Camera Talks, and film *The First Days of Life,* 22 minutes, English version of the original French film, with the famous foetal photography by Nilsson, available from Concord Films Council.

Follow up work can involve drawings, models, or paper cut outs of a few of the developmental states, always related to the condition and feelings of the mother.

i) BBC TV. *Sex Education,* Teachers notes, see page 109.
ii) Nuffield Secondary Science 3, *Biology of Man.* 1971 Longmans.
iii) Llewellyn-Jones D. 1971. *Everywoman.* Faber & Faber.
iv) Diagram group 1977. Paddington Press.
   a) *Woman's body. An Owners Manual.*
   b) *Child's body. A parents manual.*
v) Nilsson L. *A child is born.* Faber.
vi) A model: *Visible Woman,* Renwal, available from toyshops. This kit can be made up to show all internal organs in a transparent plastic female figure about 37cm high. The 'optional extra' box, contains parts to show the 7 month stage of pregnancy, a transparent womb containing a removable infant. This enables the 'upside down' baby to be clearly seen, and less able children find the 3D presentation most helpful.

Films

Films of birth often produce powerful and emotional effects, and should only be used when there is enough time afterwards to discuss them fully and 'calm down' the physiology aroused, before dashing off to the next lesson. Suitable ones are listed below.

1. *The First Days of Life* (see page 233). A 'natural' birth, with father in attendance.
2. *Having a baby* series. 5 short Trigger films made by the HEC in 1980. Free loan from Concord Films Council or the Central Film Library, as film or videos. Teachers could view them for background information. Detailed notes are available.
3. *Hello baby* 25 minutes. This starts with a natural birth and parental joy.
   joy.

Television

1. ITV *Living and Growing* series. page 109.
2. BBC Radio. *Child Care.* Age 14–16. 5 weekly programmes, 15 minutes long, to encourage discussion.
   i) *Inside.* Pregnancy and ante-natal care.
   ii) *Outside.* The father, the family, the single parent.
   iii) *Being a parent.* Breast feeding, play, emotional adaption.
   iv) *Getting help.* Community help, and post natal care.
   v) *Asking.* Pupils requests.

Chapter 11

PARENTHOOD AND FAMILY LIFE

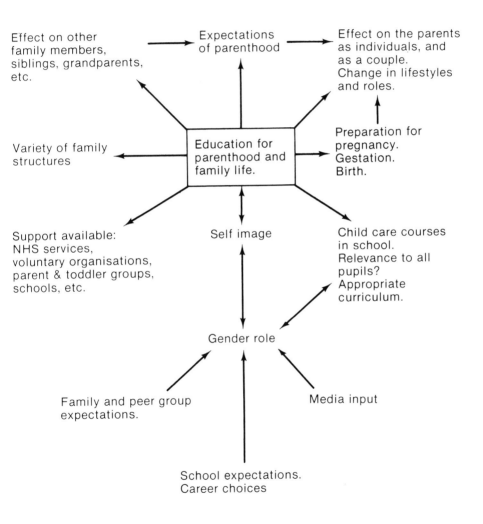

Effect on other family members, siblings, grandparents, etc.

Expectations of parenthood

Effect on the parents as individuals, and as a couple. Change in lifestyles and roles.

Variety of family structures

Education for parenthood and family life.

Preparation for pregnancy. Gestation. Birth.

Support available: NHS services, voluntary organisations, parent & toddler groups, schools, etc.

Self image

Child care courses in school. Relevance to all pupils? Appropriate curriculum.

Gender role

Family and peer group expectations.

Media input

School expectations. Career choices

A study on preparation for parenthood in the secondary school curriculum, carried out by Aston University for the DES, found that although education authorities generally view it as an area of importance they do not have specific policies for its inclusion in the curriculum. Where school courses are provided, they tend to be part of 4th and 5th year options, which are rarely taken by boys or the most able girls, and are often taught exclusively by female teachers. The majority of pupils studied in five individual schools wished to become good and responsible parents, but their attitudes to these parenthood roles were highly influenced by their perception of potential gender roles at home, or in employment [182].

The recommendations given in the study include that LEAs appoint an advisor responsible for preparation for parenthood education and that a teacher co-ordinator for that field, with appropriate status, be identified in every school. This person might then be able to ensure every child was involved in some parenthood education and the structures of option schemes could be re-examined and changed, so more boys and male teachers participated. The report also advocates a greater liaison of interested groups within the community, and proper provision for training teachers in parenthood education together with the development of more curriculum material co-ordinating the spread of subject areas usually involved. A 'National Centre for Family Life Education in Schools' might be created, the report suggests, as the social benefits of increasing parental skills could be enormous.

As the full significance of very early learning has become appreciated, the role of parents of pre-school children has been realised to be of critical importance. Arguments have been given as in the above report for work on parenthood to be done with all pupils, as the majority will eventually choose a long term relationship, or get married, and have children. (In 1975, 60% of men and 85% of women were married by the age of 25). Other pupils will in the future be involved as relatives, or in a professional caring role, or as employers, and so will benefit from an understanding of the needs of young families, and an improved image of parenthood. Full community support and positive attitudes towards families may be developed in this way. Much of the material in previous chapters is directly relevant here, particularly the choice of parenthood and the spacing of child bearing now possible.

Families

Teacher sensitivity is needed to the wide variety of family backgrounds, and cultural and social class differences in child care. A fundamental aim of parenthood courses is to raise teenagers' sensitivity to the needs of young children. In doing so they may become more aware of inadequate parenting themselves, so great tact is required.

Variations in family structure in the UK

i) The nuclear family, typified by a husband, wife and 1.87 children [165] living together in one household.

ii) Single parent families now 1 in 7 or 12.1% of families (lone mothers 10.1%, lone fathers 1.4%)

iii) Unmarried couples (cohabiting) with children. The law now recognises some rights for 'common law wives' and illegitimate children.

iv) Second marriages with or without children from the first or second marriage.

v) Married and unmarried couples choosing not to have children.

vi) Adopted and fostered children. Distinguish here the two parent roles, a) biological, and b) caring, which can be carried out by different people.

vii) Extended families, several generations, or related families, living together.

In any one school class, some children are likely to be involved in family upheavals of divorce, separation or re-marriage, so staff awareness of this is important.

Possible teaching approach

Carry out Historical, Geographical or Sociological studies of marriage and family groupings including monogamy, serial monogamy, polygamy and polyandry. For each explain the way in which partners are chosen, by individuals, or the family, and expectations of the particular kind of marriage role, for males and females. Discuss the value of nuclear families, or extended families of several generations living together, or groups of brothers and sisters, their spouses and children, compared with communal care, such as in kibbutzim, etc.

A NMGC report (August 1983) showed the majority of people in the UK expect a 'traditional' monogamous marriage and for it to last a lifetime, and believe in love, trust and fidelity. Perhaps expectations should also include the likelihood of some 'ups and downs' and the knowledge that help is available for weathering the rough patches in a marriage. Divorce now affects one in three of all UK marriages, with as many as 60% of teenage marriages ending in divorce, a rate double that of those who marry between the ages of 20 and 24. (OPCS Population Trends 32, Summer 1983)

Needs of children

Many variations of family life are seen to be possible, as discussed above. It should be explained here, that although there is no single 'correct' way of bringing up a family, certain basic needs for all children have been identified. All parents-to-be must consider how they are going to fulfill these needs. It is often the mother who provides most of them initially, but more fathers are now willing and able to become involved early on. Children up to one year old do not appear to 'prefer' being looked after by one parent or the other [166].

Physical needs

The health and safety, food, warmth, sleep, cleanliness, etc. of children must be taken care of. This area is perhaps the most easy to understand, but needs specific knowledge and skills, on the part of the parent, which are not all innate.

Emotional needs

The baby and infant needs to relate to one or two stable adults (often the mother and father) during the first four years of life at least, and preferably into puberty and after. The 'bonding' process involved in making this relationship requires adequate time being spent with the baby by this limited number of people. The security of dependable loving care also provides positive models of parenting behaviour, and examples of gender roles.

Socialisation needs

These include language development (involving talking to the baby and seeking a response), providing new play learning experiences and the opportunity for the baby or toddler to relate to a range of people, and for the child to learn about the control of behaviour (which requires appropriate parenting skills). Socialisation processes are continued by schools.

Expectations of family life

Are these the same for women and men? They arise from:

i)   previous learning as members of a family (not necessarily good images of parenting) and other socialisation processes, some at school,

ii)   romantic ideas many people have of the perfect fullfilment of parenthood and of instantly loving, obedient, dutiful children,

iii)   TV and other media presentations, increasingly influential, which often present stereotyped portrayals of family life. What might be the cumulative effects of mother-in-law and nagging wife jokes: or babies in advertisements always looking bonny, clean, cheerful, responsive . . .?

Realism is needed, and an understanding of the parenting skills to be developed, and the appropriate time and place to learn them. Whitfield [166] details some of the parenting skills often lacking, as identified by one experienced pre-school worker who found the following problems were common:

i)   late speech development in intelligent children, due to emotional disturbances at home,

ii)   parents who tried to control children only by shouting or physical means, no attempt being made by them to be patient and loving or to explain matters or provide distractions,

iii)   parents who had no understanding of what to expect at each of their child's developmental stages and ignorance of how abrupt changes in routine disturb a child,

iv)   lack of appreciation of how complex a task rearing children is,

v)   poor relationship skills with other adults which was often reflected in the parent's inappropriate behaviour with children.

The effect of children on the parents

Awareness is needed that after the initial delight of a successful birth, feelings are very often mixed. There may be anxiety about how to cope, jealousy in other family members, resentment at the enforced responsibility, the time consuming repetitive routines required, or the lack of privacy or sleep, or the expense, etc. Relationships change for a couple when an extra person is added for the first time. Adjustments are needed all round, and often a change in life style for a while. 'Togetherness' for partners needs to be positively maintained, so babysitters are essential for mental health! Individual interests and hobbies other than parenthood should be kept alive if possible.

A mother may well be tired for some time after the birth, and perhaps a little depressed on occasions, possibly due to hormonal changes. This is not inevitable, but if 'baby blues' last for more than a short time, medical help should be sought. A new father shares in the increased responsibility of parenthood, trying to relieve, help and support the mother, and also becomes involved in caring for their baby. This can sometimes make him anxious and tense, as well as pleased, proud and delighted.

Child abuse

The feelings outlined above may occur even in the very best circumstances, so it is not difficult to understand how under additional stresses and poor family relationships, some children will be 'at risk' of being abused by their parents. Everyone should be aware of the support services available for families and parents under stress. Often a phone 'Help' line is provided locally, and the NSPCC and Samaritans will always offer advice (and may also run courses for teachers).

Hughes [167] gives suggestions for specific school teaching in relationships which might lessen potential family conflict later. Positive views of parenthood and the joy and fun gained from being in contact with young children can be seen in the film *Hello baby*, on free loan from Central Film Library, or Concord Film Council. Six children aged 0–20 months are shown in sequence, interacting delightfully with their parents and siblings. The father's role is particularly emphasised (teacher's notes are available for this film).

Support for families

i) Support from other members of the family has been a traditional help service. 'Nuclear families' however, often live at some distance from their relatives, so such help may be difficult to arrange. Some 'advice' from older relatives may conflict with newer methods of care and so can be confusing. Education for grandparenthood may be required!

ii) The NHS provides post-natal care such as home visits by the midwife or a health visitor arranged automatically after a birth. Also recommended are visits to the local child clinic for checks for the baby, and contacts with other families with youngsters.

iii) Friends, and parents and toddler groups, can give encouragement and advice and offer comradeship.

iv) The National Childbirth Trust has local neighbourly groups for post-natal support for young parents, and for breast-feeding mothers.

v) The Pre-school Playgroups Association runs local groups for parents and children under five.

vi) Many local groups such as Young Wives, or the National Housewives

Register, help families with very young children make friends with others similarly placed.

vii) The National Council for One Parent Families can give expert advice to single parents.

viii) Infant schools often arrange meetings or have a 'parent and child' room and provide material for families with pre-school children.

Parentcraft education in school

Many school programmes will be tailored to specify syllabi (see page 250 and the Aston study). Cowly [168] feels that parenthood education should be about normal situations rather than problem orientated and that limited objectives should be identified and related to the needs of pupils both on a general level for all children, (on such matters as choice of marriage, parenthood and child development) and for courses for disadvantaged children who may need extra help in this area. Specific courses should also be planned for more able children, to raise the academic level of understanding of child development and family life. Perkins and Morris [169] also argue for clearly defined goals, and the need to distinguish between

i) preparing for parenthood, which they suggest would be better left until the immediate relevancy of pregnancy and childbirth, as the teaching could then be adapted to the specific needs of the parents, their relationship and accommodation, etc. (Furthermore, since baby care procedures change, these may well be different several years after leaving school) and

ii) education about child development, which would be more broadly relevant and appropriate for a school curriculum. Leach [171] emphasises the need to promote real interest in child development, to raise the status of parenthood, and provide financial and community support for those with pre-school children. She gives practical suggestions for such support. All authorities emphasise the importance of the practical involvement of pupils, with young children in play groups, nurseries, etc., so child care skills can be observed, analysed and practised. Watching parents and others interacting with young children, and afterwards discussing what happened is a very valid learning situation. Some schools have been able to set up their own playgroups and Orton [170] explains how rewarding this can be, particularly in enabling some school children to develop a successful 'teacher role' for the first time. Other schools use local facilities, and we must appreciate the increasing demands made on nursery and pre-school groups. Some cope cheerfully with a seemingly unending stream of observers and amateur helpers!

Prout and Prendergast, in a preview of the HEC *Preparation for Parenthood* project [190], explain their methodology, and suggest that curriculum development should start from an assessment of the pupils' needs and interests. They themselves found that 15 year old children do in fact understand many important aspects of motherhood and child care, and are generally realistic in their view. Pupils are, however, confused by the contradictions of their own experiences of child care, and the over-glamourised public image of motherhood.

The overall aims are to raise knowledge and interest in child development and care, and the status of parents. Raising awareness of good parenting techniques may enable such practices to be identified and appreciated in everyday life. Crying infants and cross parents draw attention too easily to the negative side which needs counterbalancing with good images. Perhaps a certain couple, Diana and Charles, will have helped to focus on the positive parenthood role in the 1980s? (Though not every family has quite such a support service available.)

Child development

Child development is well documented (see resource list) but understanding of it is sadly lacking in some adults. The authors of *Child's Body – A Parents Manual* (see book list) have arranged the sequences for each age group under the headings:

i) motor development; posture, control of limbs, sitting, crawling skills,
ii) eye and hand development; the co-ordination of these,
iii) hearing and voice; response to sounds, and language development, and
iv) play and social development; reaction to others and to the environment.

Each category of development is then expanded, and details given, for example, of the natural regular swings in behaviour from well balanced and outgoing to withdrawn and unstable. It is reassuring to parents and teachers to know of such oscillations.

Some important concepts in child development

i) It must be understood by first time parents that there are recognised stages in development, and although these do vary in timing within certain limits, they do come in sequence. Thus, children will not be able to behave in certain ways (for example show bladder control, feed themselves, remain still while adults engage in other activities) until the appropriate stage is reached. False expectations of children's behaviour causes much frustration on both sides.

ii) The inherent possibilities in the child (nature) and the environment plus upbringing (nurture) interact. We can do much about the latter (and increasingly something about the former), but every child is different, and is different again from the parents. Each child has to be reacted to as an individual. What worked in 'managing' one infant may not be successful with the next, as many parents have discovered.

iii) If you are 'nice' to children, and do 'all the right things', they are not necessarily 'nice' back again! One of the major shocks of parenting, perhaps. The need for children to test the limits of tolerance of their behaviour often develops earlier than expected. Firm, consistent control before parent explosion point is reached may avoid many battles in the future.

iv)   Child control is remarkably similar to training a dog! Patience, rewards and encouragement work best. Some commands such as 'come here', and 'stop' must be learnt early for safety reasons. It is not appropriate to withdraw love as a punishment but there should be understanding that it is possible to love but not to like one's child at certain times.

v)   The interaction of siblings must be anticipated. To have a second child 'for the first one to play with' does not always work as planned. The involvement of children in the arrival of the next is therefore very important. Jealousy and anger are normal reactions, as is a desire to return to babyhood. Many parents feel they have failed if their children do not 'get on' together, but it seems that this is a very common phenomenon. The meaning of 'equal' becomes definitive when divisions of time, attention and objects are made under family scrutiny!

Sub-themes which could be identified during child development work

i)   Groups of children might consider specific areas such as safety and the various motor skill stages in child development could be related to potential hazards. Suggest that exploration and problem solving skills (taking lids off) may come earlier than anticipated while self-feeding skills (propped up bottles?) may develop much later.

Explain that traffic 'sense' is late developing. Periferal vision is not at an adult level until about 10 years and the capacity to interpret the distance and speed of vehicles and to 'compute' the information gained is not fully developed until about 12 or so. Pupils could contact the road safety officer for details of the most vulnerable child age groups for accidents on the road, and help work out safety schemes for them. Child skills in looking after themselves appropriately could be linked with each developmental stage, but explain that learning *should* actually be allowed to take place i.e. don't blame the 'naughty table' if a toddler walks backwards into it. After rubbing the bump, explain that 'eyes are in the front, so you must always look where you are going' as overprotection is not such a good idea. The group could survey the BBC-HEC campaign *Play it Safe* which has been most successful in alerting adults to hazards in the home. A fully illustrated booklet is free, (from HEOs) and reinforces the series of 10 minute TV programmes presented by Jimmy Savile.

ii)   Physical health could be considered. First relate this to safety, as above, then suggest that preventive medicine is also vitally important as many 'modern' diseases are habit-related. Habits are learnt young, so parents of pre-school children play a critical part in their healthy upbringing, in providing a low fat, adequate fibre diet for example, and in not using drugs unless necessary, and not smoking in front of children etc. The group could collect HEC material for educating parents about these areas.

iii)   Mental and emotional health is intrinsically related to physical health. Explain the constant need for reciprocal affection, and the display of this between parents and children. Also, how to be able to say 'sorry', as no one is perfect! The basic needs of children have been mentioned (page 237), and include social health, the third side of the 'health triangle', so arranging parties and outings to help develop young children's social skills would be an appropriate activity for pupils here.

iv)   The role of parents as educators is not perceived by some parents, who do not always distinguish which part of child behaviour is learnt and which is developmental. Understanding of how learning takes place is therefore very important. Parents nowadays perhaps have less control over what their children learn as TV (requiring no literary skills) is in virtually every home. Discuss perhaps a new need for parents to discuss with children the programmes they have seen and heard, and what they thought about them, as well as being prepared to face the consequences of turning the TV off! Pupils could investigate early learning processes, and perhaps each individually help a younger child to develop a particular skill.

The sex education role of parents

For teacher preparation for this section, please read pages 11–15, and chapter 4. To enable pupils to understand the on-going nature of sex education, and the parents' role in this show a sequence of slides, from family holidays perhaps, or pictures from magazines, of young boys and girls of various ages and cultures and ask the pupils such questions as:

i)   What age do you think this child is?
ii)   Do children need to know anything about sex at this age?
iii)   When do they begin to ask questions about sex?
iv)   How do they ask them?
v)   Are they always verbal questions?
vi)   Does learning begin before they can talk?
vii)   What do small children believe about where babies come from?
viii) What may they believe if no one tells them the truth?
ix)   Does this matter?
x)   What names do children use for the sexual parts of the body?
xi)   How do they learn about the differences between boys and girls, or boys and men, girls and women?
xii)   How else do children learn about sex?
xiii) Do parents always help their children learn these things?
xiv)   Why might some parents not help, or not want them to know?
xv)   Are there some things that children could not be expected to understand at x years old?
xvi)   What are these young children learning about parenthood?
xvii) What would you say to a four year old who said
    'Why does a lady have cherries on her chest?'
    'That's a lady dog 'cos its got a pink collar on'
    'Why are those butterflies stuck together?'

How *do* children learn about life?

Group work

Make a collection of sex education books for young children (see lists on pages 34, 35, 55, 72), perhaps borrowed from local schools, libraries, or the HEO.

Groups of pupils could then look at a selection of books for various ages and assess what age each book would be suitable for. Points for them to consider might include an analysis of the pictures:

are they clear and attractive?

are there any 'hidden' messages?

how are male and female roles portrayed?

or the text; is this accurate, but suitable for the age group?

could it be read as a story?

does it use difficult medical terms?

Consider how the book could be used. Could it be:

read to the child all through at one go

or left for the child to look at alone

or read with the child?

Could a few of the pictures only be shown and comments made, or asked for or the book be used to back up learning from real life for example after seeing a new baby, or a pregnant woman, etc.?

Finally, would the book be really useful to parents, and where could it be obtained? Each group could then present their findings to the others, and an overall summary could be made of what to look for in children's books.

Further insight into sex education in the home might be developed by arranging a debate on 'Parents should be more responsible for the sex education of their children' and by cultivating an ongoing interest in sex education material, and the work of the FPIS etc.

Gender Role

One of the important aspects of parenthood is its influence on gender role, both for the parents and in the way they raise their children. The physical difference between the sexes is biologically determined for reproduction. Difference in gender (the concept of masculinity and femininity) is produced by socialisation processes starting at birth and often firmly established by the age of three years.

Research has shown it is possible to socialise these images either way, as different cultures have 'expected' different behaviour from males and females at different times in their history. Powerful political and socio-economic factors shape gender roles, but the patriarchal male-dominant system which has been the norm for so long, is now increasingly being questioned.

Attitudes to women

It has been suggested [172, 173] that women have been consistently under-valued and the work they do perceived to be of low status. Children of 5 and 6 already have this concept (see page 54). Although in 1978 41% of the British workforce was female, 40.2% of this work was part-time, and much was rated as 'secondary' i.e. more flexible and 'disposable'. The following facts are also documented [172].

i)   Women's jobs often do not reflect the level of education they have received, as they are frequently over qualified.

ii) Women tend to earn less than men with the same qualifications.

iii) Girls' education tends to be orientated towards marriage and short term work, (and the concept that their first duty is to look attractive).

iv) Women tend to consider their career prospects in relation to men and not as independent, autonomous, equal beings.

v) They may also fear that success will 'damage their image' in the eyes of males, and they will lose 'femininity' if they are 'too clever'.

vi) Attitudes are related to social class; gender role becomes more stereotyped and disparity between the sexes widens on going down the social classes.

vii) When women do work outside the home, they generally do this in addition to their home care role.

Attitudes in school

Some authorities, such as ILEA, have been trying to analyse the gender role socialisation processes in schools, and develop more truly equal opportunities in education. However, raising the expectations and performance of girls (which often begin to deteriorate at secondary level [172]) will have to be linked with a genuine change in attitude towards women workers in the industrial market, or even more frustration will be generated. It is possible that in times of high unemployment attitudes to women's work outside the home harden, as they are perceived to be competing, equally or not, for limited numbers of jobs.

It is therefore even more necessary to educate the next generation of parents, employees and employers to the potential for beneficial change, with more flexible views of both men's and women's work, particularly if these are eventually to be linked with shorter working hours for everyone.

The report on the conference *What's in it for boys?* [173] stresses the need for males to become aware of these positive benefits which in the long run will mean a reduction of the enormous pressures on them from society, and particularly from peer groups, to live up to the restricting male 'macho' image (i.e. be brave, strong, non-emotional, competitive, not admit to worries or problems, and to be able to 'take' alcohol) which can cause anxiety and the internalisation of worries and emotions in a self-destructive way. Boys also need, more than girls, to be made aware of the way they rigidly stereotype gender roles, and transmit such attitudes in a forcible way.

The report gives six guidelines for schools interested in ensuring equal opportunities in education. It makes the following suggestions.

i) Whole school policies should be developed, a group being set up to monitor sexism, make suggestions for more equal treatment of boys and girls, formulate policies and liaise with the LEA, parents, school managers, etc.

ii) Institutional self evaluation and school focussed in-service training schemes should be provided to enable teachers to evaluate their own and others' performance on 'equality' in the classroom.

iii) It is valuable to raise issues in school and try and reach uncommitted colleagues to challenge sex-stereotyping continually, and to have access to research material to strengthen arguments.

iv) There is a need for resources and support for equal opportunities from

LEAs and teachers' centres, for monitoring sexist material, for in-service or training college courses for teachers, on assertiveness or sensitivity training, and for the development of curriculum material for schools.

v) Individual initiatives by teachers, such as in using questionnaires on sex differentation in school, changing classroom practices, etc. are needed.

vi) Knowledge of work in other schools, such as on sexual harassment, primary/secondary school liaison for work on sexism, is valuable.

Subject areas

It is well known that girls have done less well in subjects such as mathematics and science, and boys in English language and literature. (Girls in 1979 had 40% more passes in 'O' level English literature than boys, with an entry difference of only 9%) [173]

The Schools Council has produced specific reports giving suggestions for change in relevant areas (see page 249).

Girls and mathematics

Schwarzenberger [174] comments on the appendix to 'Mathematics Counts' (the Cockcroft report) by Shuard: *Differences in mathematical performance between girls and boys*, saying 'Tests on children aged between 10 and 16 have shown differences between boys and girls in mathematical ability. The average performance of the boys was better overall but especially in tests involving spacial visualisation, length, area, volume, graphs, fractions, decimals, and in problem-solving generally. The average performance of the girls was better in straightforward numerical computations, especially long sums requiring patience. However, the differences are not enormous: while it is true that more boys than girls would come in the top 10% of a typical group of children, it would not be true to say that most boys perform better at mathematics than most girls.

It is possible that these differences have a biological origin, but against this they are more marked in some countries than others. The differences are more likely to spring from personal preferences and social attitudes. For example, a smaller proportion of girls than boys enter for O-level mathematics and of those with high grades a smaller proportion proceed to A-level. The result is that in 1979 nearly three times as many boys as girls entered for A-level mathematics. In the same year 50% of all the male entrants to universities in England and Wales had passed A-level mathematics, but only 25% of all female entrants. Studies in schools suggest that for the learning of mathematics, boys are more likely to attribute their successes to stable causes such as ability, and their failure to unstable causes such as lack of effort, while girls attribute their successes to unstable causes such as the effort they put into their work, and their failures to stable causes such as their lack of ability.'

Teaching approach on attitudes to gender role

This is one area where single sex classes may be beneficial for some discussions (e.g. 4 below), as otherwise previous practices may still function and boys may tend to disrupt, ridicule, dominate, or demand an unequal share of attention!

The overall aims are to identify, analyse and challenge traditional sexist attitudes and stereotyped portrayals of masculinity and femininity, and assess how much these prevent free choice of behaviour and careers for boys and girls.

Discussion, research and project areas

1. What *are* the differences between boys and girls? Pupils could research:
    i)   Physical differences – see chapter 6, (page 114) but there is an overlap in height, weight, strength, etc. between the sexes.
    ii) Behavioural differences. Boys and men tend to be more aggressive than girls and women; this could be due to socialisation processes or, after puberty, the effect of testosterone.
    iii) Differences in intellectual ability. The only differences consistently found between males and females are that males seem to have better spacial visualisation abilities than females (i.e. can think more clearly in three dimensional terms) but only by about 4% (BBC Horizon, February 21st, 1983). This may be related to certain problem solving abilities in mathematics [175].

    Females have a higher verbal ability than males e.g. in reading, comprehension, and literature.

    These differences are now decreasing [175], but research continues into their causes, which may be due to: biological differences between the sexes, such as genetic differences of the X and Y chromosomes, serum uric acid differences; differences in cerebral organisation and brain lateralisation, i.e. the specialisation in function in left and right hemispheres, or to hormonal differences. The situation is complex as some of these factors may interact. Others feel that complex educational and socialisation processes could account for the present intellectual differences between men and women.

2. Socialisation processes
    i) In the home.

    Pupils could investigate the 'pink/blue' syndrome. They could collect the 'welcome to the new baby' cards parents receive in abundance, read the definitions of boys and girls, and assess the associated picture messages or look at other 'age' birthday cards in the same way.

    They could consider ways in which parents influence gender role, such as in the way they dress their pre-school children or expect certain behaviour from girls or boys' or provide 'appropriate' toys and books, and in the way that they talk generally about males and females, and enact gender roles themselves. Pupils could look at catalogues for childrens toys, and analyse how girls and boys toys are presented in them.

    They could also consider how people other than parents influence gender role; perhaps by giving praise for 'looking pretty', or 'being strong', etc?
    ii) In school.

    A group of pupils could ask staff at local nursery or infant schools if they consider the points listed on pages 60, 61 to be important, and what gender differences are already perceived by reception class pupils. Do the teachers think these influence the childrens choice of toys and activities?

3. Research into the history of housework.

    This has been related to family productivity, the role of women, the separation of work from the home, industrialisation, wars, etc. refer to, Hill, C., 1980. *The history of the housewife* (Details and extracts from this book are given in *Class, gender and education*, [172]. A display about the history of housework could be prepared by pupils, for a parents' evening perhaps, and might lead to an interesting discussion on current practices!

4. Attitudes to the opposite sex.

i) Ascertain and discuss the differences perceived by boys and girls in each other's attributes, such as leadership, intellectual qualities, individual performances, competitiveness, importance of school achievements, subject performance and preferences, and job performance, suggestions on how to do this are given in *Humble pi* (page 249).

ii) Is it generally true, as suggested in *What's in it for boys?* (page 249) that boys in girls' groups get support and encouragement but girls in boys' groups tend to be ignored and ridiculed? Are boys more afraid of being laughed at? Why might this be?

iii) How do boys talk about girls? Does this tend to be in a rather sexist way, using stereotyped descriptions of appearance only, and suggesting that sex is performed on them ('Yer dip yer stick') rather than it being a mutual occasion?

How do girls talk about boys? Do they describe personalities as well as appearance? What do they value highly? Kindness? Thoughtfulness, being gentle? (If only boys realised how these qualities are appreciated!)

iv) Reverse role play. 'Typical' situations include secretary and boss, surgeon and theatre nurse, etc. Analyse the attitudes shown. Monitor TV for a whole day (!), consciously reversing the male/female situations and noting time spent showing 'female' cricket, football, politicians, etc., or 'male' beauty contests, etc. Note 'male' visual glamour support for comedy acts, conjurers, quiz programmes, etc. Note the ratio of male to female panelists in programmes such as 'Call my bluff', etc. Consider: Are we still in a patriarchal society? If roles were reversed, would it be seen as a matriarchal one?

5. Effect of the mass media

i) Assess the roles of males and females as presented in current rock and pop records. What attitudes do these show?

ii) Collect sexist comments from the press. For starters, use the collected Guardian material in Veitch, A. (ED.), 1981, *Naked Ape*, Duckworth, or for example the following article from the Sunday Express Magazine, March 27th 1983, on Superbird, the first USA female astronaut, which contains: 'There is no doubt that Sally Ride, brown hair, blue eyes, 5'6" tall, weighing 115lbs, born on 26th May 1951 is an unusual woman. A tennis champion in her teens, a research physicist in her twenties, an astronaut in her thirties, she seems to have defied the usual life cycles of women, even highly educated women. But last summer, on 24th July, she did something every woman can appreciate; she got married . . .'

6. The future

Are male and female roles changing? Are equal opportunities for men and women now a reality? Do roles change during a lifetime?

i) Consider the effect of

The Women's Liberation Movement,

The Sex Discrimination Act, (1975)

The setting up of the Equal Opportunities Commission,

Evidence given by Havinghurst [176] of the growth in the USA of both androgyny, i.e. having flexible and more interchangeable sex roles, and a tendency in middle age (from 50–55) for a gender role change i.e. some women become more masculine in lifestyle, some men more passive or feminine.

ii) Write an essay on 'Home life in 2020', or, 'Family resources should include time and homecare skills, and value these equally with money'.

iii) Draw up a schedule for men and women who wish to return to work outside the home, after some years of child care. What provisions could be made for them; such as retraining programmes, flexible working hours, part-time but secure work with visible promotion stages?

iv) Suggest a suitable logo for the 1980s *Be your own person?*

Resources

See pages 87, 244 and 249.

1. Schools Council Reports, in conjunction with the Equal Opportunities Commission.

i) Schools Council Programme 3. *Developing the curriculum for a changing world.*

ii) *Humble pi: the mathematics education of girls*, Eddows, M. 1983, Longmans.

iii) *Pour out the cocoa, Janet, Sexism in childrens books*, Stones, R. 1983 Longmans.

iv) *Switched off; the Science Education of Girls*, Harding, J. 1983 Longmans.

All have extensive suggestions for analysing and changing school practices, and lists of resources and background books.

v) *Equal Opportunities, What's in it for boys?* Schools Council, 1983. Report of conference held November 19th, 1982. A most valuable source of ideas, which includes situation cards for analysing staff attitudes to gender roles.

2. *Books for teachers*

i) *'Invisible Women' The Schooling Scandal*, Spender, D. 1982, Writers and Readers.

An investigation into control systems operating to prevent equal opportunities for girls in our education system.

ii) *Gender and Schooling* Stanworth, M. 1981. Women's Research and Resources Centre. A study of sexual divisions in the classroom.

3. *Books for children*

His and Hers Groombridge, J. Penguin Education Looks at masculinity and femininity, role reversal and attitudes to this.

4. *Television;* ITV *Making a living,* for 15+ *'Two women- Two men',* and *'Three women- but in whose world?'* Teacher's notes available.

Preparation for parenthood

See previous sections on the family, pages 167–169, and on gender role, 59–60 and 84–87.

1. Curriculum material.

i) Schools Council Health Education Project 5–13, 5–8 see page 72, and 9–13, see page 106.

ii) *Home Economics in Middle Years.* Schools Council Project, *Home and family,* 8–13 see page 108.

iii) *Preparation for parenthood.* National Childbirth Trust. Sections 2, *The New Family,* and 3, *Responsibilities, Commitment and Problems of Parenthood,* see page 232.

2. Material for teachers
   i) *Education for Family Life,* 1981. Open University In-Service Education for Teachers. A comprehensive pack, including school health topic survey sheets and a study book with detailed analysis of relevant syllabi and examinations at secondary level. Theme books on family responsibility and child development are being planned.
   ii) *Parenthood Education in Schools,* 1979. TACADE. Symposium papers and workshop material. Background notes give details of organisations providing parenthood education material.
   iii) *Parentcraft Education Teaching Aids.* National Association for Maternal and Child Welfare. Helpful notes and a guide to resources and courses run by the Association.

3. *Television*

ITV *'Making a Living'* series for 15+. Parenthood/Sex Roles.
   i) *Baby Love,*
   ii) *Two's company ... Three's a crowd,* and
   iii) *And baby makes two* (About single parent families). Teacher's notes give suggestions for follow up work. For radio programmes see page 234.

4. Books

For teachers:
   i) *Education for Family Life* Whitfield, R. C. 1980 Hodder and Stoughton
   ii) *The Making of the Modern Family* Shorter, E. 1977 Fontana
   iii) *The Death of the Family* Cooper, D. 1972 Penguin
   iv) *Who Cares?* Leach, P. 1979 Penguin
   v) *Growing up in a One Parent Family.* Ferri, E. National Childrens Bureau for secondary children:
   vi) *Parentcraft: childcare from birth to school* Bass, K. 1978 Cassell
   vii) *Looking at Marriage.* West, G., Loeb, J. & Beecham, Y. 1973 Nelson
   viii) *It's a Great Life* Baldwin, D. 1973 BBC in conjunction with the National Children's Home
   ix) *For better, for worse. Marriage & the Family* Gillot, J. 1971 Penguin Education

Child development

1. HEC source List. Child development.
2. Open University Publications (Ward Lock Educational)
   i) *The first years of life*
   ii) *Understanding pregnancy,*
   iii) *Your baby and you,*
   iv) *Getting ready for pregnancy.*
   v) *The pre-school child*
   vi) *Childhood 5–10*
   vii) *Parents and teenagers.*
3. HEC leaflets. Useful source of pictures, as well as information. There is a very wide variety related to child care e.g. *Your children need you, Play and things to play with* etc. contain useful multicultural illustrations.
4. HEOs have many other leaflets, provided by commercial firms, such as *It's your baby too. Advice for fathers.* Wyeth.
5. Developmental Guide 0–5, National Childrens Bureau, 1977. Handbook and charts.
6. Books
   i) *Pyjamas don't matter* Gribben T. 1979 John Murray, Realistic advice on what to expect as a parent. Humorously illustrated.

ii)   *Family feelings* Raynor C. 1977 *Understanding your child from 0–5'* Arrow comprehensive advice, incorporating HEC material. Focusses on emotions and gives specific help on such matters as loss of interest in sex after the birth.

iii)   *Child's body. A Parent's Manual.* Paddington Press, 1977 and Corgi *Then and now* Baldwin D. 1978 Longman, for children.

Chapter 12

UNPLEASANT REALITIES

Unwanted pregnancies

Counselling

In order there should be no question of pressure to have an abortion, or not, it is highly desirable that someone with an unwanted pregnancy is put in touch with a non-medical counsellor, who is able to discuss in complete confidence, in a non-directive and non-judgemental way, all the options open to her. The counsellor will need a good knowledge of the legal position and the support service, both statutory and voluntary, which would be available after any particular decision was made.

This would 'help her explore her feelings about pregnancy and related areas of her life, help her study possible courses of action (keeping, adoption or termination) and their outcomes for her, and encourage her to make her own decisions' [156] Guidance would be needed to enable a 'reasoned assessment', to be made, from a realistic viewpoint, of:

i)   the implications of becoming a parent, or a single parent, with or without support from the father of the child, or her family. The restrictions, loss of 'freedom' and complete change in life style involved in looking after young children are often not appreciated by teenagers. It can be an isolating and lonely experience.

ii)   The need for ante natal care should be stressed, especially important for teenage mothers, who may have particular difficulties.

iii)   The possibilities of accommodation before and after the birth must be discussed, (many girls think a flat, near their friends and families, will be readily available).

iv)   The provision of monetary grants, benefits and supplements (75% of single mothers are on supplementary benefit).

v)   Employment prospects, and, for schoolchildren, continuing education are other matters to be considered.

Guidelines on this last point are given in the Pregnant at School report [7], and local authorities may have made specific provisions for this.

It is also important to discuss

i)   the possibility of fostering or adoption, the arrangements which could be made, and the implications of such a step

ii) the possibility of an abortion, the risk involved, and the need for pre and post operative emotional support, and medical examination

iii) the importance of involving her family, and how dependent she may be on their help

iv) future contraception methods, and where and how these could be obtained, so unplanned pregnancies could be avoided in the future.

Schoolgirl pregnancies

In some cases a teacher may be the first person to be confided in, so it is useful to know in advance what counselling and reliable pregnancy testing services are available in the area.

Pregnancy test

This can usually be done 14 days after the first day of a missed period, but some can be earlier, at 8 days 'overdue' or less. In both cases if the test is positive, the pregnancy is confirmed, but if negative there may be advice to have a further one a few days later, in case the level of hCG in the urine has not reached a detectable amount the first time (see page 227).

A pregnancy test may be obtained:

i) free, from a general practitioner, a Family Planning Clinic, a Brook Advisory Centre or Life organisation, and some Local Authorities have special arrangements for tests for schoolgirls

ii) for a small fee from BPAS (which usually gives very quick results, some clinics providing a 'while you wait' service) and from most chemists.

All tests are done on a sample of the first urine of the morning, collected in a clean dry jar or container and labelled with name, age, address, and date of the first day of the last period.

A negative result

If the test result is consistently negative, then counselling on contraception can be suggested, and some attempt made to analyse how the initial situation arose. If a teacher suspects the girl is under pressure to have unprotected intercourse or in a situation she cannot cope with, then further help perhaps from her parents or referral for specialist counselling may be necessary.

A positive result

If the test result is positive it could be suggested first that the girl gets help from her parents, and help in telling them if necessary. This will be particularly needed if the girl does not have a good relationship with them. It can be explained that further advice in confidence, for the girl, and her parents, would be available from a sympathetic counsellor either at school or outside. This could be from a Pregnancy Counselling Co-ordinator (such as was appointed by Coventry Health Authority, to link all the relevant support services) or one from the social services, or a hospital social worker, or from specific agencies offering trained counsellors and non directive advice, such as Youth Advisory Services, Brook Advisory Centres, British Pregnancy Advisory Service or the Samaritans.

Every Authority should have a list of such agencies and their local contacts.

Confidentiality

This is obviously extremely important, as the perceived possible reaction of parents or doctors, and fear of the involvement of the police if the girl is under 16, can be overwhelming, and may mean the pregnancy is 'denied' and ignored, and help is not sought early. This is particularly likely in schoolgirl pregnancies [7] where complex emotional reactions are involved. In fact there is no legal requirement for anyone to report an offence under the 'Age of Consent 1956 Sexual Offences Act', so this need not be a deterrent to seeking help.

If the girl is willing to say who the father is, then this should be treated as confidential information and the offer of help be given to him through her. There is evidence that the needs of young fathers (most are under 19 and some still at school) have not been fully considered in the past, and support for them and their families, and a chance to be involved in the decisions being taken about the pregnancy, would be very beneficial [7].

Abortion

Abortions can be obtained, subject to the requirements of the Abortion Act from these sources.

i)   They can be obtained free, from the NHS, sometimes from outpatient day care centres. The availability varies tremendously in different parts of the country however.

   The majority of NHS services react positively to requests for the termination of schoolgirl pregnancies, so it *is* worth trying this official channel first. The Pregnant at School Report [7] recommended that all Health Authorities should ensure these were available free of charge.

ii)   Non profit-making organisations such as the British Pregnancy Advisory Service, or the Pregnancy Advisory Service, charge a fee. This varies with the stage of the pregnancy, but will be over £100. See the list of charges available from them.

iii)   Profit-making private clinics perform abortions, but the charges will probably be higher.

Some local health authorities use these organisations as their agents, the fees would then be paid by them. All independent nursing homes such as ii) and iii) offering pregnancy terminations have to be licensed and approved by the DHSS.

In 1981, 47.5% of abortions to residents in England and Wales were performed free by the NHS, 52.5% were done in independent premises, for a fee [120]. Concern has been expressed about the findings of a report by the Royal College of Obstetricians and Gynaecologists (Jan. 1984) that 1 in 5 women referred for an NHS abortion before the 12th week of pregnancy, have to wait up to 12 weeks later for the operation. There are no such delays in the non-profit making charity services.

Possible teaching approach

The subject may be raised spontaneously, or arise from press comment, or as one of the options open to Debbie (see page 221), or from discussion material listed in Resources (page 271). Questions can be answered factually, and then attitudes to abortion could be explored by using the following list of statements.

Pupils could be asked to decide which they agreed with, individually. The ticked sheets could be collected anonymously, and the results discussed by asking volunteers to argue for certain viewpoints, not necessarily those they held themselves.

With older children, speakers from organisations such as BPAS and LIFE, could be asked to take part in a debate on a 'Freedom of Choice' theme.

Discussion of the spectrum of attitudes to abortion.

How many of these statements would you agree with?

Abortions are never justified under any circumstance.

Human life begins at fertilisation together with the rights of that individual, which must be protected.

Abortions undermine respect for the sanctity of life and could lead to increasingly liberal views on euthanasia etc.

It is not justifiable to seek to alleviate social problems of over-crowding, poverty, and child abuse, by the abortion of unwanted conceptions.

No child need be unwanted, as there are waiting lists for the adoption of such babies.

Most women don't want abortions. They have them because of other people [153].

Abortion is discrimination against unborn human beings.

Abortion is not necessary.

Because abortion is legal under some circumstances it does not mean it is morally right.

Women feel a deep sense of guilt and remorse after an abortion.

Abortion is justified only for some very specific circumstances such as after a rape, or when the life of the mother is in danger.

It is justifiable to offer an abortion to a woman who has had Rubella in early pregnancy, has a high risk of transmitting a genetic abnormality, or who has had an amniocentesis test which has revealed an abnormal foetus.

Some women may feel guilty about *not* feeling guilty after an abortion.

Every case for abortion will be different and must be judged on the particular relevant circumstances.

Human life begins when the foetus can live independently from the mother.

Early abortions are acceptable, later ones increasingly disturbing from every point of view.

Abortion is justified as a support service for failed contraception and as part of total fertility control including sterilisation.

Women feel relieved after an abortion, and may then be more able to cope with a wanted pregnancy later.

A woman has the absolute right to decide whether or not she wishes to continue with a pregnancy, as it will be her body which will be affected.

The father has some rights and should be consulted about a possible abortion.

Abortion could be used as a main method of birth control in this country, as it has been in Japan, and Eastern European Countries for some time. Abortion 'on request' should be freely available.

Conclusions of such a discussion might be, people vary very much in their attitudes towards abortion, and some will always consider it morally wrong. For people who do not, then the advisability of those in need seeking an early abortion is clear. This implies early recognition and acceptance of the pregnancy, and willingness to communicate about this so help can be sought. One course of action might be to reduce the possibilities of ever being in a position of having to take a decision about an abortion, by responsible behaviour based on a good knowledge of human sexuality.

Explanations for children
The concept of an abortion on medical grounds may already have been introduced (page 98) together with the fact that some 15% of all established pregnancies will spontaneously abort or miscarry. There may be some slight consolation for those affected in the knowledge that a high proportion of such foetuses have been found to be abnormal in some way [72]. Help and support is available from the Miscarriage Association, 2 West Vale, Thornhill Rd, Dewsbury, West Yorkshire.

At this age pupils will be capable of a more detailed consideration of the physical and moral aspects of abortion. As it is one of the most controversial subjects, perhaps introduce the discussion by explaining consensus will be unlikely, and the skills of presenting arguments, and listening to other people's points of view, are ones which everyone might cultivate. It is possible of course to understand someone's beliefs but not to agree with them.

The background of the children's families will vary greatly, and some will include the experience of an abortion (there were 162 797 legal abortions for residents of England and Wales in 1982 OPCS Monitor AB 83/5 11.10.83). The teacher should take a neutral line, helping to present factual information and survey the spectrum of opinions on the subject. This can show that in a pleuralist society it is possible to accommodate extreme views, and the majority probably hold a position somewhere between them. In a Gallup National Opionion Poll in March 1982, 80% agreed with the statement 'Abortion should be a woman's choice after consultation with her doctor', 15% did not agree, and 5% did not know.

What is an abortion?
Technically abortions include the spontaneous abortions or miscarriages mentioned above, but the term is generally used to mean an artificial or induced termination of a pregnancy by the removal of the embryo (or foetus as it is called after about the 10th week of pregnancy) the placenta and membranes.

Methods used
These vary according to the length of the pregnancy, and can, technically legally be performed until the minimum age at which the foetus could be born

alive outside the mother's body. When the Abortion Act was introduced by David Steel in 1967, this was thought to be before the 28th week of pregnancy, a limit set in 1929.

It is rare however, for abortions to be done after the 24th week of pregnancy, (only 0.2% were done at this stage, whereas 79.3% were done before the 12th week of pregnancy, for women in England and Wales in 1981 [120]) as new techniques can enable some younger foetuses to survive.

An illegal, criminal or back-street abortion is one performed outside the requirements of the Act (see page 260) sometimes by unqualified non-medical people, usually for profit. Such abortions carry a high risk of shock, haemorrhage or an incomplete abortion (some material remaining in the womb), with subsequent infection. It was to try and overcome the dangers of such situations, estimated to be from about 80 000 illegal abortions in this country [81], that the act was formulated.

Post-coital methods

Opinions differ as to the exact moment that 'life' begins. Some consider this to be as soon as fertilisation occurs, others that it is not until the fertilised ovum has divided, travelled down the Fallopian tube, and actually embedded in the lining of the womb, that 'carriage' has taken place. It has been estimated that 60% of 'conceptions' do not survive the first cycle [51]. If 'morning after' or post-coital contraception is used within 3 days of intercourse, the ovum, if fertilised, could not have implanted, 'carriage' would not have taken place, and some conclude that this method cannot therefore be classified as an abortion or 'mis'carriage.

Delayed period

If a period is up to 12 days late, and unprotected intercourse has taken place previously, 'menstrual extraction' regulation is possible. This operation takes a few minutes and involves sucking out the contents of the womb with a fine flexible tube attached to a syringe or other gentle suction method. It can be done with or without a local anaesthetic at the doctor's surgery, or out patients' clinic. Prostaglandins can also be used at this stage to precipitate menstruation.

Vaginal surgery methods

These may be conducted in weeks 4 to 12 of the pregnancy.

i)   Vacuum aspiration is also a suction method, but the tube has to be slightly wider, so the cervix may first have to be stretched or otherwise opened to about the width of a finger by the insertion of a series of graded smooth metal rods, or a gently expanding stick made from seaweed (called a Laminaria tent) or by a prostaglandin analogue, used vaginally or by intramuscular injection, which softens and dilates the cervix. The operation takes about 10 minutes, under local or general anaesthetic, and the patient is often able to leave the clinic after a few hours, so 'day care' treatment is possible.

ii)   Dilation and curettage (d & c). Under a general anaesthetic the cervix is again stretched slightly (i.e. dilated) and the contents of the womb scraped out with a spoon-like curette. This method can sometimes be used after the

258

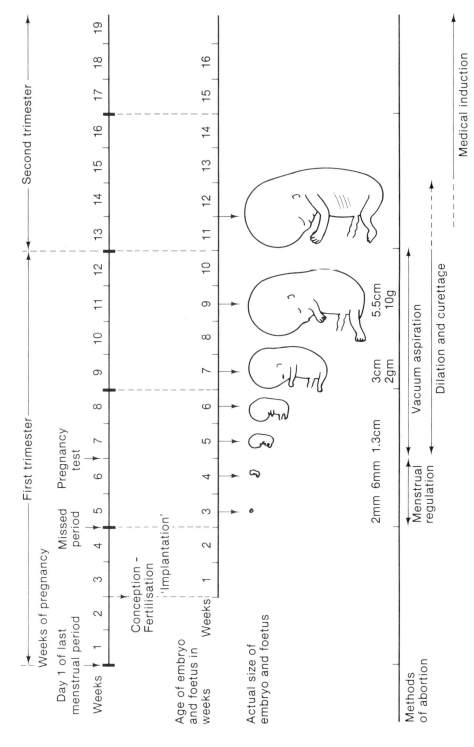

Figure 45   Development during early pregnancy and methods of abortion.

12th week of pregnancy, and may involve an overnight stay.

After twelve weeks

By this time the foetus could be too large to be extracted through an artificially dilated cervix, so a medical induction method may be used, which precipitates labour and a miscarriage. Prostaglandin hormones or other chemicals are introduced into the womb, either through the vagina and cervix, extra-amniotically, or, for later stages a fine needle is inserted through the wall of the abdomen and womb into the fluid surrounding the foetus, (i.e. intra-amniotically) and the prostaglandins are passed in. They may also be given intravenously at the same time. The foetus is subsequently 'born' in the same way as a full term delivery. This method may require a few days stay. Another technique, now much less often used, is to perform the equivalent of a Caesarian operation, called a hysterotomy (not to be confused with a hysterectomy, see page 93).

The risks

The risk for the patient, associated with the methods above, used legally, increase with the length of pregnancy. The emotional involvement and upset and sense of loss presumably also increase proportionately.

Early abortions, performed legally within the first 12 weeks of a pregnancy, have a very low risk factor, lower in fact than that of continuing with the pregnancy. USA data for 1972–75 gives mortality rates of 2 or less per 100 000 abortions up to the 10th week of pregnancy, less than 4 per 100 000 up to the 12th week, and only after the 16th week does the risk rise to 19, which is greater than that of childbirth, put at just over 12 per 100 000 births. Each week of delay after the 16th week of pregnancy increases the mortality risk by about one half [151]. Deaths from abortions in England and Wales in 1978 were given at 3.5 per 100 000, and totalled 5 [152].

When comparing the risks of various methods of birth control, the lowest level of all is achieved by the use of barrier methods (the sheath or cap plus spermicides) and early abortion as a back up procedure for contraceptive failure or patient misuse of the method [151].

The risks associated with illegal abortions are thought to be high, and in countries where abortion has been legalised, the take up of hospital beds for treating women suffering from complications following inefficient abortions, has dropped.

In the world as a whole it is estimated between 30 and 55 million abortions take place annually, about half of them performed by unskilled persons, illegally [151], when maternal mortality can be as high as 1000 per 100 000.

The long term effects

The long term effects of abortions, both physical and psychological, on subsequent pregnancies must always be considered. There were fears, for example, that repeated mechanical dilation of the cervix, as used in older procedures, could have lead to subsequent pregnancy problems. Potts and Shadbolt [155], in their critical analyses of the Wynn report [154], which documented possible adverse effects of abortion, have pointed out some of the difficulties in collecting information on this. Currently (Feb. 1984) such data available is thought to be equivocal, and not statistically significant where the abortion has been carried out by skilled doctors. The risk of a subsequent pregnancy leading to a low birth weight, premature delivery or spontaneous abortion in a woman who has previously had a vacuum aspiration is minimal [183].

The Pregnant at School Report [7] summarises evidence on the mental effects of pregnancy terminations, suggesting there are fairly consistent findings that no serious psychological harm necessarily follows. They quote a study of girls of 16 and under, who felt guilty and depressed immediately after the operation, but 6 months later were judged restored to their previous emotional health. However, they state there is some evidence the more severe psychological consequences are likely if the girl has poor relationships with her family, or is pressured into a termination. Other evidence suggests women refused an abortion are also at risk, and their children are more likely than others to suffer both socially and psychologically. Research is being done on the medical and psychological aspects of pregnancy termination, in women of all ages, by the Royal College of General Practitioners jointly with the Royal College of Obstetricians and Gynaecologists.

An abortion experience can be a motivation to use contraceptives, and studies have shown a greater uptake of such services when counselling on family planning is given in conjunction with the operation. Abortion may not be desired as a first choice when other methods of fertility control are freely and easily available, but it is desirable that women who have chosen to have one should have access to support and counselling afterwards, to enable them to come to terms with any possible feelings of grief, guilt or anger.

Legal abortion
In the United Kingdom, since 1967 abortion has been legal for any woman provided that in the opinion of two doctors (formed in good faith) it is performed for one or more of the following reasons.

The continuance of the pregnancy would involve risk:

i)   to the life of the pregnant woman greater than if the pregnancy were terminated,
ii) of injury to the physical or mental health of the pregnant woman greater than if the pregnancy were terminated,
iii) of injury to the physical or mental health of the existing child(ren) of the family of the pregnant woman greater than if the pregnancy were terminated,
iv) there is substantial risk that if the child were born it would suffer from such physical or mental abnormalities as to be seriously handicapped.

The law also states that no doctor, nurse or other worker need assist with an abortion if she/he has a conscientious objection to abortion.
Can a girl under 16 have an abortion?
Anyone under the age of 16 (conventionally, but not legally) [189] needs the consent of one of her parents or a legal guardian, before the operation is done,

unless there are very exceptional circumstances. Anyone over the age of 16 can consent to an abortion, or any other medical treatment, in her own right.

No one can be made to have an abortion if they do not wish to, the consent of the patient is taken to be of paramount importance.

Sexually transmitted diseases (STD)

The incidence of the total number of cases of sexually transmitted diseases in the UK has been rising steadily in the last decade, after a substantial increase between the 1950s and 1970s. When particular diseases are considered however, a more complex pattern emerges.

The three venereal diseases in this official category are Syphilis, which is declining in incidence, TABLE 15, Gonorrhoea, which has levelled out after reaching very high numbers, TABLE 16 and Chancroid or 'soft sore', a tropical bacterial disease causing painful genital ulcerations. This is rare in this country.

	1977	1978	1979
Gonorrhoea	65 963	63 569	61 616
Syphilis	4 780	4 866	4 385
Chancroid	49	57	49

For comparison, the total number of notifications for selected diseases in England and Wales in 1982.

Measles	94 193
Whooping cough	65 816 ('epidemic' rate)
Food poisoning	14 190
Tuberculosis	7414
Dysentery	2850

Source OPCS Monitor. Infectious Diseases. Ref, MB283/2 26.7.83. which gives a full discussion of these figures.

Factors affecting increased incidence of STDs

Some of the rise in reported cases may be due to an increased willingness of patients to come for treatment, better diagnostic techniques and services, and better contact tracing of infected individuals, and some because of a 'real' increase in incidence. There is continuing discussion about the relative importance of social and medical factors. e.g.

i)   Increased travel opportunities and anonymity when 'abroad' may lead to sexual experimentation of people of all ages,

ii)   There is more variation in the type of sexual activity, oral and anal sex also transmitting STD.

iii)   There has been a change from barrier contraceptive methods which give some protection from infection, to oral contraception or the coil, which do not. (However studies [2] [160] have found the more 'casual' the sexual encounter the less likely it is that a reliable method, or any method of contraception will be used. One study showed only 4% of those having casual sex had used any method. 96% of such people will therefore be particularly at risk of catching and transmitting STD.)

iv) Extra-marital activity has increased.

v) The number of partners any one person may have in their lifetime has increased.

vi) The total number of young people reaching sexual maturity has risen, and people are becoming sexually active earlier.

vii) Some strains of Gonorrhoea are now resistant to some antibiotics.

Table 15   Syphilis

Syphilis (The Pox)	
Incidence	In England in 1980 (158) All Ages Under 20 Under 16 Male 1,340 63 0 Female 207 59 3 The majority of cases of Syphilis (60–70%) occur in homosexual (or bisexual) men.
Cause	The spirochete bacterium *Treponema pallidum*, which has a longer incubation period than Gonorrhoea. It is detected by blood tests, as it can live in all parts of the body.
Transmission	i) Through moist mucus membrane, or damaged tissues or small breaks in the skin, through vaginal, oral or anal sex or by sexual kissing. (162) ii) Infection of a foetus is possible through the placenta. All expectant mothers having ante natal care will have blood tests which include one for Syphilis, so babies with congenital Syphilis are now rare.
Symptoms. These are the same for men and women, and occur in stages.	**Primary stage** From 10 days to 12 weeks after infection a painless sore or ulcer develops, either externally on the sex organs, the penis, labia, or anus or less often, on lip or tongue, or internally on the vagina, cervix, or rectum, where it will remain unseen. These sores are very infectious, but do heal up and disappear on their own. **Secondary stage** Some 4–12 weeks later a non irritating rash may develop on the body or limbs, lasting for some weeks. There may also be an "unwell" feeling, loss of appetite, flu like symptoms and mouth sores, and enlargement of lymph glands. These symptoms also disappear on their own, but the disease remains in a latent form which is still infectious in the early stages. It can, however, be detected by blood tests. Eventually, after many years, it may continue into the nervous system. **Tertiary stage** If this develops, damage may be caused to limbs, and joints, with ulcers forming in many sites, including the skin, or organs such as the heart or nervous system are affected causing paralysis and mental disturbance, or death. This stage is now rare, as treatment at any previous stage will prevent it. (There were 56 deaths due to Syphilis in England and Wales in 1981. OPCS Monitor Ref. DH2. 82/3.)
Treatment	Syphilis responds well to a course of treatment with antibiotics, often penicillin. The patient may be asked to come for long term follow up checks for a couple of years after the initial infection.

Table 16   Gonorrhoea

Gonorrhoea (Clap, a dose)	
Incidence	In England 1980 (158) All Ages Under 20 Under 16 Male 34,070 4,383 94 Female 20,320 6,521 305 Total cases in the UK in 1979 61,618.
Cause	A bacterium *Neisseria gonorrhoeae* Very short incubation period. Detected by microscopic examination and culture of samples.
Transmission	i) by contact of mucus membranes during vaginal, oral or anal sex, when the cervix, urethra, rectum or throat in women, and the urethra, rectum or throat in men may be infected. ii) Barlow (159) suggests that some 5% of pre-pubertal daughters of infected mothers may contract the disease from them (perhaps from damp flannels or towels) as the less acid, thin walled vagina of young girls makes them particularly susceptible to infection. iii) during birth as the child passes through an infected cervix. The baby's eyes may be affected, with resulting damage if left untreated.
Symptoms. These are different in men and women.	Women In 60% of women there are no symptoms, so they will not be aware they have the disease, nor that it is developing. In 40%, from 2 days to 3 weeks after sexual contact, there may be painful urination, an unusual vaginal discharge, a fever or 'chill' symptoms, abdominal pain, or painful joints. Men Some 10 – 15% of men have no symptoms. For the rest, from 2 to 10 days after sexual contact there may be painful urination and/or a light or heavy yellowish discharge from the penis.
Complications	In women if the disease is untreated it may cause the Fallopian tubes to become inflamed and blocked (salpingitis) possibly leading to sub-fertility, infertility, or ectopic pregnancies. If still untreated, further damage, such as to the heart, could occur. In men untreated gonorrhoea can affect other parts of the male reproductive system causing swelling and pain, and possible sterility.
Treatment	As the infective organism is a bacterium, it does respond to antibiotics. However, some strains have become partially resistant to some antibiotics, and one type produces an enzyme, ß-lactamase, which breaks down penicillin completely, making it ineffective. The number of infections in the U.K. involving this type of Gonorrhoea is still relatively small (613 cases in the second half of 1982) but is increasing. The usual treatment is a course of antibiotics, of one dose, orally or by injection, if the disease is in the early stages. Further examinations are always necessary to check the cure has been successful.

Global figures for the incidence of venereal diseases are estimated by the World Health Organisation to be 250 million new cases of Gonorrhoea, and 50 million of Syphilis each year.

Non-venereal sexually transmitted diseases

There are now a large number of such diseases, some occurring together in mixed infections, which can be difficult to isolate and diagnose, as the symptoms may overlap or mask each other. They have been called the second generation of sexually transmitted diseases, now actually more common than the 'classic' variety [54]. There is particular concern about the increase in those causing Pelvic Inflammatory Disease (PID) in women, where the infection spreads up from the cervix, and affects the Fallopian tubes, and the surrounding and supporting structures of the womb, leading to an increase in infertility and ectopic pregnancies. Also worrying is the increase in cervical cancer, where the viruses causing genital warts and herpes have been implicated.

Table 17   NSGI or NSU

Non-specific genital infection (NSGI), or non-specific urethritis (NSU)	
Incidence	New cases in the UK in 1979 were 113,138, an increase of 5,000 over the previous year. (158). It is twice as common as Gonorrhoea.
Cause	In about half the cases no particular microorganism can be detected, in others the very small bacterium *Chlamydia trachomatis,* has been found. This is difficult to detect as unlike other bacteria which will grow on culture 'plates' it only grows in living cells, so must be cultured on the yolk sacs of chicken embryos.
Transmission	By sexual means.
Symptoms	Women (NSGI) There may be 'cervicitis' and a slight increase in vaginal discharge, urethritis, and pain on urinating, or the infection may spread upwards causing pelvic inflammatory disease and salpingitis. Men (NSU) The symptoms can be rather similar to Gonorrhoea, causing urethritis, and hence, painful urination.
Complications	In women these can be those of sub or infertility caused by damage to the Fallopian tubes and the disease can also infect the eyes of a child as it is born. In men the infections may spread to other parts of the sex organs which may become inflamed and painful.
Treatment	A course of antibiotics such as tetracyclins, which may be given over several weeks. Further checks may be needed to detect and prevent the return of the infection.

Other non-venereal sexually transmitted infections

There are many other diseases which can be sexually transmitted, such as pubic lice, the insect, *Phthirius pubis,* or scabies, caused by the mite *Sarcoptes scabiei,* and several thousand cases of these are reported each year. They can be treated very effectively with ointments and lotions.

Genital warts

There were 27 654 cases of these in the UK in 1979. These are caused by the virus *Condylomata acuminata,* on the ano-genital area.

Table 18   Candidiasis

Candidiasis (Thrush)	
Incidence	In UK, 1979, 42,637 cases
Cause	A yeast-like fungus *Candida albicans* found naturally in the intestines of 70% of the population, and in the vagina of some women, without causing symptoms. It can also sometimes occur in the mouth, particularly in babies.
Transmission	This may be by direct infection from the anus, in women, or by vaginal or anal sex.
Symptoms	Women A whitish discharge from the vagina, with intense irritation and itching of the vulval area, and the perineum (area between the vagina and the anus). Men Itching and soreness of the penis, or anal region. It is more likely to infect uncircumcised men, as it can colonise the area under the foreskin, causing 'balanitis'.
Complications	In both sexes there may be an allergic reaction to the fungus, so exacerbating its effect. It can be present without causing any problems, but if a change in the acidity of the vagina occurs, perhaps because of i) the use of a broad spectrum antibiotic, ii) during pregnancy, or iii) as a side effect of some types of oral contraceptive pill, it may begin to grow freely. Diabetics may be particularly susceptible to thrush infections. Correct wiping of the vulva, always from front to back, can help prevent reinfection.
Treatment	By fungicidal pessaries, both vaginal and anal, and cream for the external growth. Drugs may also be given orally. Some women have found it helpful to aid the return to acidity in the vagina by introducing plain, live, natural yoghurt, which contains the helpful bacterium *Lactobacillus*.

They are unsightly and have recently been implicated in causing cervical cancer [191]. They can be treated with chemicals or surgery or sometimes disappear of their own accord, but they should be taken seriously and medical help sought. A regular cervical smear test might be advised for women who have been in contact with the virus.

Molluscum contagiosum

This virus is sometimes caught from swimming or Turkish baths. Small raised hard spots form on genitals, thighs, buttocks and lower abdomen. They can be removed chemically or mechanically, by a doctor.

Hepatitis

One form of hepatitis can be transmitted sexually, particularly by homosexual men during oral or anal sex [159].

Acquired Immune Deficiency Syndrome

This is rare in Britain up to now (1984) with 50 or so cases since December 1981, but an increasing number of infections have been reported in the USA, with thousands diagnosed, the majority among homosexual men. The cause is being sought, and is probably a virus or viruses, which seem to have a long incubation period, of up to 3 years. It is transmitted sexually, and possibly also through blood transfusions or the use of some blood products. Some drug addicts, using injected drugs, have also developed the disease.

The body's natural resistance to infections or cancers, seems to be affected, so the sufferer becomes prone to many diseases, which may eventually prove fatal.

Research is continuing, to elucidate the nature of the disease, and its mode of transmission, so treatment or prevention techniques may be developed.

Possible teaching approach

Please refer to the section on sexually transmitted diseases, page 99 for introductory information which could be revised at this stage. Before any of the work is undertaken, it might be helpful for members of the sex education team to liaise with staff at the nearest special clinic, They could explain confidentiality, the routine, and any commonly held myths about STDs, which might be dispelled by sound education.

The lead-in to the topic at this stage for the class should be from the social and personal relationship side, rather than the medical. The initial presentation could be the discussion of any scenario where a character has had casual sex (with a 'primary contact') perhaps while away from home, or on holiday, and has subsequently realised the possibility of being infected. The emotions and feelings thus raised can be explored, and the full implications discussed, including future relationships with the steady partner (the 'secondary' contact) if there is one. Some anger may be generated for example, and adjustments and acceptances will be required all round.

What happens at a clinic?

It may be called a 'special' or genito-urinary clinic, or be 'coded' eg. Martha and Luke, and is very often run in association with a hospital. Many people go to their own doctor first, who may diagnose and treat some conditions, but can refer a patient to a special clinic. Anyone, however, whatever age, can go directly to such a clinic for free help, advice and treatment, without a referral note or any 'permission' being necessary. The clinic addresses and phone numbers can be found in some telephone directories under Venereal Diseases, or on posters in public toilets or libraries, or by phoning a hospital or family planning clinic.

At the clinic

(See film sequence page 272.) First the patient must register with the friendly receptionist. Forms do have to be filled in, but any name and address given is in complete confidence, and a patient number may be used instead. Next comes a talk with the doctor, who will ask about any symptoms, sexual behaviour, menstrual cycle etc. The doctor will need to examine the genital area, and take samples of fluid and cells from the urethra, and possibly the rectum and throat of both sexes, and the vagina and cervix. There may be fear of such procedures so doctors stress the need to relax and that the specimen will be taken from just inside the urethra, (not the deep penile probe dreaded by the boys in the

Table 19   *TV* and *Gardnerella*

Trichomonas vaginalis (TV, Trich)	
Incidence	In the UK in 1979, 21,222 reported cases.
Cause	A minute single-celled animal, a protozoan, *Trichomonas vaginalis*, belonging to the flagellate group. It is extremely common, between 10 and 20% of women have it at some time.
Transmission	By sexual intercourse, and just possibly, by contact with damp objects, as the organism can survive for a very short time outside the body.
Symptoms	Women A vaginal discharge which smells very unpleasant, and may be frothy, and can cause soreness of the vulva and vagina. Men A thin, white or colourless discharge from the penis which may be frothy.
Treatment	This animal responds well to a course of oral drugs. Both heterosexual partners are usually treated as although the male may not show any symptoms, it is possible he might be carrying the disease.
Gardnerella vaginalis	This organism also causes a vaginal discharge with an unpleasant smell, but no irritation. Treatment is similar to that for *Trichomonas*.

Table 20   Cystitis

Cystitis	
Incidence	Over half the women in the UK suffer from Cystitis at some time in their lives, a proportion having repeated attacks. Men are only occasionally affected.
Cause	There are many possible causes, sometimes an infection, by the bacterium *Escherichia coli*, which normally lives in the rectum, or other organisms may be implicated. Friction or bruising of the urethra as may happen during sexual intercourse, or abnormalities of urethra, bladder or kidney, can also lead to cystitis. In some cases it has been suggested initial pain may subsequently lead to psychosomatic effects.
Symptoms	Inflammation of bladder and urethra, causing tenderness and pain in the abdomen, pain on passing urine, and a 'need' to pass it frequently, even if none is present. The urine may look dark, or include blood flecks from the inflammation.
Treatment	Because of the very varied reasons for cystitis, the treatment will be different for each cause. A doctor's help should always be sought. Antibiotics can be prescribed if an infection is diagnosed. To avoid bruising the urethra during sex, advice on different positions, or techniques, or the use of lubricants, may be given.
Self help	See HEC leaflet *Cystitis*.

Table 21   Genital Herpes

Genital Herpes	
Incidence	In the UK in 1981 there were nearly 12,080 cases. (Family Planning Today. First Quarter 1983) and there are an estimated 100,000 sufferers overall in this country.
Cause	A virus, *Herpes simplex* Virus, type II. This is very similar to HSV Type I, which causes cold sores on the face, or which may affect the eyes. They can overlap in infection sites, so virus from a cold sore could cause genital Herpes. The Herpes viruses are very widespread, perhaps 70–80% of the population have had them (159), and many people have developed partial immunity, or 'contain' the virus, without showing any effects, or being infectious. The 'family' of Herpes viruses, includes those causing glandular fever, chicken pox and shingles.
Transmission	By contact of mucus membranes, or through damaged skin, by genital or oral sex, or transferred on the hands to various parts of the body. It is also just possible it could be caught by contact with damp objects or towels with the virus on them. Up to 20% of Herpes infections are passed on in a non-sexual way. Herpes is transmissible to babies, as they are born, if the cervix is actively shedding the virus.
Symptoms	These are usually worse in women than in men, and tend to be worst on the first occasion. Within a few days of infection, (2–10) itching, tingling or aching of the vulva or penis may give rise to spots, developing into fluid-filled blisters. These subsequently break, leaving raw ulcers, which in some cases can be very painful. They may spread to the thighs or round the anus, or they may be internal on the vagina or cervix. In some cases there is no pain, and a woman may not be aware she has the disease. Others 'shed' the virus but have no ulcers. One of the main symptoms is pain on passing urine (which may be similar to that of cystitis). There may also be a general "unwell" feeling, an increase in vaginal discharge, or enlargement and tenderness of the lymph glands in the groin. The ulcers gradually dry up and heal, but this may take days or weeks, and the virus may then still remain in the nervous system, dormant or 'latent'
Complications	In both sexes the ulcers may become secondarily infected with bacteria. In many cases the symptoms recur, sometimes triggered by sunshine or UV lamps, stress, local irritation of the genitals, being fatigued or 'rundown', menstruation, or by having sex. Recurrent attacks are less severe, and may gradually become less frequent. The Herpes virus has been implicated in the development of cervical cancer, so any woman who has had Herpes is advised to have a cervical smear test done every year, so early detection and cure could be assured, with the new techniques, perhaps using a colposcope to examine the cervix, and excising the affected part with a laser. For infected pregnant women the baby can be delivered by Caesarian operation if necessary. A woman should always tell her doctor if she has had genital Herpes and is, or wishes to become, pregnant. The psychological effect of having this disease may be considerable, so hypnotherapy has been used to combat the stress factors which exacerbate the disease and a voluntary support group has been set up for advice and co-ordination of self help groups:– The Herpes Association, c/o Spare Rib, 27 Clerkenwell Close, London EC1 0R7.
Treatment	As Herpes is a virus, at the moment there is no specific cure. It must first be correctly identified, as not all ulcers are caused by Herpes. Antibiotics are sometimes prescribed, to clear up any secondary bacterial infections. Research is being done to find more effective drugs such as Acyclovir already available. A vaccine is also possible and one is being tested by Dr. Skinner and his research team at the University of Birmingham Medical School Virus Research Unit, and has shown most encouraging results. Other treatment concentrates on soothing and alleviating the symptoms.

Trigger film 2, page 272). A general examination will also be given, and blood and urine samples taken.

There then follows a wait of about a few hours while the quick laboratory tests are done, and specimens are stained, and examined under a microscope. Others may need to be grown in a culture before they can be identified, and these results will not be available for a few days.

Finally there is a second talk with the doctor, who may be able to make a diagnosis and give treatment immediately, or may ask the patient to come back some days later, for the diagnosis, treatment, or a check up.

Conclusion of work on STD

At the end of this work there could be a few reminders.

A certain amount of vaginal secretion is normal as it lubricates the vagina and keeps it healthy. This will vary slightly at different times in the monthly cycle, during sexual excitement, or pregnancy. Every woman learns what variation is normal for her, and it is only if this changes much, (or she knows she has been at risk of catching an STD), that help need be sought.

Explain that personal hygiene is always important, and women are particularly vulnerable to genital infections for these reasons:

i) the urethral, vaginal and anal openings are in close proximity
ii) the inner vulval area is covered by a mucous membrane (a moist skin layer, like the inside of the mouth)
iii) the urethra is relatively short, so infections reach the bladder easily
iv) the nature of the vagina provides an 'incubator' for some infections

Men, having a 'dry' genital region, and a long urethra (with the opening far away from the anus) may be less susceptible, though the region under the foreskin is moist, and may need special care.

Self assessment quiz

i) What diseases other than Gonorrhoea and Syphilis can be sexually transmitted? (*See previous list of non-venereal diseases.*)
ii) Can some of these infections be transmitted other than sexually? How? (*Self infection, from the mother, while 'in utero' or during birth or from damp objects.*)
iii) Are these diseases serious? (*They can be, if left untreated.*)
iv) Is it possible to self diagnose them?
   (*No, as no symptoms may develop, or can be similar for different infections, so need laboratory tests for accurate identification.*)
v) Can they be cured?
   (*The majority can, and Herpes becomes less of a problem with time, or a vaccine may be found.*)
vi) Can they be caught again?
   (*Yes, and again ... and again*)
vii) Can several be caught together?
   (*Yes, and may mask each other's symptoms, so expert help is needed.*)

viii) Who would be particularly at risk?
    (*Anyone having several partners, particularly in quick succession [159].*)
ix) How could they reduce the risks?
    (*By using a sheath or cap plus spermicide, washing before and after sex, urinating soon afterwards, and by having check ups every 3 months at a special clinic, or more frequently if symptoms develop.*)
x) Where can free, expert, confidential advice and treatment be obtained?
    (*GP, or special clinic.*)
xi) Does everyone going to a special clinic have a *sexually* transmitted disease?
    (*No, see answer 2, and many are not in fact infected.*)
xii) Does everyone run the risk of getting these diseases?
    (*No, it depends on the chosen life style of the person.*)

Background reading for teachers

1. *Sexually Transmitted Diseases, the facts.* Barlow D. 1979. Oxford University Press. Very readable, comprehensive and with rare humour.
2. *Herpes, the facts.* Oates J. K. 1983. Penguin.
3. *Sex with Health. Which?* Consumers Association. The Which? Guide to Contraception, Abortion and Sex related diseases.
4. *Sex and VD* Llewellyn-Jones D. 1975 Faber.
5. *Sexually Transmitted Diseases.* Oates J. K. 1979. Women's Health Concern.
6. *VD and Diseases Transmitted Sexually.* Morton R. S. 1978. Family Doctor Booklet. BMA.
7. *Understanding Cystitis.* Kilmartin A. 1975. Pan.
8. *Sexually Transmitted Diseases.* HEC Source list.
9. FPIS Leaflets.
  i) VD the facts.
  ii) HEC set, *What you should know about sexually transmitted diseases,* (Gonorrhoea, Syphilis, Urethritis, viral infections and infestations, vaginal health and discomfort.)
  iii) *Cystitis. What you should know about it.*
  iv) 1982 Fact Sheets F1(3) *Facts about teenagers* F3(11) *Sexually Transmitted Diseases and Contraception.*
10. Brook Advisory Centre Information sheet 1983. *Genital Herpes.*
11. *Sexual infections.* Sugrue D. and Clayton J. An excellent well illustrated booklet in colour. Obtainable from West Midlands Regional Health Authority, 146 Hagley Rd, Birmingham, B16 9PA

Discussion material on STD

1. Health Education 13–18 (see page 49) 1982. Schools Council and HEC. Level 2 14–16 years *What would you do ... about sexually transmitted diseases?* The unit provides background notes for teachers, and two case histories, of situations as outlined above. Worksheets, and drawings of the characters, which could be used in role play, are included.

2. Posters from Project Icarus. A set of 8 black and white posters, a selection of which could be used as flexible discussion starters with older children, or youth groups, or to illustrate points arising from other material. Discussion can include the reasons why it was felt important to produce the posters in the first place, and whether the term STD will replace VD in general use.

i) *In the Spring a young man's fancy ... lightly turns to thoughts of love.* Picture of a youth, face blanked out, leaving a special clinic. Possible discussion points. Why might the face have been covered? Is confidentiality of treatment so important? What sort of responsibility is he showing by going to a clinic? Could he go to any special clinic, even outside his area? (*Yes*) Would he need a letter from his doctor? (*No.*) Is his partner, so 'lightly' encountered, likely to need help? Why? Do the seasons, or weather, affect sexual desire? (See Parkes ref 61). Does 'desire' have to be satisfied at once, or do other factors matter too?

ii) *One place you won't catch VD* Picture of a lavatory. Discussion of VD implies Gonorrhoea and Syphilis, which do not survive outside the body, so cannot be caught from lavatories. Some other STDs, such as Trichomonas, can survive in films of water for a short time, so if in contact with the moist vulval area it is *just* possible it might cause an infection. Men are much less vulnerable in this respect.

iii) *Isn't this nice? Just you, me ... and seventy million gonococci*
Picture of a couple in the grass. Discuss the following
Can you tell if someone's got an STD?
(Not always, some have *no* symptoms, and do not know themselves).
Do 'nice' people have STD?
(*Yes, if they have been 'at risk'. Clinic patients include all social classes and professions. Famous people who had these diseases include Schumann, Moliere, Gaugin, Boswell and Baudelaire, and, presumably, their less famous partners.*)

iv) *Here today ... Gonorrhoea tomorrow*
Picture of bare feet of couple on the grass.
The higher the number of sexual partners, and the shorter the time between them, the more likely it is an STD will be transmitted. There is an 'incubation' period for all diseases, and some people could be *pre*-symptomatic but still infectious.
What other risks might this sort of life style have? (Emotional as well as physical)

v) *VD: the cheapest form of contraception*
No picture, statement only. The long term effects of untreated STDs, particularly of PID should be discussed, N.B. VD can't be 'cheapest' because contraceptives are free.
How could it be very 'expensive' in the long run, in terms of relationships?

vi) *VD: as common as measles*
Statement only, no picture. Compare the figures for the incidence of VD and measles. (page 261) Discuss the effects of the measles vaccination. Are there likely to be vaccines against STDs? Research continues on these, but the task has proved difficult because the body does not produce any useful immune reaction to these infections, with the exception of Herpes (page 268).

vii) *VD: Something to keep in the family*
Picture of a new born baby. Discuss the risks of a woman with STD infecting her baby during pregnancy by the disease passing through the placenta, as in Syphilis, or during the birth process e.g. Gonorrhoea, Chlamydia, Herpes. Such complications can be avoided through ante-natal care, and honesty with the doctor, and in not running the risk of catching the diseases in the first place.

viii) *Five reasons ... why Sandra Croft may have VD*
Picture of a young woman, and five male signatures. Discuss the risks of having several sexual partners particularly if they themselves also have several partners. What is the chance of a woman showing no symptoms? Might Sandra wish to have a family later? How might her present behaviour affect that wish?

All the Icarus posters have extra information at the bottom, and the statement 'If you put yourself at risk, have a check up. It makes sense to make sure.'
3. Sound tape. *The X factor.* 24 minutes. 1971. Infotape from E.J. Arnold. A tape cassette of the relationship conflicts generated when a contact slip is received by one member of a group. Teaching notes available.

Films

1. VD Trigger films. *Attitudes to Health and Sexually Transmitted Diseases.* Made for the HEC by Concord Films Council. Three 6 minute, 16mm, films, to stimulate discussion. Extensive teachers' notes, with facts about STD, and guidance on how to use the films are available.
   i)   Film One: *Janet*
        Janet feels unwell, but is persuaded to go to school, where she seems to cope. We do not know why she might be unwell, or if she is 'spoofing'.
   ii) Film Two: *Rupert*
        A discussion between classmates liberates ancient myths about STDs, but enables Rupert to get himself to a special clinic. Some descriptions of symptoms and procedures are vernacularly graphic, so provide reassurance at this point by describing actual clinic routines (see page 266).
   iii) Film Three: *Sue*
        Rupert has been asked to contact Sue, as a possible source of his infection. He does so, though rather indiscreetly tells three other people in the process. Why might he have 'confessed' his secret in this way? Is it fair to Sue, to do so, or ought everyone to be more open about having these diseases?
2. *Casual encounters of the infectious kind* 16mm colour. 1979. Boulton Hawker and Oxford Health Authority Concord Films Council. Comprehensive teacher's notes provided.
   i) Part 1. *The facts about sexually transmitted diseases* 25 minutes. A non-moralising factual account of all major STDs, illustrated by diagrams, commentary, and simulated interviews with 'ex patients'.
   ii) Part 2. *A check up at the clinic.* 26 minutes. A most useful sequence showing a young woman, Linda, (played by a social worker) attending a special clinic. All stages are shown including a pelvic examination (viewed from the head of the patient), and the test material being stained and examined in the laboratory. These films are very suitable for older children, 15 +, but are best used separately, as they are rather long for a full discussion afterwards, if used together.
3. *VD – Attack Plan* 16mm colour. 16 minutes. Walt Disney Productions. Guild of Sound and Vision. A lively approach with VD germ 'troops' being briefed for their attack, aided by shame, fear and ignorance. This is usually enjoyed and is 'non threatening' to staff or pupils. It would be useful as lead in or summary material but perhaps consider that children often feel cheated if 'the *only* thing *we* had was a *cartoon* on' ... STD or contraception etc,

Resources for teaching about unwanted pregnancies

Essential reading as background information for teachers. *Pregnant at School Report* [7]
Also most helpful are these booklets from Coventry Health Authority:
i) *Pregnant? Problems? Help?*
ii) *Information and guidelines for those working with pregnant schoolgirls, and schoolchild parents and their families.* Some of this booklet is only relevant to Coventry, but it does cover comprehensively, the general approach, legal considerations, financial support, educational, health and social services provision and possible support from voluntary organisations for pregnant schoolgirls.

Booklet ... *Mixed feelings* Mira Dava. Channel 4 Broadcasting support series PO Box 4000 London W3 6XJ

British Pregnancy Advisory Service, material
1. Booklets
    i)   *Abortion, the next steps.* July 1974. A discussion of the report of the Lane Committee on the working of the Abortion Act.
    ii) Doggett. M. *Post coital contraception.* August 1982.
2. Leaflets
    i)   *Introducing the British Pregnancy Advisory Service.*
    ii) *Pregnant?*
    iii) *Unwanted pregnancy and abortion, questions and answers.*
3. Document. *Pregnancy Counselling: Some questions and answers.*
4. Film. Suitable for staff, or 6th formers, and available from Concord Films Council. *A Question of Understanding*, 28 mins. Colour, 16mm. Two case histories of women seeking a pregnancy termination.

Brook Advisory Centre material
Three papers on Teenage Pregnancy by Simms M. and Smith C.
Part I. *Ten Schoolgirl Mothers* Detailed studies of 10 teenagers who kept their babies, suggesting the 'motherhood role' is the only one perceived and attainable by some young girls under certain circumstances.

Part II. *Teenage mothers and abortion* A report suggesting some teenagers would have liked the choice of an abortion rather than continue with their pregnancy.

Part III. *Teenage mothers and adoption* The experiences of teenage mothers who considered having their babies adopted.

Family Planning Information Service material
Fact sheets
i)   HI(34) *Abortion in Great Britain* Jan. 1982.
ii) H2(8) *Abortion statisitcs.* Jan. 1982.

Abortion
1. Anti-abortion material can be obtained from:
    i)   LIFE, 7 Parade, Leamington Spa, Warwickshire.
    ii) Society for the Protection of the Unborn Child (SPUC) 94 Brechin Place, London SW7.
    iii) Lifeline Pregnancy Care, 53 Victoria Street, London SW1.
2. For pupils, the booklet, *Abortion*, Brook Advisory Centres Education and Publications Unit. Updated 1983. A balanced view of abortion, giving discussion points for and against, a reading list, and abortion statistics.
3. Audio-visual material
    i)   BBC, Radio. *Make Up Your Mind.* For age 15+ Five programmes discussing the ethics of using new scientific knowledge, such as the possibility of an abortion after an amniocentesis test has disclosed a foetal abnormality. Teacher's notes available.
    ii) TV. *Scene* 14–16 A series of plays and documentaries on controversial subjects, including one on an unwanted pregnancy. Teacher's notes available.
    iii) TV, *General studies* for Age 16–19 A series which includes two episodes on life and death before birth, covering foetal development and the issues of abortion. Teacher's notes available.

REFERENCES

[1] Education Act (1980) Publication of information (Section 8) Hansard. House of Commons. 30th June 1980.

[2] Farrell'C. (1978) *My Mother Said ... the way young people learn about sex and birth control.* London. Routledge & Kegan Paul.

[3] Barnes D. *From communication to curriculum.* Penguin.

[4] Zelnik, M. & Kim, Y.J. (1982) *Sex Education and its Association with Teenage Sexual Activity, Pregnancy and Contraceptive Use.* Family Planning Perspectives 14.3 May/June 1982.

[5] Ashken, I.C. & Soddy, A.G. *Study of pregnant school-age girls.* British Journal of Family Planning 980. **6**. pp.77–82.

[6] OPCS. Office of Population Censuses and Surveys, Information Branch (Dept. M) St. Catherines House, 10 Kingsway, London WC2B 6JP.

[7] *Pregnant at School* (1979) Joint Working Party on Pregnant Schoolgirls and Schoolgirl Mothers. National Council for One Parent Families.

[8] Schools Council Health Education Project 5–13 (SCHEP) (1977) London. T. Nelson & Sons.

[9] *Health Education 13–18* (1982) Schools Council and Health Education Council Project. London. Forbes.

[10] *Sex Education* (1974) Teachers' Advisory Committee Report, Liverpool Education Committee.

[11] Balding, J.W. (1979) *Health education topics and their relative importance to parents, pupils and teachers* 1979 Monitor No. 52. TACADE.

[12] National Council for Civil Liberties (1975) *Homosexuality and the teaching profession.* NCCL Report No. 8.

[13] *Woman's Own* magazine (May 23rd 1981) *Teenage Sex Dilemma. What you think.*

[14] Dawkins, J. (1967) *A Textbook of Sex Education.* Oxford Basil Blackwell.

[15] Film *Then One Year* British Version Boulton-Hawker Films Ltd., from Concord Films Council Ltd.

[16] *Loving and Caring* Family Planning Association and Health Education Council. 'Trigger' film in five parts. Central film library or Concord Films Council Ltd.

[17] Reid, D. (1982) School sex education and the causes of unintended teenage pregnancies, a review. Health Education Journal, March 1982.

[18] Kirkendall, L.A. (1965) *Sex Education. SIECUS Study Guide No. 1.* Sex Information and Education Council of the US.

[19] Kirby, D. (1980) The effects of School sex education programs: a review of the literature. Journal of School Health. Dec. 1980. pp.559–563.

[20] Rogers, R. (1974) *Sex Education Rationale and Reaction.* Chapter 14. Cambridge University Press.

[21] Williams, T. & Williams, N. *Personal and Social Development in the School Curriculum.* Health Education Project 13–18. Schools Council and Health Education Council

[22] Walters, J. & Walters. L.H. (1983) *The Role of the Family in Sex Education.* Journal of Research & Development in Education 16.2.1983.

[23] Lambert, L. & Pearson, R. *Sex Education in Schools.* Journal of the Institute of Health Education. **15** 4–11.

[24] Stanworth, M. (1981) *Gender and Schooling. A study of sexual divisions in the classroom.* Women's Research and Resources Centre.

[25] Francome, C. (1983) *Unwanted pregnancies amongst teenagers* Vol 5. pp 139–143. Journal of Biosocial Science.

[26] Ripley, G.D., Burns, C. & Dickinson, V.A. (1971) *A Survey of Sexual Knowledge and Attitudes in Borehamwood.* The Practitioner. **207** 1971. pp.351–360.

[27] Gagnon, J.H. & Simon, W. (1973) *Sexual Conduct,* London, Hutchinson.

[28] Schofield, M. (1965) *The Sexual Behaviour of Young People.* London, Longman.

[29] Newcastle-upon-Tyne Health Education Study Group *How are you man?* (see page 17). Newcastle Education Department.

[30]   Cowley, J., David, K. & Williams, T. (Ed.) (1981) *Health Education in Schools* London Harper & Row.

[31]   CEM (1976) *Discovering life through Growing Up* Vol. III, No. 2. Spring term 1976 Christian Education Movement.

[32]   TACADE (1981) *Free to choose. An Approach to Drug Education.* Pack of 10 units.

[33]   Dunnell, K. (1979) *Family Formation 1976.* Office of Population Censuses and Surveys. London. HMSO.

[34]   Emery, M. (1980) *The theory and practice of behaviour change in the school context.* International Journal of Health Education **23** (2) 1980 116–125.

[35]   Baldwin, J. & Wells, H. (1979) *Active Tutorial Work Books 1–5.* A five year programme of pastoral work for tutorial periods. Lancashire County Council. Blackwell. Available from TACADE.

[36]   Rice, W. (1981) *Informal methods in health and social education.* TACADE.

[37]   Evans, M. (Ed.) (1981) *Health Education in Secondary Schools: 10 Case studies.* TACADE.

[38]   Christopher, E. (1980) *Sexuality and Birth Control in Social and Community Work.* London. Temple Smith.

[39]   Sathar, Z.A. (1983) Birth spacing and Childhood mortality IPPF Medical Bulletin 17 No. 4. August 1983.

[40]   If only We'd known 3 part Trigger film. Spastics Society & HEC. Free loan from Concord Films Council or Central Film Library.

[41]   Schools Council Working Paper 57 (1976) Health Education in Secondary Schools. London. Evans/Methuen Educational.

[42]   Burkitt, A. (1980) *Learning to live with sex.* Family Planning Association.

[43]   Jackson, S. (1978) *On the social construction of female sexuality.* Women's Research and Resources Centre Publication.

[44]   Kreitler, H. & S. (1966) *Children's concepts of sexuality and birth.* Child development. **37** (1966) pp.363–378 and in Rogers, see ref. 20.

[45]   Chandler, E.M. (1980) *Educating Adolescent Girls.* London George, Allen and Unwin.

[46]   British Pregnancy Advisory Service (BPAS) 1976 Annual Report.

[47]   Brook Advisory Centres. Annual Report (1980–81) p.7. *Trends in teenage pregnancies 1970–1979 England and Wales.*

[48]   Dallas, D.M. (1972) *Sex Education in School and Society.* National Foundation for Education Research.

[49]   Rudduck, J. (Ed.) *Learning to teach through discussion.* Book and tape. Centre for Applied Research in Education. University of East Anglia.

[50]   Dalzell-Ward, A.J. (1974) *A Textbook of Health Education* for students in Colleges of Education, teachers and health educators. Tavistock.

[51]   Tanner, J.M. (1978) *Foetus into Man.* London. Open Books.

[52]   Kinsey, A.C., Pomeroy, W.B. & Martin, C.E. 1948 *Sexual behaviour in the human male.* Philadelphia. W.B. Saunders.

[53]   Goldman, R. & J. (1982) *Children's Sexual Thinking.* London. Routledge and Kegan Paul.

[54]   Catterall R.D. (1981) *Biological Effects of Sexual Freedom.* The Lancet. Feb. 7th 1981.

[55]   Lifeskills Associates Ashling, Back Church Lane, Leeds.

[56]   Trigger films *Attitudes to Health and Sexually Transmitted Diseases.* Three 6 minute films, *Janet Rupert* and *Sue.* HEC and Liberation Films.

[57]   School Broadcasting Council (1971) *School Broadcasting and Sex Education in the Primary School.* London. BBC publications.

[58]   Fogelman K. (Ed.) (1976) *Britain's 16 year olds.* London. National Children's Bureau.

[59]   Clarke L. (1982) *Teenage Views of Sex Education.* Health Education Journal. **41** (2) 47–51.

[60]   Spender, D. (1982) *Invisible Women.* London. Writers & Readers

[61]   Parkes, A.S. (1976) *Patterns of Sexuality and Reproduction.* Oxford University Press.

[62]   Oubridge, J. (1983) *Personal communication.*

[63]   Health Education Council and The Spastics Society. *Teachers' Notes* for the film *If only we'd known.* Health Education Council.

[64]   1956 Sexual Offences Act, Sections 5 and 6.

[65]   Report (Sept. 1979) *Towards healthy babies.* The Spastics Society.

[66]   Collins, W.P. (1982) *Ovulation prediction and detection.* IPPF Medical Bulletin. **16**, 5th Oct. 1982.

[67]   Doggett, M. (1982) *Postcoital Contraception.* BPAS.

[68]   Photopack Kit and Tapes. *Who are YOU staring at?* Community Service Volunteers and Mental Health Film Council.

[69] Barlow, D. (1981) *Sexually Transmitted Diseases, the Facts.* Oxford University Press.
[70] Study day report *Sexually Transmitted Diseases.* West Midlands Regional Health Authority.
[71] Roberts, C.J. & Lowe, C.R. (1975) Lancet **i**, 498.
[72] Lauritsen, J.G. (1982) *The Cytogenetics of spontaneous abortion.* Research into reproduction. **14**, 3rd July 1982.
[73] Douglas, J.W. & Ross, J.M. (1964) *Age of puberty related to educational ability, attainment and school leaving age.* Journal of Child Psychology & Psychiatry 5, pp.185–196.
[74] Mussen, P.H. & Jones, M.C., (1957) *Self-conceptions, motivations and interpersonal attitudes of late and early maturing boys.* Child development **28** pp.243–256.
[75] Eveleth, P.B. & Tanner, J.M. (1976) *Worldwide Variation in Human Growth.* London. Cambridge University Press.
[76] *Ortho Pelvic Model.* Ortho Pharmaceutical Ltd. Saunderton, High Wycombe, Buckinghamshire.
[77] Hite, S. (1977) *The Hite Report.* Summit Books. (Paul Hamlyn Pty. Ltd.)
[78] Which? publication, (1969) *Infertility* Consumer Association.
[79] *Religions and Cultures.* A guide to patients' beliefs and customs for health service staff. Lothian Community Relations Council, Edinburgh.
[80] Report. (1976) *Britain's Sixteen-Year-Olds* National Children's Bureau, London.
[81] Derek Llewellyn Jones (1971) *Everywoman.* Faber & Faber.
[82] National Opinion Poll Survey (1980) *Prevalence and some effects of period pains among women aged 15–44 years in the United Kingdom.*
[83] Dalton, K. (1978) *Once a Month.* Fontana.
[84] Godelieve, C.M.L., Christiaens, Sixma, J.J. & Haspells, A.A., (1982) *Morphology of haemostasis.* Research & Clinical Forums. **4**. 4
[85] Rees, M.C.P., Chimbira T.H. & Anderson A.B.M. & Turnbull A.C. (1982) *Menstrual blood loss, measurement and clinical correlates.* Research & Clinical Forums. **4**.4 pp.69–77.
[86] Anderson A.B.M. *The role of prostaglandin synthetase inhibitors in gynaecology.* The Practitioner.
[87] Brain Behaviour Research Centre. Sonora State Hospital USA.
[88] Rybo, G. (1982) *Variations of menstrual blood loss.* Research and Clinical Forums. **4**.4 pp.81–88.
[89] Anderson A.B.M., Turnbull A.C. (1978) *Treatment of menorrhagia with a prostaglandin inhibitor.* Research & Clinical Forums. **1**.2 pp.83–87.
[90] Dalton, K. (1977) *The Pre-menstrual Syndrome and Progesterone Therapy.* Heinemann.
[91] Davis, P.D., Chesney, P.J., Wand, P.J. & La Venture, B.S. (Dec. 1980) *Toxic-Shock Syndrome.* The New England Journal of Medicine. 303.25. pp.1429–1435.
[92] Anon. (1982) *The Premenstrual Syndrome.* Research in Reproduction. 14.1.
[93] Morris, D. (1978) *Manwatching.* Triad/Granada.
[94] School's Council Moral Education Curriculum Project (1974) Lifeline. Longmans.
[95] Dobson, J.C. (1979) *Focus on the Family,* film Series. Word Incorporated.
[96] Bostrom, C. *Study Guide to Focus on the Family. Christian World.*
[97] Sorensen, R.C. (1973) *Adolescent Sexuality in Contemporary America: Personal Values and Sexual Behaviour, Ages 13–19* Harry N. Abrams.
[98] Aitken, P.P. (1978) *10–14 year-olds and alcohol.* Vol III. HMSO Edin. Scottish Health Ed. Unit.
[99] Bewley, B.R. & Bland, M (1978) *The Child's image of the young smoker.* Health Education Journal 37.4
[100] The Diagram Group (1977) *Woman's body. Paddington Press.*
[101] Masters, W. & Johnson V. (1966) *Human Sexual Response.* Little, Brown & Co.
[102] Kaplan, H. (1974) *The New Sex Therapy.* Brunner/Mazel-Quadrangle.
[103] Anon. *Human sexual behaviour at different stages of the menstrual cycle.* Research into Reproduction. **10**.1. Jan 78. IPPF.
[104] Wagner N.N. *Counselling in Sex Education* FPA.
[105] Kinsey, A.C. et al (1953). *Sexual Behaviour in the Human Female.* W.B. Saunders & Co.
[106] *Homosexuality. A fact of life.* A teachers' guide (1978). Campaign for Homosexual Equality.
[107] FPA *Men, sex and contraception.* Family Planning Association.
[108] Anon. *Sex education for boys growing up.* Catholic Marriage Advisory Council.
[109] Hite, S. (1982) *The Hite Report on Male Sexuality.* Macdonald.
[110] *Report of the Committee on Homosexual Offences and Prostitution* (1957). HM. Stationery Office.

[111] Hooker, E. *The Adjustment of the Male Overt.* Journal of protective techniques. Vol. 21.

[112] West, D.J. in *Psychosexual Problems* (1976). Ed. Milne, Hugo, Hardy Shirley J. Bradford University Press.

[113] Stoppard M *Everywoman's life guide.* Family Planning Association

[114] NCVYS *Report of the working party on young people and Homosexuality* (1976) National Council for Voluntary Youth Services.

[115] Dannecker, M. *The Ordinary Homosexual.*

[116] Maddox, B. (1982) *The Marrying Kind.* Granada.

[117] Haupt, A. & Kane, T.T. (1978) *Population Handbook.* Population Reference Bureau USA.

[118] April 1982 *World Population Data Sheet* Population Reference Bureau Inc. Washington DC. USA.

[119] Kendall, M. (1979) *The World Fertility Survey: Current Status and Findings.* Population Reports of the John Hopkins University, Series U, No. 3, July 1979.

[120] OPCS Monitor Legal Abortions (1981) Ref. AB82/5. 7 Sept. 1982. Office of Population, Censuses and Surveys.

[121] Cartwright, A. (1978) *Recent Trends in Family Building and Contraception.* Studies on Medical and Population Subjects No. 34. OPCS.

[122] Bone, M. (1978) *The Family Planning Services. Changes and Effects.* HMSO.

[123] Lambert, J. (1971) *Survey of 3000 Unwanted Pregnancies.* British Medical Journal. **4** pp.156–160.

[124] (1982) *Sex education in Schools – Responsible Society. What every parent should know.*

[125] Dominian, J. (1979) *Who Divorces?* Routledge & Kegan Paul.

[126] Zabin, L.S., Kantner, J.F. and Zebnik M. (1979) *The risk of adolescent pregnancy in the first months of intercourse.* Fam. Plann. Perspectives **11**. No. 4.

[127] Anon. *Number of sex partners not increased by giving contraception to teens* (1978) Fam. Plann. Perspect. 10(6) 369. Nov/Dec.

[128] Chester, J. (1980) *Twenty-Seven Strategies for Teaching Contraception to Adolescents.* Journal of School Health, Jan. 1980.

[129] Ory, H.W. (1982) *The Non-contraceptive health benefits from oral contraceptive use.* Fam. Plann. Perspectives **14**.4 July Aug. pp.182–184.

[130] RCGP *Oral Contraception Study* (1977) British Med. J. **2** .9 p.47.

[131] Vessey, M. (1982) The Lancet 10.4.82.

[132] Anon. (1982) *Trials of the ovulation method of natural family planning.* Research in reproduction. 14. No. 3. July 1982.

[133] RGGP Oral Contraception Study (1981) *Further analysis of mortality in oral contraceptive users.* Lancet 1981. **ii** pp.451–546.

[134] Vessey, M., Doll, R., Peto, R., Johnson, B. & Wiggins, P. (1976 Oct) *Long term follow-up study of women using different methods of contraception: an interim report.* Journal of Biosocial Science, **8**(4) pp.375–427.

[135] Population Report Series A. No. 6 (1982 May/June) A pp.189–222, *Oral Contraceptives in the 1980s.*

[136] Christopher, E. (1983) Novum 22 (Feb. 1983) *Family planning Today – an Overview.* Some personal and psychological factors in contraceptive use. Schering.

[137] British Organisation for NON-Parents. BM Box 5866. London WC1N 3XX.

[138] Wynn, M. & Wynn, A. (1982) *Comment.* Family Planning Today. 3rd Quarter. 1982. FPIS.

[139] FPIS Fact Sheet GI (38) (Jan. 1982) *Perinatal and Infant Mortality.*

[140] Social Services Committee on Perinatal and Neonatal Mortality. Second Report. 19.6.80.

[141] Holland, M. (1979) *Towards Healthy Babies.* The Spastics Society.

[142] DHSS (1975) *Report on Confidential Enquiries into Maternal Deaths in England and Wales.* 1970–1972. London HMSO.

[143] (1982) *Maternity Care in Action. Ante Natal Care.* HMSO.

[144] Wynn, A. & Wynn, M. (1982) *'Prevention of Handicap of Early Pregnancy Origin. Some evidence for the value of Good Health Before Conception.* Foundation for Education and Research in Childbearing.

[145] OPCS. Monitor DH3 82/2.

[146] Rodmell, S. & Smart, E. (1982) *Pregnant at Work.* OU and Kensington, Chelsea and Westminster Health Authorities. Hounslow Health Education Unit.

[147] Boyd, C. (1982) BBC. TV. That's life *Having a baby.* Spastics Society.

[148] Perkins, E.R. (1980) *The Pattern of Women's Attendance at Antenatal Classes. Is this good enough?* Health Education Journal **39**.1.

278

[149]   Slater, P.J.B. (1981) *Baby knows best: the physiology of pregnancy and lactation.* Journ. Biol. Ed. **15**.1. Spring 1981.

[150]   Leboyer, F. (1974) *Birth without violence.* Fontana.

[151]   Tietze, C. & Lewit, S. (1978) Abortion. People **5**.2. 4–6. IPPF.

[152]   Abortions Statistics. Fact Sheet H.2 (8) Jan. 1982. FPIS.

[153]   1983. *Two million too many.* Leaflet published by Life.

[154]   Wynn, M. & Wynn, A. (1973) *Some consequences of Induced Abortion to Children Born Subsequently.* London Foundation for Education and Research in Childbearing.

[155]   Potts, M. & Shadbolt, R. (1973) *Longterm side effects of abortion.* Family Planning July 1983.

[156]   *Pregnancy Counselling: Some questions and answers.* BPAS.

[157]   BAC Booklet *Abortion.* Updated 1983. Brook Advisory Centre. Education and Publications Unit.

[158]   (1982) *Sexually Transmitted Diseases and Contraception.* FPIS Fact Sheet F.3 (11)

[159]   Barlow, D. (1981) *Sexually Transmitted Diseases. The facts.* Oxford Uni. Press.

[160]   Lambert, J. (1971) *Survey of 3000 Unwanted Pregnancies.* British Medical Journal. 16.10.71.

[161]   Morris, D.F. (1982) *Sexually transmitted diseases in the UK.* Novum 20. August 1982. Schering.

[162]   (1982) *Sexually transmitted diseases. Report of a study day on Sexually Transmitted Diseases. Prevention and Cures.* West Midland Regional Health Authority.

[163]   Wright, J.T. et al (1983) *Alcohol consumption, pregnancy and low birth weight.* Lancet 1983. 1.663.

[164]   National Council of Women (1980) *The Fetal Alcohol Syndrome.* National Council of Women.

[165]   OPCS Monitor (21.06.83) *General Household Survey.* Preliminary results for 1982.

[166]   Whitefield, R.C. (1980) *Education for Family life* Hodder and Stoughton

[167]   Hughes, J. (1979) *A Child Care View* Parenthood Education in Schools TACADE

[168]   Cowly, J. (1979) *Some final considerations.* Parenthood Education in Schools TACADE

[169]   Perkins, E.R. and Morris B. (1981) *Should we prepare for parenthood?* Health Education Journal 40.4

[170]   Orton, A. (1979) *Parentcraft-A Teachers View.* Parenthood Education in Schools TACADE.

[171]   Leach, P. (1979) *Who Cares?* Penguin.

[172]   MacDonald, M. (1981) *Class, Gender and Education.* OUP

[173]   Conference Report (1982) *Equal Opportunities. Whats in it for boys?* Schools Council

[174]   Schwarzenberger, R. (1983) Science Education Department, University of Warwick Personal communication.

[175]   Levine, D.U. and Ornstein, A.C. (1983) *Sex differences in ability and achievement.* Journal of Research & Development in Education, 16.2. pp.66–72.

[176]   Havinghurst, R.J. (1983) *Sex Role Development.* Journal of Research & Development in Education 16.2 p.60–65

[177]   Simms, M. and Smith, C. (1983) *Teenage Mothers and their partners.* Institute for Social Studies in Medical Care.

[178]   Government Survey, (July 1983) *Young people in the eighties.* HMSO.

[179]   Ellis, B. (1983) *What do you remember about the area before the school was built?* Teaching Geography, Volume 8, Number 4, 1983.

[180]   Pike, M.C., Henderson, B.E. & Krailo, M.D. et al. *Breast cancer in young women and use of oral contraceptives: possible modifying effect of formulation and age at use.* The Lancet. Oct. 22nd 1983.

[181]   Vessey, M.P., Lawless, M. & McPherson, K., et al. *Neoplasia of the cervix uteri and contraception; a possible adverse effect of the pill.* The Lancet. Oct. 22nd 1983. General Practitioner, 6.1.84.

[182]   Grafton, T., Smith, L., Vegoda, M. & Whitfield, R. (1983) *Preparation for parenthood in the secondary school curriculum* report for DES by Dept. of Educational Enquiry, University of Aston, Birmingham, August, 1983.

[183]   IPPF International Medical Advisory Panel report. IPPF Medical Bulletin Vol. 18, No. 1, February 1984.

[184]   Hall, R. (1984) *Changing Fertility in the Developing World, and its Impact on Global Population Growth.* Geography Volume 69, Part I, January, 1984.

[185]   *The Pill in Perspective.* Symposium held in London on December 15th, 1983, organised by

Schering Chemicals, Wyeth Laboratories & Organon Laboratories.

[186]   World Fertility Survey (1981) Annual Report, 1981 Voorburg International Statistical Institute.

[187]   Crisp, A.H., Palmer, R.L., and Kalucy R.S. (1976), British Journal of Psychiatry **126**. 549.

[188]   Wood, N. (1983) *HMI find few schools earmark time for sex education.* Report of HMI Survey of primary schools in Avon. Times Ed. Supp. 29.4.83.

[189]   *Freedom to choose?* Social Work Today 16.4.84

[190]   Prout A., Prendergast S. *Parenthood: what pupils know and what they learn.* Education and Health. Vol 2 No 3. May 1984

[191] Rebora A., Borghi S, and Basso G. *Warts and cervical cancer.* The Lancet. 26.5.84.

Appendix 1

Family Planning Association, regions

i) North of the Thames
Regional Administrator
FPA
38b St. Peter's Street
Bedford MK40 2NN
Tel: Bedford (0234) 62436

ii) South east England
Regional Administrator
FPA
13a Western Road
Hove
East Sussex
Tel: Brighton (0273) 774075

iii) South west England
Regional Administrator
FPA
53a Bridge Street
Taunton
Somerset
Tel: Taunton (0823) 72759

iv) Wales
Regional Administrator
FPA
6 Windsor Place
Cardiff
Tel: Cardiff (0222) 387471

v) Eastern England
Regional Administrator
FPA
20a Bridewell Alley
Norwich NR2 1SY
Tel: Norwich (0603) 28704

vi) Midlands
Regional Administrator
FPA
7 York Road,
Birmingham B16 9HX
Tel: Birmingham (021) 454 8236

vii) North west England
Regional Administrator
FPA
9 Gambier Terrace
Liverpool 1
Tel: Liverpool (051) 709 1938

viii) Yorkshire and the North east
Regional Administrator
FPA
17 North Church Street
Sheffield S1 2DH
Tel: Sheffield (0742) 2191

ix) Scotland
Regional Administrator
FPA
4 Clifton Street
Glasgow G3 7LA
Tel: Glasgow (041) 333 9696

x) London
Regional Administrator
FPA
160 Shepherd's Bush Road
London W6
Tel: London (01) 602 3804

xi) Northern Ireland
Regional Administrator
FPA
47 Botanic Avenue
Belfast BT7 1JL
Tel: Belfast (0232) 25488

Appendix 2

Abbreviations used

ATW	Active Tutorial Work
BAC	Brook Advisory Centre
BMA	British Medical Association
BPAS	British Pregnancy Advisory Service
CVS	Community Volunteer Service
DES	Department of Education and Science
DHA	District Health Authority
DHSS	Department of Health and Social Security
FPA	Family Planning Association
FPIS	Family planning Information Service
HEC	Health Education Council
HEO	Health Education Officer
HEP	Health Education project 13–18
ILEA	Inner London Education Authority
IPPF	International Planned Parenthood Federation
IUD	Intra Uterine Device
LEA	Local Education Authority
PAS	Pregnancy Advisory Service
PTM	Photographic Teaching Materials
NCW	National Council for Women
NHS	National Health Service
NMGC	National Marriage Guidance Council
OPCS	Office of Population Censuses and Surveys
RCGP	Royal College of General Practitioners
RHA	Regional Health Authority
SCHEP	Schools Council Health Education Programme 5–13
STD	Sexually Transmitted Disease
TACADE	Teachers Advisory Council on Alcohol and Drug Education
VD	Venereal Disease

Appendix 3

Education officers of independent television

Education Officer
Anglia Television Limited
Anglia House
Norwich. NOR 07A
(East of England Region)
Tel: 0603 615151

Schools Liaison Officer
Border Television Limited
Television Centre,
Carlisle. CA1 3NT
(The Borders and Isle of Man Region)
Tel: 0228 25101

Education Officer
Central Independent Television plc
Central House
Broad Street
Birmingham. B1 2JP
(Midlands Region)
Tel: 643 9898

The Education Officer
Channel Television
St Helier
Jersey. C.I.
(Channel Islands Region)
Tel: 0534 73999

Education Officer
Grampian Television Limited
Queen's cross
Aberdeen. AB9 2XJ
(North East Scotland Region)
Tel: 0224 53553

Education Officer
Granada Television Limited
Deansgate
Manchester. M60 9EA
(Northern Region)
Tel: 061 832 7211

Education Officer
HTV
Television Centre
Cardiff. CF1 9XL
(Wales and West of England Region)
Tel: 0222 21021

Asst. Education Officer
HTV
Television Centre
Bath Road
Bristol. BS4 3HG
(Wales and West of England Region)
Tel: 0272 779975

Head of Education
Scottish Television Limited
The Gateway
Edinburgh. EH7 3AH
(Central Scottish Region)
Tel: 031 556 5372

Asst. Head of Education
Scottish Television Limited
Cowcaddens
Glasgow. G2 3PR
(Central Scottish Region)
Tel: 041 332 9999

Education officer
Thames Television Limited
149 Tottenham Court Road
London. W1P 9LL (London Region)
Exec Producer Schools:
Tel: 01 388 5199

Education Officer
TSW Limited
Derry's Cross
Plymouth. PL1 2SP
(South West Region)
Tel: 0752 69311

Education Officer
TVS
Northam
Southampton. SO9 5HZ
(South of England Region)
Tel: 0703 28582

Education Officer
Tyne Tees Television Limited
The Television Centre
City Road
Newcastle upon Tyne. NE1 2AL
(North East Region)
Tel: 0632 610181

Education Officer
Ulster Television Limited,
Havelock House
Ormeau Road
Belfast. BT7 1EB
(Northern Ireland Region)
Tel: 0232 28122

Education Officer
Yorkshire Television Limited
The Television Centre
Leeds. LS3 1JS
(Yorkshire Region)
Head of Education:
Tel: 0532 438283

Appendix 4

Useful addresses

BAECE
(British Association for Early Childhood
Education)
Montgomery Hall
Kennington Oval
London SE1 5SW

BBC School Broadcasting Council
The Langham
Portland Place
London W1A 1AA

Camera Talks Ltd
31 North Row
London W1E 5EZ

Central Film Library
Chalfont Grove
Gerards Cross
Bucks SL9 8TN

Concord Films Council Ltd
201 Felixstowe Road
Ipswich IP3 9EJ

Education and Health
(Journal of the HEC Schools Health
Education Unit)
University of Exeter
Heavitree Road
Exeter EX1 2LU

Equal Opportunities Commission
Overseas House
Quay Street
Manchester M3 3HN

ICARUS
Project Icarus
Raglan House
4 Clarence Parade
Southsea
Hants PO5 3NM

Lifeskills Associates
Ashling
Back Church Lane
Leeds LS16 8DN

MENCAP
National Headquarters
123 Golden Lane
London EC1

National Childbirth Trust
9 Queensborough Terrace
Bayswater
London W2 3TB

National Council for One-Parent Families
255 Kentish Town Road
London NW5 2LX

NCCL
National Council for Civil Liberties
21 Tabard Street
London SE1

National Council of Women
34 Lower Sloane Street
London SW1

Ortho-Pharmaceutical Ltd
PO Box 79
Founderton
High Wycombe
Bucks HP14 4HJ

Osmiroid Educational
Osmiroid Works
Gosport
Hants

RSPCA Education Department
Causeway
Horsham
West Sussex R812 1HG

School Natural Science Society
Publications from:
The Association for Science Education
College Lane
Hatfield
Herts AL10 9AH

The Spastics Society
12 Park Crescent
London W1N 4EQ

For details of more organisations, including the FPA, HEC, BPAS and others, please see pages 45 to 49.

Index